HUMAN
STERILIZATION

HUMAN STERILIZATION

A Conference
Sponsored by

International Institute
for the Study of Human Reproduction
College of Physicians and Surgeons of
Columbia University

and

Center for Population Research
National Institute of Child Health
and Human Development

Edited by
RALPH M. RICHART, M.D.
and
DENIS J. PRAGER, Ph.D.

With Forewords by
Philip A. Corfman, M.D.
and
Raymond L. Vande Wiele, M.D.

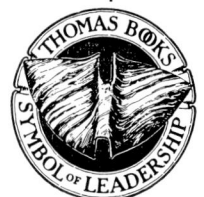

CHARLES C THOMAS • PUBLISHER
Springfield • Illinois • U.S.A.

Published and Distributed Throughout the World by
CHARLES C THOMAS • PUBLISHER
BANNERSTONE HOUSE
301–327 East Lawrence Avenue, Springfield, Illinois, U.S.A.
NATCHEZ PLANTATION HOUSE
735 North Atlantic Boulevard, Fort Lauderdale, Florida, U.S.A.

1972, CHARLES C THOMAS • PUBLISHER

ISBN 0–398–02388–3

Library of Congress Catalog Card Number: 78–165895

With THOMAS BOOKS *careful attention is given to all details of manufacturing and design. It is the Publisher's desire to present books that are satisfactory as to their physical qualities and artistic possibilities and appropriate for their particular use.* THOMAS BOOKS *will be true to those laws of quality that assure a good name and good will.*

Printed in the United States of America

BB-14

CONTRIBUTORS

Oscar Aguero, M.D.

Director of Obstetrics and Gynecology
Concepcion Palacios Maternity Hospital
Caracas, Venezuela

Donald W. Baker, B.S.E.E.

Technical Director
Bioengineering Division
University of Washington
Seattle, Washington

Ray G. Bunge, M.D.

Professor of Urology
College of Medicine
University Hospital
Iowa City, Iowa

Ronald A. Chez, M.D.

Chief of the Pregnancy Research Branch
N.I.C.H. & H.D.
Bethesda, Maryland

Martin J. Clyman, M.D.

Associate Clinical Professor of
Obstetrics and Gynecology
Mt. Sinai School of Medicine
New York, New York

Philip A. Corfman, M.D.

Director, Center for Population Research
National Institute of Child Health and Human Development
Bethesda, Maryland

B.S. Darbari, M.D.

*Assistant Commissioner of the Ministry of Health
Government of India
New Delhi, India*

Francis J. Fry, M.S.

*Interscience Research Institute and Bioacoustic Laboratory
University of Illinois
Urbana, Illinois*

Celso-Ramon Garcia, M.D.

*Professor of Obstetrics and Gynecology
Hospital of the University of Pennsylvania
Philadelphia, Pennsylvania*

Motoyuki Hayashi, M.D.

*Professor of Obstetrics and Gynecology
The University School of Medicine
Tokyo, Japan*

J.F. Hulka, M.D.

*Associate Professor of Obstetrics and Gynecology
University of North Carolina
School of Medicine
Chapel Hill, North Carolina*

Robert E. Innis, M.S.

*Senior Physicist
American Optical Corporation
Research Laboratory
Framingham Centre, Massachusetts*

Wen H. Ko, Ph.D.

*Professor of Engineering
Division of Electrical Sciences
Case Western Reserve University
Cleveland, Ohio*

Contributors

Kenneth A. Laurence, Ph.D.

Associate Director
Biomedical Division
The Rockefeller University
New York, New York

Hee Yong Lee, M.D.

Director, Department of Urology
College of Medicine
Seoul National University
Seoul, Korea

Fred Leonard, Ph.D.

Scientific Director
Biomechanical Research Laboratory
Walter Reed Army Medical Center
Washington, D.C.

Frederick W. Martens, Jr., M.D.

Clinical Assistant Professor of
Obstetrics and Gynecology
Cornell University Medical College
Assistant Attending Obstetrician and Gynecologist
New York Hospital
New York, New York

F.C. McLeod, B.S.E.E.

Research Associate, Veterinary College
Cornell University
Ithaca, New York

K.H. Moon, M.D.

Assistant Professor of Urology
University of Iowa
College of Medicine
Iowa City, Iowa

Robert S. Neuwirth, M.D.

Director, Obstetrics and Gynecology
Bronx-Lebanon Hospital Center
Bronx, New York

D.N. Pai, M.B., B.S.

Professor of Preventive and Social Medicine
Seth G.S. Medical College
Director, Family Planning, Maternal and Child Health
Municipal Corporation of Greater Bombay
Bombay, India

Lelia V. Phatak, M.D.

Director–Principal
Safdayang Hospital
New Delhi, India

Denis J. Prager, Ph.D.

Director
Battelle Population Study Center
Human Affairs Research Centers
Seattle, Washington

B. Rakshit, M.D., F.R.C.O.G.

Director and Professor
Department of Obstetrics and Gynecology
R.G. Kar Medical College
Calcutta, India

John W. Ratcliffe, M.D.

Chief Advisor
East Pakistan Research and Evaluation Center
Dacca, East Pakistan

Ralph M. Richart, M.D.

Professor of Pathology
College of Physicians and Surgeons
Columbia University
Director Pathology and Cytology Laboratories
Obstetrical and Gynecological Division

(The Sloane Hospital for Women)
Presbyterian Hospital
New York, New York

Stanwood S. Schmidt, M.D.

Research Associate
Department of Urology
University of California
School of Medicine
San Francisco, California

Sheldon Segal, Ph.D.

Director, Biomedical Division
The Population Council
The Rockefeller University
New York, New York

Anna L. Southam, M.D.

Program Officer
The Ford Foundation
New York, New York

C.H. Swope

Senior Physicist
American Optical Corporation
Research Laboratory
Framingham Centre, Massachusetts

Horace E. Thompson, M.D.

Director, Obstetrical and Gynecological Service
Denver General Hospital
Denver, Colorado

Stephen C. Woodward, M.D.

Associate Professor of Pathology
Georgetown University
Washington, D.C.

Jaime Zipper, M.D.

Associate Professor of Physiology
University of Chile
Santiago, Chile

FOREWORD

The Center for Population Research was established in the National Institute of Child Health and Human Development in order to advance progress in the sciences relevant to solution of population problems. Special attention is given in this effort to the development and evaluation of fertility regulating techniques, which together would assure that each couple could choose among many effective methods in spacing or limiting its family.

Sterilization is an important technique of fertility regulation. Like other methods, it should be assessed and improved in order to be most useful to those for whom it is the method of choice. We were therefore pleased to join with the International Institute for the Study of Human Reproduction in the sponsorship of this Conference on Human Sterilization which was held on October 28–31, 1969 in Cherry Hill, New Jersey.

The structure of the conference demonstrates the wide range of disciplines required for a careful examination of this topic. The participants included clinicians, public health officials, sociologists, biologists, physicists and engineers, and particular effort was made to foster communication among the disparate fields represented.

The conference was helpful to the Center in formulation of its research activities in the area of sterilization, an area which accounts for an increasing share of our program.

PHILIP A. CORFMAN

FOREWORD

The premise that led to the organization of the Conference on *Human Sterilization* held on October 28–31, 1969, in Cherry Hill, New Jersey, was albeit in a restricted way, very much the same as the premise that was in Dr. Howard C. Taylor's mind in conceiving the International Institute for the Study of Human Reproduction. The subject of Human Reproduction stretches across the full range of human knowledge, biology, physics, psychology, social sciences, and even philosophy and religion, and in creating the International Institute for the Study of Human Reproduction, Dr. Taylor wanted to bring together, under one roof and to integrate into one unit, a group of investigators devoted to the study of all these aspects of human reproduction.

In organizing this Conference on *Human Sterilization,* Dr. Ralph Richart, who is head of the Division of Reproductive Morphology of the International Institute, felt strongly that if progress is to be made it will be necessary to go beyond the skills of the medical profession.

Participating in this Conference were physicians, engineers, instrument makers, sociologists, demographers, etc., and the reason for the success of this Conference must be found in this multidisciplinary approach. Most of us feel that newer, simpler and cheaper methods of sterilization are going to play an increasing role in programs of population control, and the International Institute for the Study of Human Reproduction takes pride in the results of this meeting.

RAYMOND L. VANDE WIELE

PREFACE

Sterilization as a means of limiting family size has increasingly become accepted during the last fifty years. The recent experience in large scale, national population control efforts undertaken during the last decade indicate that the techniques for male sterilization are adequate. The major problems would appear to be individual motivation and health care delivery. For women, however, motivation appears to be a lesser problem but the current techniques of female sterilization require expensive equipment, are time-consuming, and must be undertaken by highly skilled professionals who, in many regions, are in short supply for treating the ill and cannot easily be spared for preventive medicine.

The Conference on Human Sterilization was organized to assess the role of sterilization today and in the future as a population control method. The emphasis was on exploring new ideas for improving the techniques of human sterilization by bringing past and present experience together with new experimental approaches. The conference was interdisciplinary and provided an opportunity for investigators from the physical and biological sciences to exchange ideas and to set up avenues for collaboration. The invited papers covered a wide range of topics and stimulated the formal discussion which has been abstracted in the proceedings and the many individual informal discussions which are not recorded but are probably one of the most productive phases of expert conferences.

The conference did not yield immediate new methods or techniques for performing sterilizations, new ways to motivate men or women to accept sterilization or even a philosophical agreement regarding the proper role of sterilization in population control programs. It did bring together a group of investigators who reviewed the current state of the art and, if it stimulates new work resulting in even a single new approach towards alleviating the urgent problem of controlling the growth of our population, it will have achieved an important goal.

RALPH M. RICHART
DENIS J. PRAGER

CONTENTS

	Page
Contributors	v
Foreword—Philip A. Corfman	xi
Foreword—Raymond L. Vande Wiele	xiii
Preface	xv

I FOREIGN PROGRAMS
Howard C. Taylor, Jr., Moderator

Chapter

1. Indian Vasectomy Camps—*D.N. Pai* 5

2. Tubal Ligation Program in India—*B.S. Darbari* 12

3. Tubal Ligation in Caracas, Venezuela—*Oscar Aguero and Leopoldo Cardenas-Conde* 18

4. Male Sterilization in East Pakistan—*John W. Ratcliffe, A.H.G. Quddus, and H.T. Croley* 23

5. The Korean Vasectomy Program—*Hee Yong Lee* 38

6. The Use of Learning Aids in Human Sterilization Programs—*Ronald A. Chez* 48

   Discussion: Foreign Programs 53

II PERMANENT STERILIZATION
Ralph M. Richart, Moderator

7. A Modified Operative Technique for Vasectomy—*Hee Yong Lee* 71

Chapter	Page
8. Vas Reanastomosis Procedures—*Stanwood S. Schmidt*	76
9. Evaluation of the Optimal Time for Tubal Ligation—*Lelia V. Phatak*	86
10. Tubal Sterilization by Operative Culdoscopy—*Martin J. Clyman*	93
11. Nonpuerperal Sterilization by Laparoscopy—*Robert S. Neuwirth*	101
12. Oviduct Anastomosis Procedures—*Celso-Ramon Garcia*	116
Discussion: Permanent Sterilization	129

III BIOENGINEERING TECHNOLOGY (A)
Denis J. Prager, Moderator

13. Visualization of Soft Tissue Structures: Principles and Limitations—*F.C. McLeod*	143
14. Polymer Implants—*Fred Leonard*	155
15. Ultrasonic Surgical Techniques—*Francis J. Fry*	160
16. Applications of Ultrasonics in the Study and Control of Population Processes—*Donald W. Baker*	166
Discussion: Bioengineering Technology (A)	175

IV REVERSIBLE STERILIZATION
Ralph M. Richart, Moderator

17. Reversible Vas Occlusion by Intravasal Thread—*Hee Yong Lee*	193
18. Tubal Sterilization with Clips—*Motoyuki Hayashi*	201
19. Temporary Occlusion of the Ductus Deferens—*K.H. Moon and Ray G. Bunge*	204

Chapter	Page
20. THE SCOPE OF LIQUID PLASTICS AND OTHER CHEMICALS FOR BLOCKING THE FALLOPIAN TUBE—*B. Rakshit*	213
21. OCCLUSIONS OF THE VAS DEFERENS WITH SILASTIC—*Kenneth A. Laurence*	222
DISCUSSION: REVERSIBLE STERILIZATION	229

V BIOENGINEERING TECHNOLOGY (B)
Denis J. Prager, Moderator

22. FIBER OPTICS FOR VISUALIZATION AND ILLUMINATION—*Robert E. Innis*	245
23. PRODUCTION OF CLINICALLY USEFUL INTERACTIONS OF LASER RADIATION WITH TISSUE—*C.H. Swope*	254
24. TISSUE RESPONSES TO POLYMERIC IMPLANTS: THE CYANOACRYLATES—*Stephen C. Woodward*	264
25. MICROELECTRONICS AND IMPLANT INSTRUMENTS—*Wen H. Ko*	276
DISCUSSION: BIOENGINEERING TECHNOLOGY (B)	294

VI NONSURGICAL STERILIZATION
Sheldon Segal, Moderator

26. ATTEMPTED CRYOSURGICAL CLOSURE OF THE FALLOPIAN TUBES—*Frederick W. Martens, Jr.*	305
27. CAUTERIZATION FOR TUBAL STERILIZATION—*J.F. Hulka and K.F. Omran*	313
28. TUBAL STERILIZATION BY CORNUAL COAGULATION UNDER HYSTEROSCOPY—*Motoyuki Hayashi*	334
29. CHEMICAL AGENTS FOR TRANSVAGINAL STERILIZATION—*Jaime Zipper, M. Medel, E. Stachetti, L. Pastene, M. Rivera and R. Prager*	339

Chapter	Page
30. TRANSVAGINAL DELIVERY OF STERILIZING CHEMICALS— *Horace E. Thompson, Thomas Moulding, Charles Dafoe and Dale L. Osterling*	353
31. EXPERIMENTAL STUDIES OF FALLOPIAN TUBE OCCLUSION—*Ralph M. Richart, Robert S. Neuwirth and Howard C. Taylor, Jr.*	360
DISCUSSION: NONSURGICAL STERILIZATION	368
32. SUMMARY AND DIRECTIONS FOR THE FUTURE—*Anna L. Southam*	377
Name Index	383
Subject Index	387

HUMAN
STERILIZATION

I   FOREIGN PROGRAMS

Howard C. Taylor, Jr., *Moderator*

Chapter 1

INDIAN VASECTOMY CAMPS

D.N. PAI

The global problem of population has engaged the efforts of both scientists and community workers in a search for a solution. In order to be successful, any contraceptive method must not only be safe and effective, but also be acceptable to the masses and implementable on a large scale.

India's problems of population are vast. Tradition, poverty, illiteracy, transportation and communication barriers, and poor health services all militate against continuing motivation towards family restrictions. One-shot procedures, like intra-uterine contraceptive devices and sterilization are considered suitable in light of our demographic problems. India's rural masses are scattered in 560,000 villages in which 80 percent of the population resides, 61.4 percent of these in huts and slums.

Although about 12 percent of married couples in the United States are sterilized, in the Greater Bombay area more than 20 percent are sterilized. In order to reach the objective of reducing the birth rate by 1978, 100 million target couples must be reached. Table 1-I summarizes the number of sterilizations performed in India from 1956 through 1969.

TABLE 1-I

Year	Number of Sterilizations*
1956	7,153
1957	13,736
1958	25,148
1959	42,302
1960	64,338
1961	104,585
1962	157,947
1963	170,246
1964	269,575
1965–1966	670,823
1966–1967	887,368
1967–1968	1,839,811
1968–1969	1,649,686

* From 1956 through 1969 there were a total of 5,902,708 sterilizations.

Statewide acceptance of sterilization (vasectomies and tubectomies) is presented in Table 1-II and statewide distribution of sterilization by vasectomy is presented in Table 1-III.

TABLE 1-II
ACCEPTANCE OF VASECTOMY AND TUBECTOMY BY STATES IN ORDER OF DECLINING ACCEPTANCE (1956–1964)

	Sterilizations	Vasectomies	Tubectomies
	Maharashtra	Maharashtra	Assam
	Madras	Madras	Gujarat
		Punjab	
	Gujarat	Mysore	Bihar
	Kerala	Kerala	Mararashtra
Totals	884,972	605,720	279,252
Improvement Index (1964/1956)	37	67	23

The following states recorded poor performances: Uttar Pradesh, Bihar, West Bengal, Andra-Pradesh, and Orissa.

The population of India ranges between 500 and 550 million, but the fact remains that there are 100 million target couples to be reached in 560,000 villages. Of these 100 million target couples there are 56 million couples with three or more children. Among the couples who had vasectomies performed 70.8 percent had three children or less, whereas 29.2 percent had four or more children.

TABLE 1-III
STERILIZATIONS IN INDIAN STATES, PAKISTAN, AND OTHER COUNTRIES

Locale	Percent of Sterilizations
Maharashtra	70.3
Gujarat	6.8
Uttar Pradesh	5.7
Andhra Pradesh	4.4
Mysore	3.9
Madras	2.7
Goa	1.2
Other States and Territories	4.3
Pakistan	0.3
Other Countries	0.4

Motivation is of the utmost importance in the continuation and implementation of a contraceptive program. Intra-uterine contraceptive devices are of importance because they are one-shot procedures. The program of intra-uterine contraceptive device insertion has not been of noticeable success, however, and the rate of IUCD insertions has shown a downward trend. Sterilizations at first showed a tremendous increase, but the trend reversed, and from 1968 to 1969 the number of sterilizations declined (Table 1-I).

When the acceptability of vasectomies is compared with that of tubal ligation, it can be seen that vasectomies are about two and one-half times more acceptable than tubectomies (Tables 1-II, 1-IV, 1-V).

TABLE 1-IV
STERILIZATIONS IN MAHARASHTRA

Year	Sterilizations	Vasectomies	Tubectomies
1965–1966	51,412	32,585	18,827
1966–1967	65,614	43,374	22,240
1967–1968	332,329	286,867	45,462
1968–1969	273,034	206,584	66,450

This trend is related to the scarcity of institutional facilities in India, which, in effect, decreases the opportunities for the performance of tubal ligations. Thus, the capacity for the implementation of a vasectomy program is much greater. This being the case, vasectomy is the procedure of choice at the present time.

TABLE 1-V
STERILIZATIONS IN GREATER BOMBAY

Year	Sterilizations	Vasectomies	Tubectomies
1965–1966	2,806	503	2,303
1966–1967	3,525	485	3,040
1967–1968	64,408	53,193	11,215
1968–1969	46,348	32,730	13,618

The sterilization program, as well as the vasectomy program has been most successful in Maharashtra (Tables 1-II, 1-III, and 1-IV). The number of camps for sterilization was increased substantially. These figures are most meaningful since the population of Maharashtra is 10 percent of that of India as a whole.

A large number of the births in Maharashtra occur in families with three or more children. About 41 percent of the births in 1967 fell into this category. The fact that 45 percent of the births in 1964 were to families with three or more children most certainly indicates that the sterilization program has had some impact.

If an 80 percent effective contraceptive method is used by 20 percent of the population, the birth rate would be reduced by about 9 percent. However, if a 20 percent effective contraceptive method were used by 80 percent of the population, the reduction in birth rate would be only about 4 percent. The necessity of a highly effective contraceptive method is self-evident, and there is no doubt about the efficacy of sterilization.

The data on the sterilization program in Greater Bombay are presented in Tables 1-V and 1-VI. At first, the acceptability of

TABLE 1-VI
VASECTOMIES PERFORMED IN CAMPS IN GREATER BOMBAY

Date	Number of Vasectomies
February, 1967	89
March, 1967	164
April, 1967	179
May, 1967	239
June, 1967	244
July, 1967	1,373
August, 1967	3,960
September, 1967	6,230
October, 1967	6,106
November, 1967	5,572
December, 1967	6,255
January, 1967	7,180

tubectomy was substantially higher than that of vasectomy, but starting in 1967 the situation reversed itself dramatically.

At first the number of sterilizations showed a dramatic increase, but in 1968–1969 a decline was shown. Of these sterilizations performed, the number of tubectomies has increased, while the number of vasectomies has declined. It would be of importance to determine if this situation is attributable to a completion of the "backlog" cases or to some deficiency in the vasectomy camp program.

Sterilization camps are, in essence, temporary field facilities for family planning; they are established where regular services are not available. They permit the extension of specialized services to remote areas. Vasectomy camps were the first to be organized. The initial success achieved in Maharashtra and Madras has led other states to adopt vasectomy camp programs.

Later these facilities were extended to the insertion of intrauterine contraceptive devices and the performance of tubal ligation.

The increase in India's sterilization program can be attributed to the camp program. Six million sterilizations were performed in India as of March 31, 1969; this is a most impressive figure.

There are various types of camps in which vasectomy facilities are maintained at some delivery stations and community locations. There are temporary camps which are established for from ten to fifteen days and there are camps which only exist for a single day. Recently we have started a program of performing vasectomies on a bus which has been specially equipped for that purpose. This permits instant motivation and in one month some three thousand sterilizations have been performed in this manner.

During 1967–1968 there were 15,000 camps where 150,000 vasectomies were performed. The data for vasectomy camps in Greater Bombay are presented in Table 1-VI.

The so-called helper system has been of tremendous importance in this program. Regular family-planning workers were involved in only about twenty-six percent of these sterilizations. The majority of the sterilizations were motivated by others. It is most necessary to involve the total community in the program and to motivate everyone to be interested in and concerned with population control.

Religion appears to be a factor in the acceptance of sterilization. Acceptance of sterilization is greatest among Hindus, less among Muslims, and least among Christians. In Maharashtra the population is 82 percent Hindu, 7.67 Muslim, and 1.42 percent Christian. Of these, 90 percent of the Hindus have accepted sterilization, while only 5.57 percent of the Muslims and 0.45 percent of the Christians have done so. In Greater Bombay the Muslims represent 13 percent of the population and the Christians only 4.8 percent. In the first year of the sterilization program it was accepted by 8 percent of the Muslims and 1.5 percent of the Christians. In the following year a family planning acceptance was 10 percent for the Muslims and 2.5 percent for the Christians.

A demographic study of 32,967 vasectomy patients was undertaken, and some interesting data emerged.

The residence of 61.4 percent of the couples is in huts and slums, while only 38.6 percent live in other domiciles.

The average age of the husband was 38.5 years, with 79.3 percent falling into the 20 to 45 year age range. The average age of the wife is 31.5 years, with 92.2 percent falling in the 20 to 40 year age range.

The average number of living children among our vasectomy patients is 3.1, while among tubectomy patients it is 4.5 or possibly higher. The general figure for average number of living children for vasectomy patients is purported to be 3.5, but I do not know on what data this figure is based. Among these children the average of males is 1.8, of females, 1.3. This is a factor worthy of consideration, for family planning is not usually considered in India unless a couple has two sons; this is a limiting factor for the sterilization program and family planning in general.

The average monthly income of families in our sample was 114.5 rupees, with 88.5 percent earning under 200 rupees, 8.3 percent earning 200 to 299 rupees, and only 3.2 percent with incomes above 300 rupees. The average is about 15 American dollars per month.

Among our 32,967 vasectomy cases, 80.6 percent of the husbands were illiterate, as were 88.4 percent of the wives.

Unskilled workers formed 57.7 percent of our sample. The occupational distribution of the other cases was as follows: skilled workers, 7.4 percent; service workers, 15.5 percent; production workers, 6.1 percent; clerical workers, 0.7 percent; sales personnel, 3.7 percent; business personnel, 3.9 percent; workers in the primary sector, 1.7 percent; unemployed, 2.3 percent; and beggars, 0.4 percent.

A considerable amount of effort is required to make the family planning program a success. The sterilization program is very poorly accepted in Uttar Pradesh, but residents of Uttar Pradesh who are in Bombay accept our services. Also, persons from other countries come and utilize our services, which are entirely free.

Most people are weary of the socioeconomic pressures forced upon them, and if the sterilization program has a good method, a skilled approach, and convenient service it will gain still greater acceptance.

One of the existing problems is complications, which in our program exist at a rate of 1 percent. Immediate complications are hematoma, infection, and testicular tenderness and pain. Later complications include sexual weakness and impregnation of the female due to failure of the surgical procedure.

Perhaps one of the factors in the decline of the sterilization rate is due to defects in the present program. Once these are eliminated, the program should gain greater acceptance among the masses and can be implemented on a still larger scale.

Chapter 2

TUBAL LIGATION PROGRAM IN INDIA

B.S. DARBARI

Sterilization is one of the most important methods available to the public for family planning. To date, experience has shown that, if accepted by the target population, sterilization can have a significant effect in reducing the birth rate. However, it cannot alone meet the needs of population control, for there is the necessity for contraceptive practices for spacing of children. Education campaigns directed towards the acceptance of sterilization should be undertaken by developing nations; ultimate goals should be sterilization after a couple has two children, and most definitely after three children.

Acceptance of sterilization increases as prospective parents become convinced that their existing children will get the best of possible care. Accordingly, nutritional, health, and innoculation programs have been integrated with the family planning units. Acceptance of sterilization increases where family planning services are coordinated with other health services.

Table 2-I shows the sterilization trend in India since 1956.

TABLE 2-I
STERILIZATION IN INDIA 1956 TO 1969
(MALE VERSUS FEMALE PERCENTAGES)

Year	Males (Percent)	Females (Percent)
1956	33.5	66.5
1957	30.2	67.8
1958	36.5	63.5
1959	41.7	58.3
1960	58.4	41.6
1961	61.1	38.9
1962	71.1	28.9
1963	67.3	32.7
1964	74.6	25.4
1965	84.2	15.8
1966 (January to March)	90.2	9.8
1966–1967	88.5	11.5
1967–1968	89.6	10.4
1968–1969	82.6	17.4
Overall	83.6	16.4

It will be noted that over 15 percent of the eligible couples have been sterilized in India, and it is hoped that this percentage can be increased.

It will also be noted that before 1960, tubectomy was the sterilization method of choice, but after 1960, vasectomy increased in popularity considerably. About 11.7 sterilizations per thousand population have been performed so far. Statewide distribution of sterilizations per thousand are the following: Tamil Nadu, 21.3; Maharashtra, 20.3; Orissa, 15.3; Kerala, 15.4; Punjab, 12.7; Gujarat, 13.7; Mysore, 11.9; Madhya Pradesh, 12.9; and Andhra Pradesh, 12.6. It is of interest to note that most of these states are below average in intra-uterine contraceptive device insertions.

It has been estimated that about 10.6 percent of eligible couples currently are preventing pregnancy with sterilization. Pregnancy prevention by the combined program of sterilization and IUCD use is utilized by 13.5 percent of the couples, while 1.5 percent rely on more conventional contraceptive devices.

Demographic characteristics of women undergoing tubectomy vary from state to state. In Maharashtra 78 percent of the tubectomies were done on women between the ages of 26 to 35. In the Kolar District the median age of sterilized females was 31–32 years, while between 72 to 78 percent of the women were 25 to 34 years of age. Of the 400 tubectomies performed, the age distribution was as follows: 0.5 percent, 15 to 20 years old; 15.0%, 21 to 25 years old; 53 percent, 26 to 30 years old; 25.7%, 31 to 35 years old; 5.5%, 36 to 40 years old; and only 0.3% were 41 years old or older.

Other figures for the tubectomy cases in the Kolar District show that 0.3% of the women had 1 living child; 6.7% had 2, 20.5% had 3; 25.0% had 4 children, 10.0% of the women had 5 children; and 28.5% of the women had 6 children. In Western nations women who undergo tubectomy usually have between 6 and 7 living children.

The religious distribution of the cases was as follows: 77.5% Hindu; 7.0% Muslim; 1.3% Christian; and 15.2% others. Almost 80 percent of the sterilized females have primary level education; 31.8% were literate, while 68.2% were illiterate. Occupations ranged from agricultural and household (93.7%), laborers (5.5%), to officials (0.8%).

SURGERY

There should be no postoperative effects of tubectomy, either in menstrual history or sexual response, which if anything, should be improved by the removal of the fear of an unwanted pregnancy. In practice, there are a larger number of psychosomatic disturbances following tubectomy than there are after vasectomy.

Reconstruction of the divided tubes is a major surgical procedure requiring skillful manipulation; less than half the reconstructions are successful. As more time elapses between the original tubectomy and the reconstruction procedure, the chances of success diminish; the fact that such women are nearing menopause may play a part in these results.

Sterilization may be done by the abdominal or vaginal route, and, although there are various acknowledged methods of tubal sterilization, the Pomeroy method is generally preferred. The operation can be performed at any time, although postpartum surgery is more economically advantageous. The vaginal route is preferred because postoperative hospitalization and convalescence are minimal. However, this technique requires special instruments and great surgical skill.

The following are some of the recognized methods of tubal sterilization.

Pomeroy Technique

This procedure of midway division and tubal ligature is simple and is usually preferred because of its speed and absence of sequelae. The technique can also be performed by the vaginal route.

Irving Procedure

This is probably the most dependable tubectomy technique, especially when performed in conjunction with cesarean section. There is a low failure rate, but the technique is technically difficult, takes an appreciable length of time, requires a large incision, and often leaves two permanent tender areas on either side of the uterus.

Madlener Operation

This procedure of crushing an angle of the tube and ligating the crushed portion has been used extensively. The method is simple, gives fair security, and is indicated when there is marked vascularity in the tubal area. The Walthard modification in which the crushing and ligation includes a large tubal loop may jeopardize ovarian circulation and is contraindicated.

Tubal Cauterization

Included in this classification is intra-uterine tubal cauterization and permanent sterilization by tubal electrocoagulation.

Other surgical procedures include the Aldrige method of temporary surgical sterilization, cornual resection, the Shirodkar method, and total salpingectomy.

DELIVERY OF SERVICES

About 90 of 180 couples of reproductive age in a population of 1,000 are eligible for family planning. Calculations indicate that about 13.5 percent of the eligible couples are protected; 10.6 percent by sterilization, and 2.9 percent by the use of intra-uterine contraceptive devices. If the estimated birth rates for 1951 to 1961 are reduced by the eligible couples protected, the birth rate of 41.7 for 1951–1960 should have been reduced to 37.6 in 1967–1968.

At the present time sterilization facilities are provided by 4,042 nonmobile and 410 mobile units. The 1966 facilities consisted of 192 mobile units and 2,324 nonmobile units.

CONCLUSIONS

By making certain assumptions concerning age distribution, fertility, and mortality rates, the number of births prevented by all contraceptive methods may be calculated. Results of of these calculations are shown in Table 2-II.

Without family planning, the general fertility rate in India is 195 per 1,000 women of child-bearing age; this conforms to the officially estimated birth rate of 41.7 from 1951–1960. If the number of births prevented by family planning are substracted birth rate estimates would be as follows: 1965–1966, 39.8; 1966–1967, 39.2; and 1967–1968, 38.5. This agrees substantially with the birth rate of 37.6 calculated on the basis of protected couples.

TABLE 2-II
MILLIONS OF BIRTH PREVENTED ANNUALLY BY CONTRACEPTIVE METHODS

Year	Sterilization	IUCD Insertions	Other Contraceptives	Total
1965–1966	.2005	.0066	.0023	.2094
1966–1967	.3153	.1552	.0539	.5244
1967–1968	.4962	.3246	.0773	.8981
1968–1969	.8472	.4412	.1282	1.4166

For the last two years the number of sterilizations has increased. It is calculated that one sterilization prevents 1.5 births; one IUCD insertion, 0.5 births; and use of regular contraceptives, 0.125 births. Sterilization would thus appear to be the method of choice in population control. Each year the number of births prevented has increased, with that, the expenditure per preventive intervention has declined. Except in certain psychological conditions, sterilization has no detrimental effect on physical, mental, or sexual processes. Its chief advantage is that it is a one-time procedure and insures permanent results.

The philosophy of the family planning program is to provide services close to residence areas, thus ensuring maximum, immediate motivation. Although the number of sterilization centers is large, it is manifestly impossible to provide services for each and every one of the 560,000 villages and 3,000 towns and cities. Therefore, a strategy has been developed to cater to the needs of the population.

The plan is twofold. In addition to centers for vasectomies, both static and mobile, there will be field hospital facilities for tubectomies located at central points in order to provide services for a number of villages. Provision has been made to provide for expenses incurred in traveling to facilities and loss of wages during postoperative periods. The need for this reimbursement will diminish as services expand into the peripheral areas.

Since one-third of the country's population lives in fifty-one districts, about one-fourth of the eligible couples could be provided for by provision of facilities in these areas. Also, organized groups could bring a sizeable number of eligible couples into the program. Industry has recognized the relationship between family size and the efficiency and productivity of the workers. Over sixty industrial concerns in India provide incentive money to have their employees undergo sterilization.

Although sterilization remains the most effective family planning method, there is a need for a strong service program which also dispenses intra-uterine contraceptive devices and conventional contraceptives. The place of oral contraceptives in rural family planning programs is small because of the large margin of error. There is need for high motivation for sterilization. However, the lasting results and definite impact on fertility provide for great acceptability. Also, economic problems in rural areas can be alleviated by planning only for the number of children that can be supported.

Acceptance is aided by the large number of satisfied individuals who have been sterilized and can vouch for its effectiveness and efficiency. Experience has shown that when a sterilized person talks to others he has a great influence upon the acceptance of the program. People are usually most influenced by friends, relatives, and neighbors in their home settings, and this factor should play an important role in the increase in the acceptance of sterilization as a family planning method.

Chapter 3

TUBAL LIGATION IN CARACAS, VENEZUELA

OSCAR AGUERO AND LEOPOLDO CARDENAS-CONDE

There is no special program for tubal ligation in Caracas, or in Venezuela as a whole. The procedure is unlawful in Venezuela because it affects the permanent reproductive capacity of the individual. However, tubal ligation is being used with increasing frequency in both hospitals and private practice, in spite of the establishment of family planning clinics in Caracas in 1963.

Data on tubal ligations performed in the main obstetrical hospitals in Caracas follow.

Concepcion Palacios Maternity Hospital

About seventy percent of the deliveries in Caracas and its environs take place in this institution; it is a free hospital and caters to the lower socioeconomic groups of the population.

During the period from 1939 to 1968 there were 832,395 admissions; of these 728,400 were for deliveries (including cesarean section), abortion, and ectopic pregnancies. In this same period, 6,974 tubectomies were performed, representing 8.3 per thousand admissions and 9.5 per thousand pregnancies. From 0.8 tubectomies per thousand admissions in 1939 (0.9 per thousand pregnancies), the frequency rose to 18 per thousand admissions in 1968 (20.6 per thousand pregnancies). The number of tubal ligations performed in 1939 was two; in 1968 it was 1,084 (Figs. 3-1 and 3-2).

This increase in the number of tubectomies has resulted from the liberalization of indications for its performance. These data are summarized in Table 3-1. The attitudes of medical personnel have been changing during the last eight or ten years, and tubectomy is often performed along with a cesarean section in a multigravida. These factors help to explain the increase in

Tubal Ligation in Caracas, Venezuela

TUBAL LIGATION IN "CONCEPCION PALACIOS" MATERNITY HOSPITAL
——— By 1000 Admisions
------ " " Pregnancies

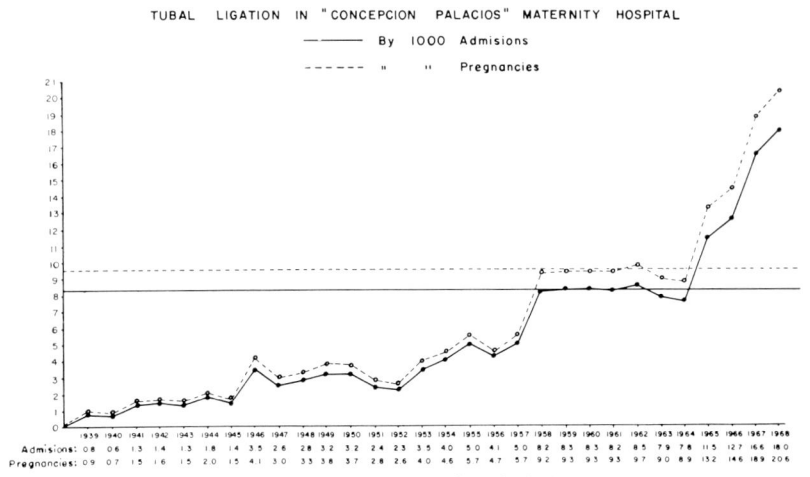

Figure 3–1. Frequency of tubal ligations.

TUBAL LIGATION IN "CONCEPCION PALACIOS" MATERNITY HOSPITAL
——— By 1000 Admisions
------ " " Pregnancies

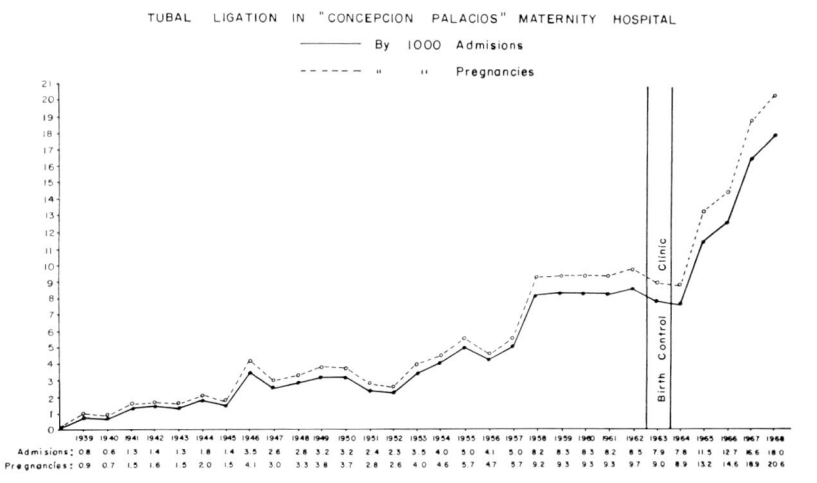

Figure 3–2. Frequency of tubal ligations before and after birth control clinic establishment.

TABLE 3-I
INDICATIONS FOR TUBAL LIGATION—1939–1968

Date	Previous Cesarean Section (in percent of cases)	Multiparity	Other
1939–1950	67.7	3.7	28.6*
1959–1965	38.1	50.2	11.7
1966–1968	39.0	47.5	13.5

*This includes 34 cases with pulmonary tuberculosis and 12 cases with toxemia or hypertensive disease.

tubectomies in spite of the existence of a very active family planning clinic. As of May, 1969, 17,227 women have attended the clinic: 16,227 are using intrauterine contraceptive devices, 913 are using oral contraceptives, and 87 are using other methods.

Criteria for the number of cesarean sections required to justify surgical sterilization have varied through the years. When the program was begun, tubectomy was permitted at the second and third section. Although we generally still ligate during the third section, additional pregnancies were permitted in 604 cases. Tubal ligation was performed during the fourth section in 558 cases, in forty-four cases during the fifth section, and in two cases during the sixth section.

Similarly there have been variations in the criteria for the number of living children before surgical intervention. Although, in general, we use surgical sterilization after the eighth child, many cases have been ligated after the fourth pregnancy.

In 5,355 cases tubectomy was performed during cesarean section, repair of uterine rupture, or other surgical procedures; in 1,619 cases it was performed postpartum or postabortion.

Policlinica Caracas Maternity Hospital

This is a private institution in which there were 24,965 deliveries and 597 tubal ligations from 1949 through 1963. For each thousand deliveries, there have been 23 tubectomies; 10 per thousand deliveries in 1949–1951, and 30 per thousand in 1962–1963. Indications for these 597 sterilizations were the following: previous cesarean section, 316; multiparity, 218; toxemia and hypertensive disease, 19; Rh negative blood tests, 12; neuropsychiatric conditions, 4; varicose veins, 4; urovaginal or rectovaginal fistula, 4; uterine myoma, 2; ectopic pregnancy, 2; uterine rupture, 2; other, 9. Previous cesarean section is the criterion for 52.9 percent of the tubal ligations, while multiparity accounts for 36.9 percent.

In private practice multiparity criteria vary with the individual physician; in this particular series 12 percent of the cases had seven or more children. Of these 597 tubectomies 407 (68.1%) were performed during cesarean section and 190

(31.8%) postpartum or unrelated to pregnancy. Failures were about 0.5 percent.

Other Hospitals

Table 3–II presents the data on tubal ligations in other hospitals in Caracas; while Table 3–III presents tubal ligation data from other countries. The tables show a wide variation in

TABLE 3-II
TUBAL LIGATIONS IN OTHER CARACAS HOSPITALS

Hospital	Period	Pregnancies	Tubectomies	Tubectomies per Thousand Pregnancies
Concepcion Palacios	1939–1968	728,400	6,794	9.5
University	1956–1966	28,365	305	10.7
Social Security	1963–1969	52,592	907	23.1
Policlinica Caracas*	1949–1963	24,965	597	23.9
Medical Center*	1959–1968	10,783	104	9.4

* Private Hospitals

TABLE 3-III
TUBAL LIGATIONS IN BELGIUM, GERMANY, AND THE UNITED STATES*

Period	Deliveries	Tubal Ligations	Tubal Ligations per Thousand Deliveries	Data From
Belgium				
1947–1960	11,620	59	5.0	Bourg
1950–1960	9,000	23	2.5	Gosselin
1951–1960	12,111	364	30.0	Yokaer
1957–1960	4,568	24	5.2	Dussart

Period	Deliveries	Tubal Ligations	Tubal Ligations per Thousand Deliveries	Data From
Germany				
1959	13,000	130	10.0	Ruther

Period	Deliveries	Tubal Ligations	Tubal Ligations per Thousand Deliveries	Data From
United States of America				
1940–1952	32,721	462	14.0	Sacks
1949–1959	16,072	551	34.0	Powell
1949–1963	22,425	1,146	51.0	White
1949–1963	1,700	120	70.0	Goddard
1950–1959	22,727	355	15.0	Samuels
1953–1963	43,819	547	12.0	Beacham
1962–1963	8,564	325	37.0	Radman
1962–1963	8,977	409	46.0	Starr

* Reproduced from: Aguero O.: *Rev Obst Ginec Venezuela*, 26:641, 1966.

tubectomies, reflecting the range of criteria; it is interesting to note the differences between the two private hospitals in Caracas.

In spite of the fact that tubal ligation is unlawful in Venezuela, there is an increasing trend towards its use. Criteria are changing and reflect a rather liberal attitude towards tubal ligation among the physicians of Caracas.

Chapter 4

MALE STERILIZATION IN EAST PAKISTAN

JOHN W. RATCLIFFE, A.H.G. QUDDUS, AND H.T. CROLEY

Pakistan is divided into two provinces separated by India. This causes administrative problems in the family planning program, since the central government offices are located almost entirely in West Pakistan. East Pakistan is a province which is about twenty percent of the total area of Pakistan, but contains about fifty-six percent of the population, approximately seventy million people. The population density is quite high and makes the family planning program a most critical one for both the survival and the advancement of East Pakistan.

The national family planning program began in East Pakistan in July, 1965. Heavy emphasis was given to intra-uterine contraceptive devices in the Third Five Year Plan[1] and it was considered to be the contraceptive method most likely to result in program success. Since the implementation of the program, the majority of official time, effort, and expenditure has been devoted to furthering acceptance of the IUD among the female population.

However, the Third Five Year Plan did provide for an incentive program associated with vasectomies. The physician was given 15 rupees, while 20 rupees were given to the patient. The spectacular and unexpected rise in vasectomy rates in East Pakistan since 1965 might be directly related to this incentive payment.

Figure 1 shows the trend in sterilization and IUD use in East Pakistan from 1965 through 1969. In the last quarter of 1966 there were 14,000 vasectomies as opposed to 63,000 IUD insertions per quarter. Vasectomy reached a peak in 1968–1969, when 125,327 sterilizations were done in comparison to 102,746 IUD insertions.

Although sterilization was recognized in the Third Five Year Plan as the most efficient method of contraception,[1] this aspect

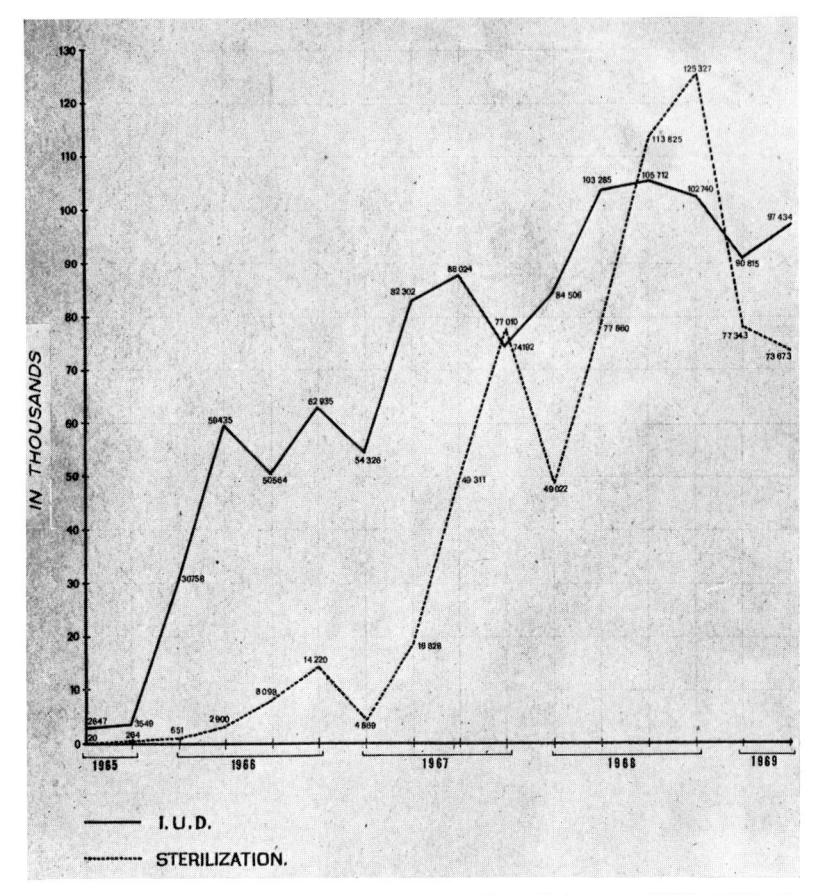

Figure 4–1. Sterilization and IUD Use in East Pakistan, 1965–1969. Statistics by quarterly totals. Tubeligations are included in the vasectomy statistics, but comprise less than 1% of the total effort. East Pakistan Family Planning Board, *Progress Report in Family Planning*, Dacca, July, 1965 through June, 1969.

of the program was viewed as a relatively minor adjunct to the total family planning scheme. Although sterilization has been available prior to 1965, it had proved to be singularly unpopular in Pakistan[1] and there was little reason to expect any radical reversal of that trend. Nevertheless, it was considered that sterilization as a method could not be ignored. Monetary incentives for sterilization were provided and a national target of 90,000 sterilizations was established for the period 1965 through 1970.

However, by the autumn of 1967, it had become obvious that the response to this new approach by the male population of East Pakistan was clearly exceeding the expectations of the program planners. In spite of its inability to compete with the IUD in terms of availability, publicity, and national program emphasis, vasectomy was making a strong bid to become the most popular contraceptive method in East Pakistan.

PURPOSES AND PROCEDURES

At this point, the East Pakistan Research and Evaluation Centre (EPREC), with the approval and cooperation of the East Pakistan Family Planning Board, decided to undertake a research study of the vasectomy program in East Pakistan. In addition to the collection of data necessary to evaluate the contribution of male sterilization as a program method, i.e. demographic characteristics of vasectomy adopters, it was thought an attempt also should be made to identify those factors responsible for the spreading interest in, and rapidly increasing acceptance of, male sterilization. It was reasoned that knowledge regarding such factors could well be of vital importance to those directing Pakistan's family planning program. Identification of those features which exert great appeal in East Pakistan could have immediate program implications in West Pakistan, where the present acceptance level of vasectomy is still relatively low. Moreover, an examination of the motivational factors involved might well provide insight into program factors which eventually could be applied with positive effect to other aspects of the total program.

Although it is possible to assume that the incentive fee incorporated in the program was directly responsible for the increased vasectomy rate, the lack of concomitant interest in West Pakistan, with an identical program, casts doubt upon this assumption. Possibly the increase in acceptance might be due to some communication factor peculiar to East Pakistan. In order to minimize the chance of excluding some factor vital to the success of the program, a fact-finding team was sent into the field for informal studies. The recommendations of the team led to investigations in four major areas: demographic characteristics of vasectomy adopters; motivation underlying the decision to adopt vasectomy; sources of information regarding sterilization; and postoperative experiences of the patients, including sexual satisfaction and side effects.

Trained investigators were sent to twenty-four government vasectomy clinics in three districts of East Pakistan to obtain information from clients at the time of sterilization. Supplementary information was also obtained from attending physicians and the accompanying vasectomy agents. The research data were collected through interviews in Bengali from pretested interview schedules which contained a combination of open-end and fixed-alternative questions. The interview data were obtained between the months of January and April of 1968.

CHARACTERISTICS OF THE VASECTOMY PATIENTS

Interviews were attempted on a total of 618 vasectomy cases. Two clients refused to complete the interview, and three fully completed interview schedules were destroyed accidentally. Half of the study population of 613 sterilized males were interviewed before the operation, and the other half were interviewed postoperatively.

The religious distribution of the group was 91 percent Muslim and 9 percent Hindu. The occurrence of these religions in the population at large is 80 percent and 18 percent respectively.[2] Muslims are thus overrepresented in the study population.

The most common occupations reported were day laborer (62%) and landed farmer (14%).

Table 4-I gives the distribution of the population by monthly income. Reported client earnings are as follows: less than 50 rupees, 29%; less than 100 rupees, 75%; and less than 150 rupees, 96% (about thirty American dollars per month). Comparable data for the total population of East Pakistan[3] indicate that the lower income groups are heavily overrepresented among the study population. Of the total population 9% earned 50 rupees

TABLE 4-I

MONTHLY INCOME OF 613 VASECTOMY CLIENTS IN EAST PAKISTAN COMPARED TO THE AVERAGE PROVINCIAL INCOME DISTRIBUTION*

Income in Rs. p/mo	Vasectomy Clients N = 613	%	East Pakistan % Rural	% Urban	% Combined
0– 49	179	29.2	9.0	5.0	8.8
50– 99	283	46.2	33.8	23.3	32.7
100–149	125	20.4	23.9	24.3	24.5
150–199	17	2.8	15.5	12.7	15.3
200–249	3	0.5	7.8	8.4	7.8
250–299	1	0.2	4.2	7.1	4.4
300–399	5	0.8	3.0	4.9	3.1
400–499			1.4	4.5	1.6
500–699			0.9	4.5	1.0
700–899			0.3	2.0	0.4
900+			0.2	3.3	0.4
Total	613	100.1	100.0	100.0	100.0

* Taken from Bergan, A.: Personal Income Distribution and Personal Savings in Pakistan, 1963/1964, In *The Pakistan Development Review*, Vol. VII, No. 2, Summer, 1967.

per month and 65% earned less than 150 rupees. These data, along with reported occupations, indicate that vasectomy patients are drawn largely from the lower socioeconomic classes.

The mean reported age for vasectomy cases is 45.6; while the mean age of their wives is 33.3. If the female reproductive period is presumed to end at the age of 45, then each vasectomy reported in the study provides almost twelve couple years of protection for unwanted childbirths. Correcting these figures for mortality yields nine couple-years of protection. These figures are based on the supposition that each operation was both successful and irreversible. The number of births prevented by vasectomy is officially estimated as three. Comparable data on the IUD collected in 1967,[4] show the mean age of East Pakistan females who accept this device as 30.4 years. This could mean that the IUD has a greater appeal among younger couples; however, it could also indicate the use of the IUD as a child spacing device.

The mean number of living children for the study population was 4.6; this family is composed of a mean of 2.4 sons and 2.2 daughters. Comparable data of IUD users[4] show the mean number of children as 4.56: 2.41 sons and 2.16 daughters. The differences between these figures are insignificant and suggest that family characteristics of couples who employ vasectomy and IUD insertion are very similar.

Table 4-II shows the distribution of patient's wives by the sex of the living children. It does suggest that, at least at lower reproductive levels, the sex of the children does influence the decision to undergo sterilization. Although these findings do not agree with comparable data from Kerala State, India,[5] they are certainly not unexpected. Among Pakistan's eligibility require-

TABLE 4-II
DISTRIBUTION OF 613 VASECTOMY ADOPTERS BY NUMBER AND SEX OF LIVING CHILDREN

Number of Female Children	Number of Male Children									Total
	0	1	2	3	4	5	6	7	8	9	
0		1	6	8	2	4	2				23
1		16	87	43	23	6	1				176
2	3	44	84	41	25	5		1			203
3	2	34	40	34	15	1	2	1			129
4	1	12	19	13	4	2				1	52
5		8	7	5	1						21
6	1	1		2	1	1					6
7		1									1
8			1								1
9											
10			1								1
Total	7	117	244	147	71	19	5	2		1	613

ments for sterilization are three living children, with a minimum of one son. The table indicates that this criterion is not adhered to in all cases.

The mean reported age of the youngest child of the study population was 2.1 years. This indicates that the average patient's wife is well within her reproductive period. This has been corroborated by the findings of a later study.[6] In addition, this mean age suggests that a reduction in presently reported family size from infant and child mortality is very likely.

MOTIVATIONS IN VASECTOMY ACCEPTANCE

Data concerning the extent of client information about vasectomy and other contraceptive methods are of importance. The extent and kind of this information clearly can influence the decision to accept sterilization.

Ninety-three percent of all clients interviewed reported being unaware of any other method of contraception. If this is true, it implies that an enormous number of persons are not being reached by present family planning communication approaches in East Pakistan; whether family planning messages reach this group but are not understood, or whether this group have no access to media which carry family planning messages is not known. Findings of other studies indicate general widespread knowledge of family planning methods among both rural and urban populations of East Pakistan.[7,8]

Patients were also asked about what rumors they had heard about vasectomy. The question *What do people say of the operation after they have had it?* produced the following answers: 56 percent said they had heard that it was a minor operation producing no problems or that the subjects were pleased with vasectomy; 32 percent had heard no rumors; 31 percent heard that the surgery resulted in sexual rejuvination; and 2 percent reported hearing negative comments.

When asked about the reason for accepting vasectomy, 94 percent of the patients said it was to prevent having children, and 13 percent* said it was for the incentive fee.

When the reasons for vasectomy acceptance were compared by income group, no significant differences were found. This was contrary to expectations, since it had been anticipated that the incentive fee as a motivating factor would vary inversely with reported income. No significant difference between reasons for acceptance were found between those individuals interviewed preoperatively and postoperatively.

With regard to the single most important benefit derived from the vasectomy operation, 88 percent of the clients mentioned childbirth prevention, 7 percent mentioned money, and 3 percent thought it was health improvement. Of the 540 clients who wished to stop having additional children, 89 percent stated that they wished to do so in order to improve, or at least stabilize, family economic conditions.

When the patients interviewed preoperatively were compared

---

* Total percentage exceeds 100 because patients were permitted to give more than one response.

with those interviewed postoperatively on their opinion of the single most important benefit of vasectomy, a significant difference was found (P = 0.05). The postoperative interview group was less likely to give *money* as a response than were the preoperative group; this suggests that money tends to be deemphasized as a motivating force either because surgery has been undergone or because of some factor in the operative situation.

In hopes of finding an indirect measure of motivation or providing a check on reported factors, data were obtained on the time elapsed between first awareness of vasectomy as a method of contraception and actual sterilization. A total of 13 percent of all clients came to the clinic for surgery on the day they first became aware of the method. However, 77 percent of the patients took a week or longer to decide, and over 53 percent took a month or longer. Of those reporting a time lag, 41 percent said it was time taken to consider the decision, 29 percent said they had been engaged in other tasks, and 14 percent that it was due to fear of the operation.

It was found that those individuals who indicated that *money* was the single most important benefit differed significantly in time elapsed between hearing of the operation and its actual performance from those clients who considered that the benefits were other than financial (P = 0.001). Fully 50 percent of the *money* clients came for surgery on the day they first learned of vasectomy, while only 10 percent of those who wished to stop childbirth came on the first day.

The above data lead to the tentative conclusion that vasectomy patients can be separated into three groups, according to reasons for acceptance. There appears to be a small group of males who adopt sterilization only for the protection it provides against childbirth; this group is probably similar in size to the group of vasectomy acceptors recorded prior to the initiation of the Third Five Year Plan and probably would have accepted vasectomy without the incentive fee. A second small group appears to undergo vasectomy strictly for immediate monetary gain, e.g. 7 percent of our sample who reported that their single major reason for vasectomy acceptance was money. The third group, the great majority of sterilization patients, appears to consist of those who accept for a *combination* of factors: immediate financial gain (more charitably, no immediate loss of income) *and* permanent protection from unwanted children who might threaten the economic stability of the family.

SOURCES OF INFORMATION ON VASECTOMY

It was found that 48 percent of the study population first learned about vasectomy from *agents*. Agents are unofficial, non-program personnel who spread vasectomy information, actively recruit potential patients, and accompany patients to the clinic to offer support during surgery. For these services, the agent generally receives, in the form of a *finder's fee*, a portion of the client's 20 rupee incentive payment. Although 38 percent of the respondents reported friends and neighbors as primary sources of information, 69 percent of the patients reported that agents were involved at some point in the decision-making process.

These findings provide some insight into a factor that is considered to be largely responsible for East Pakistan's unique program experience in sterilization. Personal communication and recruitment are undertaken by a group of entrepreneurs who came into existence spontaneously as an outgrowth of the vasectomy incentive program.* At the time of this study, agents of this type did not exist in West Pakistan, although about 652† sterilizations were performed per month. In contrast, during the same period, some 16,341 sterilizations were performed monthly in East Pakistan. The unique nature of East Pakistan's vasectomy program is not due solely to the fact that there are agents associated with the program. In India, Madras State employed agents for their vasectomy program in 1965–1966.[9] East Pakistan is unique in that the vasectomy agents are not official program employees; rather, they are private citizens who, for a relatively small incentive fee, have served in such a manner as to complement public efforts in male sterilization programs. At the time

---

* It is likely that the cultural differences which exist between East and West Pakistan are responsible for this, but in what manner and to what degree are unknown.

† This is the average monthly performance during the first quarter of 968, the same period during which the study data were collected.

of this study, awareness of the existence of these agents among official program personnel was limited generally to the grass roots level.

In order to understand these agents, EPREC conducted a concurrent study focusing on vasectomy agents.[10] The more important of the two major findings was that, of the 155 agents interviewed, 21 percent were female. In what is considered a conservative Muslim society, such a fact is startling. It is widely believed that the women of East Pakistan, particularly rural women, are too conservative to talk even with their own husbands about family planning. The study tends to refute this belief by revealing that women can, and indeed do, approach men on such a delicate issue as sterilization. The study also revealed the fact that fully 39 percent of the male agents had undergone sterilization. This was considered to be an invaluable asset, for the agent could act as a satisfied customer recommending a product he himself had found to be useful.

In an attempt to measure the influence of the agent upon the patient's decision, agent involvement and elapsed time between client awareness and adoption of sterilization were compared. It seemed reasonable to assume that clients who had an agent involved would show less elapsed time than those clients who reported no agent involvement. In other words, it seemed that the agent's influence upon the client could be estimated roughly by the reduction in time lag between individual awareness and action. However, cross-tabulation of the data showed that agent involvement does not significantly affect the time lag between knowledge of vasectomy and actual surgery. This is extremely important, because it suggests that agents generally do not, or cannot, exert great pressure upon individuals and force them to make quick and ill-considered decisions.

FOLLOW-UP OF A SAMPLE OF THE STUDY POPULATION

A sample of 135 vasectomy cases (22% of the original population of 613) was given follow-up interviews after at least three months had elapsed since surgery. This was done to determine the incidence and types of postoperative side effects and satisfactions based on a relatively short-term experience.

Side effects were reported by 42 percent of the patients: 77 percent, simple pain; 52 percent swelling; 39 percent, physical weakness.* The overwhelming majority of these symptoms were reported as both minor and temporary.

In terms of changes in sexual life following sterilization, 59 percent of the patients reported no change, 29 percent had decrease in sexual desire, 9 percent reported increased physical desire, and 2 percent reported physical weakness. Similar findings resulted from a postvasectomy study on another district of East Pakistan.[11] Since it was thought that postoperative complications might influence psychological reactions to the surgery, a comparison was made between postoperative side effects and changes in marital relations (Table 4-III). Of the 56 clients who

TABLE 4-III
DISTRIBUTION OF REPORTED CHANGES DUE TO STERILIZATION BY PRESENCE OR ABSENCE OF POST-OPERATIVE SIDE-EFFECTS

Change Due to Steriilzation	Post-Operative Side Effects					
	Present		Absent		Total	
	N = 56	%	N = 79	%	N = 135	%
No Change	23	41.1	56	70.9	79	58.5
Sexual Desire Decreased	25	44.6	14	17.7	39	28.9
Sexual Desire Increased	6	10.7	6	7.6	12	8.9
Physical Weakness	2	3.6	1	1.3	3	2.2
Wife Dead/Divorced**	2	3.6	2	2.5	4	3.0
Others**	2	3.6	1	1.3	3	2.2
Total	60	107.2*	80	101.3*	140	103.7*

Probability levels based on chi squares: $P \angle .01$.
* Percentage exceeds 100 because the client was allowed to give more than one response.
** These cells were excluded from the chi square comparison.

reported postoperative side effects, 45 percent had a decrease in sexual desire. Of the 79 patients who had no postoperative side effects, only 18 percent reported decreased sexual desire. Increases in sexual desire were reported by 11 percent of the group with sequelae, while 8 percent of the group with no side effects reported increased libido (this difference is statistically significant-$P = 0.01$).

* The percentage total exceeds 100 because more than one response was permitted per person.

With regard to satisfaction with sterilization as a method of contraception, 85 percent were satisfied, 13 percent were not satisfied, and 2 percent had no opinion. Of the 17 patients who were dissatisfied with vasectomy, only 2 agreed on a reason (the inability to have children), while the other 15 clients each expressed a unique reason for dissatisfaction.

CONCLUSIONS

In the first quarter of 1968, East Pakistan Research and Evaluation Center (EPREC) conducted a study of the vasectomy clients in East Pakistan. Field work was conducted in vasectomy clinics in Dacca, Mymensingh, and Noakhali districts. The sample consisted of 613 males: about half were interviewed preoperatively, the remainder postoperatively.

Statistics regarding the number of sterilizations performed make it clear that East Pakistan's vasectomy program is contributing substantially to the family planning program. The present study, a measure of the effectiveness of vasectomy, provides a basis for assessing that contribution with some accuracy. Each vasectomy recorded here has provided an average of almost twelve couple-years of protection; the official estimate of the number of births prevented by each vasectomy is three. The economic approach to contraception in Pakistan's incentive approach appears to be vindicated by the clients themselves: 80 percent of the individuals in this survey indicated that prevention of unwanted childbirth could achieve or maintain the economic stability of the family.

Vasectomy seems to attract clients largely from the lower socioeconomic groups of East Pakistan. In terms of education, income, and probably occupation, the more disadvantaged groups are overrepresented in the study population. This population was also disadvantaged in that they lacked alternatives to sterilization, for 93 percent of the study group knew of no contraceptive methods other than vasectomy.

Unofficial vasectomy agents have been sources of information on sterilization for the majority of acceptors. The relatively small incentive fee offered has produced a large number of private citizens who have made it their business to complement governmental efforts in male sterilization. These entrepreneurs can be found wherever there are vasectomy prospects. The lower socio-economic groups, who appear to be outside the mainstream of official communication, seem most responsive to this highly personalized face-to-face approach. The present vasectomy rate in East Pakistan is a tribute to these volunteer agents and to the effectiveness of their methods.

One of the criticisms often directed against the vasectomy program is that prospects are dupes of the agents and may be unaware of either the nature or the implications of the procedure. Although we found client knowledge at the time of surgery sufficient to vindicate the average agent, no doubt there are some who are less scrupulous in their techniques.

The key to the average agent's success, his unofficial private status, is also a form of protection from official discipline for the deviant agent. Official registration of all vasectomy agents might improve recruiting tactics; however, this study indicates that truly effective agent control will result only from control of the vasectomy physicians. There are several reasons for this. There are hundreds of physicians involved in the vasectomy program, but there are thousands of agents; it is easier to control the few than the many. The physician is always the final judge of the agent's recruiting technique, since he is in a position to ascertain the extent of knowledge of the patient. Also, if the physician refuses to operate on uninformed applicants, the deviant agent will be forced to change either his methods or his occupation. Since vasectomy physicians are registered participants in the official program, they are liable to disciplinary action if they deviate from the program. For these reasons, it seems clear that regulation of official physicans would be a simple and effective method of regulating the actions of the agents.

Another criticism of Pakistan's vasectomy program has been that the incentive fee is all-important and that the prospective patient considers no other factor. This study indicates that this is not true in the majority of cases; in fact, the data suggest that the incentive fee is a necessary, but usually not sufficient, reason for the continued high rate of sterilization. The 20 rupee fee is clearly influential enough to precipitate action among those who wish to stop further childbirth, but it does appear to initiate action among many of those who desire more children.

Prior to this study, it was thought that side effects associated with sterilization in East Pakistan were nonexistent; this was often given as a major reason for the success of the program. On the contrary, our data show that a significant number of vasectomy patients do have postoperative sequelae. They also show that postoperative side effects and postoperative changes in sexual desire are related. This relationship should be explored more thoroughly; it suggests that a reduction in physical postoperative side effects might result in a reduction in postoperative psychological side effects which appear to affect the marital relations of a significant number of patients.

REFERENCES

1. Ministry of Health, Labor and Social Welfare, Government of Pakistan: *Family Planning Scheme for Pakistan During the Third Five-Year Plan.*
2. Office of the Census Commissioner, Home Affairs Division, Government of Pakistan. *1961 East Pakistan Census* Vol. 2, Population pp. 11–110, 11–111, IV–86, IV–87.
3. Bergan, A.: Personal income distribution and personal savings in Pakistan, 1963/64. *Pak Devel Rev, VII,* No. w, Summer, 1967.
4. Croley, H.T., Miller, R.A., and Haider, S.J.: National IUD retention survey in East Pakistan—a preliminary report. *Pak J Fam Plan,* 2: 23, 1968.
5. Haynes, M.A., Immerwahr, G.E., George, A., and Nayar, P.S.J.: A study on the effectiveness of sterilization in reducing the birth rate. *Demography,* 6:1, 1969.
6. Siddiqui, K.A., and Sadik, N.: Unpublished, Karachi, The Pakistan Family Planning Council, p. 6.
7. Zaidi, W.H.: A survey of attitudes of rural population on family planning. *Technical Publication No. 8,* Comilla, East Pakistan, Pakistan Academy for Rural Development, 1961.
8. Roberts, B.J., Yaukey, D., Griffiths, W., Clark, E.W., Shafiullas, A.B.M., and Huq, R.: Family planning survey in East Pakistan. *Demography,* 2:82, 1965.
9. Repetto, R.: A case study of the Madras vasectomy program. *Studies in Family Planning,* The Population Council, No. 31, May, 1968, p. 8.

10. Quddus, A.H.G., Ratcliffe, J.W., and Croley, H.T.: The unofficial vasectomy agent of East Pakistan. *Pak J Fam Plan*, 3:17, 1969.
11. Islam, A.I.M.M.: A follow-up study of vasectomy. Unpublished paper presented at the Sixth Biannual Seminar of Research in Family Planning, Karachi, April, 1969, p. 6.

Chapter 5

THE KOREAN VASECTOMY PROGRAM*

HEE YONG LEE

Korea has an area of about 220,000 square kilometers and is divided into eleven provinces. The population is approximately 30 million, and population density is 257 individuals per square kilometer. The natural population growth rate is 2.7 percent. Annual per capita income is around 140.00 dollars and the literacy rate is 80 percent.

Two consecutive five-year family planning programs have been established by the government; in addition, there are family planning clinics in health centers throughout the country. The family planning program is organized, administered, and evaluated by the Ministry of Health and Social Affairs (MCH, FP Section); the governments of the eleven provinces; the 189 health centers; and 1473 township and small city offices.

There are 2,370 full-time field workers, mostly women, in the program. In addition, there are 11 mobile vans providing IUD and vasectomy services for remote villages without doctors. The vans are staffed with a physician, a nurse, a health educator, and a driver. The Planned Parenthood Federation of Korea is the most active voluntary organization supporting the national program.

The targets of the federal program during the period between 1962 and 1971 is 150,000 vasectomies, 150,000 users of traditional contraceptives, and the insertion of one million intra-uterine contraceptive devices.

Korea has adopted voluntary sterilization by vasectomy as an accepted method of birth control because it has been used clinically for more than sixty years and it is a safe, reliable, comparatively inexpensive and minor procedure.

* Portions of this paper have been adapted from Lee, Hee Yong: Studies on Vasectomy. III. Clinical studies on the influence of vasectomy. *Korean J Urol*, 7:11, 1966.

From 1962 through 1968, about 120,000 men were vasectomized by the free government service; the ratio of achievement to goal is about 92 percent (Table 5-I). In addition, it is estimated that there were more than 35,000 privately performed vasectomies during the same period.

Free vasectomies are performed by about 500 private physicians; they have been trained in a vasectomy program and designated to perform sterilizations by the government. Most of the physicians are not specialists in either urology or surgery. They are distributed evenly by provinces. The government pays the selected physicians $3.30 per vasectomy. In addition, each

TABLE 5-I
GOVERNMENT SUBSIDIZED VASECTOMIES

Year	Target	Achieved	Ratio of Target to Achieved (in percent)
1962	3,413	3,413	100.00
1963	23,000	19,866	86.00
1964	28,296	26,256	92.00
1965	15,000	12,855	85.00
1966	20,000	19,942	99.00
1967	20,370	19,677	96.00
1968	18,000	15,988	88.00
TOTALS	128,079	117,997	92.00

patient is paid $3.30 to compensate for transportation charges and loss of work fees. Private surgeons usually charge at least 20 dollars for vasectomy.

The criteria for free government-subsidized vasectomy are the following: three or more living children, regardless of sex; a low income, attested to by a local official; agreement of the spouse; or the existence of a severe physical or mental handicap in one of the marital partners.

It is desirable to have the applying couple undergo a psychiatric screening interview. Also, information concerning the male reproductive system and vasectomy should be supplied to the applicants. A typical examination might include the following information.

PRINCIPLES OF MALE STERILIZATION

The male reproductive organs might be compared to two types of factories. One is the testis, which produces male hormone and spermatozoa; the other is the accessory sex glands, which produce seminal fluid. The male hormone circulates through the blood vessels. Sperm are transported through the vas deferens to a depot called the ampulla. The seminal fluid is excreted through the urethra to the *baby factory,* sperm are carried in this fluid. If all of these routes are interrupted, castration results. Vasectomy only blocks the vas. There is a big difference between castration and vasectomy. Vasectomy has no effect on male hormone or seminal fluid; it consists only of closing the two small ducts (the vasa) through which the spermatozoa pass. Since no organs or glands are removed, sterilization is unlikely to affect sexual activity.

VASECTOMY PROCEDURE

The length of the incision is about the width of a finger nail. The surgery takes about the amount of time needed to smoke one cigarette. Only a limited amount of work is permitted for the first two days after surgery. When the operation is completed, it does not mean that the patient is sterilized; the reservoirs are filled with sperm and conception can occur. Intercourse must be undertaken with adequate protection until six ejaculations have followed the surgery.

EFFECTS OF VASECTOMY

The seminal fluid (semen) of a nonvasectomized man might be compared to an ordinary watermelon with seeds, while the semen of a vasectomized patient is like a seedless watermelon. The two fruits are quite similar in all respects, the only difference is the presence or absence of seeds. A seedless watermelon is convenient to eat; a vasectomized man is not inconvenienced in sexual relations.

RELATIONSHIP BETWEEN AGING AND PHYSIOLOGICAL SEXUAL POTENCY

The peak age for physiological sexual potency is generally considered to be twenty in males and thirty in females. The average age of vasectomized men is forty, while the average age of wives is thirty-five. At forty, most Korean males are exhibiting a decline in sexual potency, while women of thirty-five are likely to be sexually energetic. Vasectomy patients might exhibit a degree of impotency attributable to the aging process and not to the surgery.

An analysis was made of 3,413 vasectomies done under government subsidy before 1962 and these data were compared with those obtained from 320 private cases who underwent surgery before 1964.

The most common reason for requesting sterilization was large family size (60.8% in the private group and 43.0% in the subsidized group). Economic factors were a consideration in 30 percent of private sterilizations and 27 percent of governmentally sponsored surgery. In the subsidized group, a substantial number of men underwent vasectomy because of the physical illness of their wives (20.0%); this probably resulted from repeated, induced abortions. The private cases cited physical illness as a reason in 5.6 percent of the cases for wives and 1 percent of the cases for husbands. It is of interest to note that 7.5 percent of the husbands in the subsidized group cited their own physical illness. Eugenic factors were mentioned in 2.6 percent of the private cases and 0.3 percent of the subsidized cases. No reason was given by 2.2 percent of the subsidized patients.

The occupations of the sterilized men are shown in Table 5-II. Among the private patients, commercial workers and government officials are the most common occupations because these patients

TABLE 5-II
OCCUPATIONS OF VASECTOMY CASES

Occupation	Private Group (percent)	Subsidized Group (percent)
Agriculture	5.8	27.3
Government official	24.0	24.0
Commerce	26.0	15.1
Private company official	15.4	9.9
Labor	6.7	6.5
Engineering	2.9	5.5
Teacher	2.9	5.3
Social worker	0.0	0.4
No occupation	10.6	4.1
Miscellaneous	5.7	1.9

live in Seoul or its environs. Among the subsidized patients, agricultural workers and local government officials are prominent because this is a nationwide sample.

The time intervening between marriage and vasectomy is shown in Table 5-III. The private patients were married for from

TABLE 5-III
LENGTH OF MARRIAGE BEFORE VASECTOMY

Years	Private Group (percent)	Subsidized Group (percent)
1–10	10	9.6
11–15	53	27.8
16–20	31	38.6
21–25	4	14.8
More than 26	1	3.0
Miscellaneous	—	5.3
Mean	13.6 years	16.7 years

3 to 29 years before vasectomy, the mean length of time was 13.6 years. The marital life of the subsidized cases varied from 2 to 30 years; the mean duration of marriage was 16.7 years. These data indicate that private patients apply for sterilization earlier in their married lives than do subsidized ones.

Table 5-IV shows the age distribution of males and females

TABLE 5-IV
AGE DISTRIBUTIONS OF COUPLES IN SAMPLE

Age Group	Private Group Husband %	Private Group Wife %	Subsidized Group Husband %	Subsidized Group Wife %
20–30	5	24	1.4	8.9
31–35	29	45	14.1	37.9
36–40	33	25	39.3	40.2
41–45	25	6	30.3	11.6
46–50	7		11.2	0.6
More than 51	1		2.9	0.4
Miscellaneous			0.8	0.4
Mean	39 years	34 years	40 years	36 years

among both private and subsidized vasectomized families. The average age of males in the private group is 39 years, that of their wives 34 years. In the subsidized group the average male age was 40 years, while the average female age was 36 years. In those cases where sterilization was performed on husbands of women over 51 years old, it might be presumed that the reason for sterilization was physical illness or extramarital relations, for women of this age are usually beyond childbearing.

The mean number of living children for the subsidized vasectomy patients was 5.3, that of the private patients, 4.7. These data are presented in Table 5-V.

TABLE 5-V
NUMBER OF OFFSPRING AT TIME OF STERILIZATION

Number of Children	Private Group (percent)	Subsidized Group (percent)
0	0	2.0
1	0.5	0.2
2	4.0	1.4
3	17.0	9.8
4	33.0	22.8
5	26.0	26.6
More than 7	19.5	37.2
Mean	4.7 children	5.3 children
Boy	2.4 children	3.1 children
Girl	2.3 children	2.2 children

The educational background of the private patients was as follows: 1.5 percent, no schooling; 11.8 percent, grammar school; 21.0 percent, middle school; 35.5 percent, high school; and 30.2 percent, college. As might be expected, the educational background of the patients undergoing subsidized vasectomy is somewhat lower. In this group 6.1 percent had no schooling; 34.7 percent, grammar school; 29.2 percent, middle school; 17.4 percent, high school; and only 11.0 percent went to college.

The monthly incomes of both types of vasectomy patients are shown in Table 5-VI. Among the private patients, the average income was $25.84; the subsidized patients averaged $11.14 per month. Thus, the private patients earn more than twice as much as the subsidized patients.

TABLE 5-VI
MONTHLY INCOMES OF VASECTOMIZED CASES

Income Range (in hwan)	Private Group (in percent)	Subsidized Group (in percent)
Under 3,000	6.8	46.2
3,001–5,000	29.0	25.3
5,001–7,000	17.4	13.2
7,001–10,000	15.8	7.1
More than 10,001	5.6	1.0
Not stated	25.4	7.2
Average Monthly Income (in hwan)	6,950	2,840

The average time lost from work in the subsidized group ranged from one to thirty postoperative days (8.3 day average). In the private patients, time lost varied from one to twenty days, an average time loss of 1.8 days.

The sexual effects of vasectomy are difficult to determine, for quantitative estimation of sexual drive is most difficult to document. The patient's responses to our questions of the sexual effects of vasectomy are shown in Table 5-VII. Private patients reported the following: 81.36 percent saw no change; 13.64 per-

TABLE 5-VII
VASECTOMY AND SEXUAL ACTIVITY

	Private Group			Subsidized Group			Not stated
	No change	Increase	Decrease	No change	Increase	Decrease	
Sexual Activity (in percent)	81.36	13.64	5.0	71.14	14.2	11.42	3.4
Libido	73.3	22.7	4.0	69.1	17.1	11.4	2.5
Erection	81.4	13.5	5.1	77.4	10.6	9.5	2.6
Coital Time	82.7	12.0	5.3	60.1	25.8	12.8	1.4
Ejaculate Volume	92.7	3.3	4.0	79.3	4.4	9.4	7.1
Sexual Feeling	76.7	16.7	6.6	69.8	13.1	14.0	3.2
Sexual Feeling of Wives	87.6	12.3	0.1	71.2	14.7	9.9	3.0

cent had an increase in sexual drives; and 5.0 percent experienced a decrease. The results were different among the subsidized cases: 71.14 percent reported no change; 14.2 percent experienced increased sexual drive; and 11.42 felt a decrease in libido.

More than 87 percent of the wives of the private vasectomy patients felt no change in sexual drive, while 71.2 percent of the wives of the subsidized patients said the same. Very few of the wives of the private patients complained about the effect of vasectomy on sexual relations, but about 10 percent of the wives of the other patients had some complaints. It is interesting to note that both husbands and wives in the subsidized group complained about the loss of sexual drive to a similar extent. This is difficult to interpret, for it might be expected that wives would enjoy sexual relations more when the inhibitory fear of unwanted pregnancy was eliminated.

Table 5-VIII compares the frequency of sexual intercourse in the preoperative and the postoperative periods. In the private patients, coitus took place on an average of 1.95 times per week preoperatively, while 1.88 was the average for the postoperative period. In the subsidized group, a similar change is evident, with an average sexual activity of 2.27 times per week preoperatively compared to 1.99 times postoperatively.

The postoperative frequency of coitus showed a slight decrease from its preoperative frequency; this might be attributable to psychological factors and male preclimacteric. It will be noted that the subsidized group engaged in intercourse more than did the private patients.

TABLE 5-VIII
FREQUENCY OF SEXUAL INTERCOURSE PREOPERATIVELY VERSUS POSTOPERATIVELY

Weekly Intercourse Frequency	Private Group Preoperatively	Postoperatively	Subsidized Group Preoperatively	Postoperatively
1	37.6	42.4	26.1	33.8
2	34.4	33.6	27.8	26.5
3	10.4	9.6	21.9	13.9
4	4.8	5.6	5.8	4.1
5	3.2	2.4	3.2	1.9
6	0.8	0.8	1.6	1.1
7	0.0	0.0	0.2	0.2
Not stated	8.8	5.6	13.4	18.7

The effect of vasectomy on general health appears to be minimal; 83 percent of the private patients and 70 percent of the subsidized patients noticed no change. In fact, 11 and 16 percent, respectively, reported an improvement in general health. Only 6 percent of the private patients noted a decline in general health; however, 11 percent of the subsidized patients did.

Immediate sterilization does not follow vasectomy, for the ampullae still contain sperm. It takes from five to nine ejaculations following surgery to assure a sperm-free ejaculate. Occasional, nonmotive spermatozoa do not pose any problem. Since there are individual variations in ampulla size, microscopic examination for sperm is the only real test for safety.

If a patient is anxious for immediate sterilization, the vas may be lavaged with a spermicidal solution. Rivanol (0.2%) or potassium permanganate (0.1%) are suggested.

Spontaneous reanastomosis of the vas occurred in 1.1 percent of the subsidized patients and in 0.8 percent of the private patients. When sperm persist following vasectomy, spontaneous recanalization may be expected. The exact mechanism of this phenomenon is unknown; it is possible that an excessively tight ligature might cut through the vas and be accompanied by spermatic granuloma formation.

Vasectomy is merely the closure of the vasa and does not involve the removal of any organs or glands; and changes in either sexual activity or general health should not be anticipated. Unfortunately, sterilization is often confused with castration; this misapprehension can be a factor in the occasional sterilization neurosis. Of the 1,100 men sterilized by the government in 1962, 26 such cases were reported.

Psychiatric examinations were conducted on 20 postvasectomy cases who had somatic and psychiatric problems. The control group for this study consisted of 200 males of similar backgrounds; they had not undergone vasectomy.

The chief complaints of the neurotic group were the following: loss of libido; decreased erection potential; lowered semen volume; premature ejaculation; unpleasant orgasm; decreased coital frequency; moist perineal sensation; discomfort, weakness and fatigue; headache; lumbago; joint pain; low spirits, melancholy, depression, and hypersensitivity; insomnia; memory loss; and so forth.

The men were interviewed individually and were given the Minnesota Multiphasic Personality Inventory (MMPI), which was revised for Koreans by Dr. C.K. Lee.

Physical examination revealed normal findings. The scrotal contents were normal; and although no significant indurations were palpable in the operative area, the patients were very sensitive to palpations.

In every clinical scale, with the exception of the masculinity-femininity index, the vasectomy cases exhibited a higher mean than the control group. The scales include the following: hypochondria; depression; hysteria; psychopathic deviation; paranoia; psychasthenia; schizophrenia; hypomania; social introversion; anxiety; and internalization.

These findings indicate the possibility that the sterilized group have tendencies to be depressed, tense, unhappy, anxious, obsessive-compulsive, lack initiative and efficiency; in general, they appear to be dependent, tend to act out difficulties, and internalize problems. Of course, the fact that these men did not undergo preoperative psychiatric examinations limits the usefulness of the findings.

Male sterilization has been motivated by reasonable considerations and patients have been relatively free of unconscious neurotic fears about the operation. Unfortunately, in a few cases, vasectomy can have profound emotional impact. There is an element of self-destruction linked with self-castration, and this occasionally carries over into unconscious reasons for undergoing sterilization. It is interesting to note that men who have become sterile through disease or accident seldom develop personality disorganizations.

The frequency of sterilization neurosis in our sample indicates that preoperative psychiatric screening is necessary in order to eliminate, as much as possible, postoperative psychiatric problems.

Chapter 6

THE USE OF LEARNING AIDS IN HUMAN STERILIZATION PROGRAMS

Ronald A. Chez

In addition to the technical aspect of medical aid, several other important therapeutic steps must be undertaken by or with the patient. Almost all of these procedures involve communication, one area of which is learning aids. For example, the patient whose fertility is going to be limited must be motivated to take the first step. The motivation must be understood and reinforced, i.e. the patient must be educated. Actual therapeutic contact must be meaningful; the patient must be informed about what is happening and what is to be expected. Postcontact relationship must be supported and follow-up must be emphasized, i.e. the patient must be helped to learn.

Human sterilization workers understand this and do make contact with patients. However, professional time and effort is applied to repetitive performance of these tasks on a one-to-one basis; these jobs could be done better either by other personnel or by the use of learning aid equipment. The object of this chapter is to review types of learning aids and principles of their use.

To discuss the physiological basis and sequelae with thirty or forty patients a day is time-consuming, tedious, and by virtue of repetition, frequently neither complete nor concise as the day progresses. In addition, two possibly invalid assumptions are involved: a) the patient is receptive, comprehends, is comfortable in the situation, and can communicate; b) the professional can both listen and communicate. When a professional spends time in repeated communication with the patient, he is actually depriving the client of potential individual attention.

Learning aids are valuable in that they permit the student or learner to initiate the learning process, to proceed at his own pace, and to repeat as often as he likes. By complementing the professional-patient relationship, they free the professional for individual therapy.

What factors should be considered in the choice of learning aids? Learning aids can entertain and set a mood; they can motivate, help in learning, inform, and test.

Therefore, it is most important to define objectives. Some objectives are so diffuse that they are meaningless and do not permit accurate evaluation. For instance, the objective "to encourage the patient to be sterilized" is very different from "to have the patient sterilized at the center on ABC Street." Also, "to inform the patient about family planning" differs from "to direct the patient to XYZ Clinic for advice on contraception." Definition of the target population is an important step in defining objectives. Many aids relate optimally to only one group and are not as applicable to others; therefore, the population should be defined in terms of literacy, age, religion, occupation, etc.

Then it is necessary to determine which aid is most appropriate. Most available learning equipment is oriented towards three senses: hearing, sight, and touch. Occasionally smell and taste are stimulated. Appropriateness also refers to reproducibility of the material. Factors to be considered regarding equipment are the following: cost, cost of operation, availability, ease of operation, portability, and frequency of repair and breakdown record.

Communication by the written word is everywhere; magazines, pamphlets, brochures, signs, and posters are ubiquitous. They rely only on the sense of sight and do not necessarily require literacy. Advantages of this learning method are that it is portable, usually inexpensive, is readily produced, and it requires no personnel. A disadvantage is that, once published in abundance, these products are difficult to edit and can be disconcertingly permanent.

Pictures, as opposed to the written word, are becoming increasingly popular. Populations of certain countries are visually oriented because of exposure to movies, television, slides, billboards, and picture magazines. Whenever visual media are being used, the degree of visual literacy of the population must be considered, i.e. the ability of the viewer to recognize the picture and to conceptualize from it. Interpretation of visual matter is related to previous experience and intellectual competency. Because patients can distort what is being shown, it is necessary to determine if the remembered image corresponds to the original. Visual equipment media are slide projectors and motion picture projectors, both of which can be relatively expensive. The fundamental question in deciding between slides and movies is, "Is motion required?" Motion is needed when an action-oriented act is being demonstrated, e.g. surgery. Movies are wasted when they are used for films, charts, or tables; in general, they are expensive to make and reproduce and distribution and editing can be difficult. Slides do not present these problems.

Learning aids stimulating the sense of hearing are radios and reel or cassette tape recorders. Earphones permit limited application and loudspeakers a broader distribution. Sound use permits the speaker to use vocal nuances, and background effects can be employed. A solution for the limitations of review possibilities is to have brochures accompany the presentations.

Audio-visual equipment stimulates both sight and sound. Visual material can be on slides, film strips, movies, or videotapes; sound can be on separate tapes or combined with the visual material. The necessity of motion must be determined in this case also. It is a waste of a movie to film a lecture. With slides and film strips, the picture can coincide with the sound automatically, or the viewer can initiate the sound track. Motion picture film sizes include 8 mm, super 8 mm, and 16 mm. The first two sizes can be used in projectors with loop cartridges; these cartridges eliminate direct handling and threading of film and rewind automatically. This type of equipment has certain variations: the use of magnetic versus optical sound; playing time of cartridges; built-in versus non-built-in viewing screens; reversibility and stop action features; and print cost. Cartridge projectors are relatively portable, expensive, and effective; the most frustrating thing about them is the differences in cartridges from one manufacturer to another. Some objections to the use of 16 mm projectors are the need for a relatively well-trained projectionist, and the cost of the equipment and of production and reproduction of the films. This, in effect, reserves the 16 mm film projector for use with audiences and not with individuals. Equipment that does not require a cartridge has become available recently. Ideally, audiovisual instruction should be accompanied by a written card or brochure to enable review and enhance recall.

In some parts of the world television is available both on a closed circuit and open circuit (broadcasting) basis. Although the initial cost of equipment and repairs is very high, this medium is attractive because of portability, production ease, and ability to record spontaneous events. One difficulty with television can be its very availability, which may permit poor preparation, sloppy techniques, and amateurish efforts. Although the tape is easily erased, spot editing is almost impossible except for professionals. Televised material can be detrimental to the learner unless it is produced with attention and care.

Models take advantage of the sense of touch; they permit three-dimensional reality testing and allow the learner to make comparisons. Although original production costs of models can be high, reproduction is frequently inexpensive where large numbers are involved. A model need not be elaborate. Anatomic accuracy is not often necessary and the model need not be either lifelike or an exact rendering of the subject.

Practical considerations of budget and equipment availability determine which method is best. The most important determinant must always be the nature of the material that is available or will be produced. It is one thing to have funds or the knowledge of the availability of learning aid equipment, it is another to have suitably designed media. Because an individual has an educational interest in one area, it does not necessarily mean that he will be well suited to produce learning aids. Persons whose interests or background are too diverse from the target population should be avoided. Frequently students can produce excellent aids for their peers. In general, the best method is the one that the learner decides to use; there is an advantage in having multiple media available for learner selection.

Whatever the method or approach, it is critically important to pretest the learning material with a selected population sample. Evaluation of whether the objectives are being met is most necessary. Does the aid communicate; is it in good taste; is it technically satisfactory; is there learner acceptance and identification; is the material in proper context; is there professional follow-up support? These are some of the questions which must be evaluated as an integral and essential part of all studies.

Increased use of learning aids for sterilization prospects can be anticipated. Attention to definition of target population, desired objective, and anticipated behavior change are important in evaluation of success. Attention to these details will result in improved delivery of services and more effective utilization of the physician-patient contacts.

DISCUSSION: FOREIGN PROGRAMS

Howard C. Taylor, Jr., *Moderator*

Dr. Taylor opened the discussion by asking for specific questions relevant to Dr. Pai's presentation.

Dr. Pai pointed out the recognized fears that existed in the Indian vasectomy program: fear of sex injury and fear of loss of either spouse or children. They were able to eliminate the sexual fears by explaining that vasectomy is a very safe and simple operation. In so far as fear of loss of family is concerned, they try to explain that recanalization can be done if necessary. He noted that a public newsletter was issued explaining that if sterilization reversal were desired it would be made very readily available. He continued that of the 100,000 vasectomies performed in India during the last two and a half years, only 135 patients wanted recanalization in spite of the information on and availability of the procedure. Of the 135 cases requesting recanalization, a hundred had the procedure performed. Of the hundred recanalizations, 90 men showed a high, positive sperm count. Ten of the wives of the recanalized men became pregnant and five delivered infants. Dr. Pai considered that these figures indicated that there was a favorable chance for pregnancy when a male had his sterilization reversed.

Dr. Tietze questioned the dictum that vasectomy was an operation solely on the vasa and that no other structures or functions were affected. If this is so, he speculated on the discrepancy between normal (number and characteristics) sperm and number of pregnancies. He felt that something else must be missing to account for the low impregnation rate and he wanted to know why most of the wives did not become pregnant within a year or so.

Dr. Hulka wanted to know if reversibility was a function of the duration of the occlusion; in other words, would reversibility be more successful if performed closer to the postsurgical period.

Dr. Pai said that reversibility was indeed related to the duration of the occlusion.

Dr. Bunge took exception to the assessment of male potential on number of sperm alone. He felt that among other characteristics of importance was the number of living forms present and that the number of abnormal sperm and the type of activity were also of importance.

Dr. Schmidt said that he did not think that there was less likelihood of successful reanastomosis after twenty years as far as testicular sperm production was concerned. However, he pointed out, that with the passage of time there was greater danger of the formation of a spermatic granuloma with subsequent occlusion of the ducts.

Dr. Corfman wanted to know what proportion of tubectomies were done under regional versus local anesthesia.

Dr. Darbari replied that the majority of tubectomies were performed under spinal anesthesia, but he had found instances where local anesthesia with premedication was used, and some states in his country used general anesthesia. But by far the greatest number of operations were done under spinal anesthesia. He went on to say that the physicians performing the surgery were trained in spinal anesthesia techniques; however, in certain outlying districts trained technicians in local anesthesia were well experienced and qualified to do tubectomy with local anesthesia.

Dr. Darbari described the local anesthetic technique as follows. Good muscular relaxation is necessary for local anesthesia; the patient must be well prepared and should be given a tranquilizer the night preceding surgery. Two hours preoperatively a tranquilizer is given; if necessary, in combination with another drug. Then surgery is started. Since it is of the utmost importance that the patient be fully relaxed the skill of the surgeon is vital.

Dr. Phatak commented that the anesthesia used for tubectomy varied very much in the whole of India. General anesthesia is preferred because most women are not very happy with local anesthesia and tend to react sharply to what is happening around them unless they are absolutely determined on local anesthetics. She said that although she knew what was happening in Delhi, she was not certain of the anesthesia of choice in all of India and would be inclined to agree with Dr. Darbari that a large percentage of tubectomies were performed with spinal anesthesia. She concluded by saying that local anesthesia for tubectomy was indeed most dependent on the individual skill of the surgeon.

Dr. Clyman wanted to know the morbidity and mortality rates for tubal ligation performed under spinal anesthesia.

Dr. Darbari said that he had no figures with him on morbidity but that not one death in his series followed spinal anesthesia.

Dr. Taylor said that he recalled the central government of India provided a certain number of extra beds to maternity hospitals maintaining a certain rate of postpartum sterilization.

Dr. Darbari explained that the Indian government set aside a certain percentage of beds for tubectomies; in fact, he said the demand for beds for sterilization patients had been increasing at such a rate that the percentage was being revised. He cited as a hypothetical example that a state that might have had an allotment of 200 beds might be demanding 500 beds for tubectomy patients. He felt it was necessary to supply these additional demands, for, if additional facilities were not provided, the success of the sterilization program would be jeopardized.

Dr. Taylor commented on the impressiveness of total figures and asked for an estimation of the number of special beds that had been provided in India for postpartum female sterilization. He wanted to know if the number would be in the hundreds or in the thousands.

Dr. Phatak replied that hospitals requesting special beds were required to promise to terminate twenty percent of the deliveries with tubectomy; the maximum number of beds permitted to date has been about twenty per hospital. She added that this was what was anticipated and the total number of beds allowed should be about two thousand. She felt that, more important than providing beds, was the provision of a special maternity surgical department for tubal sterilization.

Dr. Tietze recommended that hospital administrators and chiefs of services should report tubectomy incidence in terms of parity, relating it to number of deliveries at the same parity.

It was his opinion that this would permit inter-hospital comparisons and be a more helpful manner of data presentation.

Dr. Phatak agreed with this proposal and thought that postpartum data would be forthcoming from all hospitals.

Dr. Waterman requested more information on the legal aspects of sterilization in Caracas. He wanted to know if sterilization was the only illegal birth control method, and if loops, pills, and other devices were in this category.

Dr. Aguero said that the government had accepted a birth control clinic program which included intra-uterine contraceptive devices, pills, etc., but there was neither publicity nor a policy for birth control. The government just accepts contraception, including contraception by tubal ligation. In fact, he stated that there was a population officer in the Ministry of Health to take care of birth control, but the methods had not been accepted publicly.

Dr. Waterman wanted to know if there is a specific law that says that these things are illegal.

Dr. Aguero said there was a law that stated very clearly that anyone performing an operation limiting the capacity of the patient to reproduce could be prosecuted.

Dr. Waterman wanted to know if surgery was the only thing mentioned.

Dr. Aguero said yes.

Dr. Corfman wanted to know if the insertion of an intra-uterine device was considered to be an operation.

Dr. Aguero said it wasn't yet.

Dr. Taylor then requested discussion on Dr. Ratcliffe's presentation on vasectomy in East Pakistan.

Dr. Corfman wanted to know if any data were obtained on individuals who regretted having undergone vasectomy.

Dr. Ratcliffe said it was most difficult to measure the regret factor, since the concept was too sophisticated for rural Pakistanis. He had pretested a number of questions on the regret factor and found that they were not understandable; therefore, he kept to the simple satisfaction or dissatisfaction queries.

Dr. Corfman then wanted to know what discussion there was of the fact that fifty percent of the patients who were sterilized on the same day were those who were sterilized for money.

Dr. Ratcliffe said he did not know. He said that there were two follow-up studies in progress: one year postsurgery and eighteen months postsurgery. He said he was hoping that a cross-check of these study groups would show that the patients who had surgery for money were less satisfied than those who underwent vasectomy to stop childbirth. He hoped that information would emerge on these factors, but the study period has been too short to date.

Dr. Darbari wanted to know what had been done with vasectomy in West Pakistan. He said that he was under the impression that population control in West Pakistan had been confined to intra-uterine devices and wanted to know the reason for this.

Dr. Ratcliffe felt that one of the reasons for the low vasectomy rate in West Pakistan was the lack of agents. He said official agents, who get 2½ rupees for finder's fees, operate nationwide, but that the program just had not caught on in West Pakistan. He said he did not know why this was so or why the vasectomy rate in West Pakistan was around five to six thousand a month, while that for East Pakistan was about thirty-five to thirty-seven thousand a month. He said he was sure that cultural differences existed between the two regions, but he could not speculate on any other reasons for lack of vasectomy acceptance for he had not done anything in West Pakistan.

Dr. Wood inquired if there was prevasectomy psychological screening in either Pakistan or India or if any man who was brought into the clinic was automatically vasectomized.

Dr. Ratcliffe responded that psychological screening was nonexistent but that other screening criteria were employed. The patients are required to have at least one son who has reached the age of five and are supposed to have a total of three living children. The consent of the wife is obligatory, but no signature is required. He said he did not know about the situation in India.

Dr. Wood wanted to know if patients were told of the possibility of postoperative surgical problems.

Dr. Ratcliffe responded that this topic was not discussed at the clinics.

Dr. Pai said that he was not informed about the screening program in all of India, but that the procedure in Bombay was efficient. Total responsibility for patient screening rests with the physician performing the surgery and such criteria as age, number of children, and procedure explanation are totally within his province. In four known situations where the physician did not fulfill his responsibility, he was permanently prohibited from performing vasectomies. He did agree with Dr. Ratcliffe that prevasectomy psychological screening was not emphasized to the proper extent but took issue with the idea of official finders in the Indian vasectomy program.

Dr. Pai went on to explain that finders do exist, but that they are voluntary and do not have official status. In the Greater Bombay area the finder's fee is 2½ rupees, but in Maharashtra the finder's fee is 10 rupees. He said that he had done a study of 2,700 finders and found that men who had undergone vasectomy performed best in this capacity; he found that ninety percent of the finders studied could bring in about two or three cases. He felt that the mercenary element had been overemphasized, for although the fee made it worthwhile for a vasectomized patient to try to convince others, it was not the only factor involved. For example, his study found that sixty percent of the finders lived within a one-mile radius of the patient. In other words, they were friends or neighbors and the idea of just bringing a patient in for the fee involved did not play such an important role.

Dr. Ratcliffe said that what he meant by India's *official* promoters was the fact that once there are promoters or finder's fees then the promoter angle is being worked officially. He said that Dr. Rapeto, in studies of the Family Planning Council in Madras State, said they were official.

Dr. Pai commented that the runners got the money but were not official; they are not what you call *establishment*.

Dr. Ratcliffe said it might be a question of semantics but, if the government provided a finder's fee, there would be finders. He continued by saying that the government of Pakistan did not consider the 20 rupee incentive fee in the same manner that Americans would. The government considers the decision to undergo sterilization a drastic one, and it is recommended that postoperative patients do not resume work for at least three days. The 20 rupee fee can be considered as recompense for convalesence; it is true that the rest period is not always taken, but the government still makes restitution for money lost. This is a less harsh way of looking at the incentive fee.

Dr. Darbari answered Dr. Pai's question on psychological screening for vasectomy by explaining that they employed a block system of screening in India. Field workers for the family planning program approach every household and, after obtaining data on the family, decide which individuals are eligible for vasectomy. If the couple has two or three children, sterilization is considered. At this stage it is not known if the man is psychologically fit for vasectomy, but as a second stage procedure a health educator has an interview with the husband.

At this point, the individual is about ready for surgery. He consults with the physician, who will not operate on more than twenty cases per day. The physician scrutinizes the patient and attempts to determine if he can withstand surgery well or if there will be postoperative sequelae. In spite of these presurgical precautions, postoperative complications and maladjustments do occur.

Dr. Tietze wanted more information from Dr. Ratcliffe about the agents. He wanted to know what proportion of the agents made fees their main source of livelihood and, if they did, how their incomes compared with that of their neighbors. He said he was particularly interested in the twenty percent of the agents who were women, and wanted to know more about the type of individuals they were.

Dr. Ratcliffe said that a little over a third did vasectomy procurement on a full-time basis. However, the other agents used the occupation as a fill-in for times when they were not harvesting, business was slack, and so on.

He said that the income of all the agents had increased when they changed from their previous occupations to client-finding, but the change was not significant. He was interested in the fact that agents worked until they earned enough to satisfy their family's needs and then they stopped. He did not know if they paced their work because they have just a certain number of friends and neighbors to whom they are forced to limit their procurement. Previous occupations of agents were landed farmers, service trades, or business; day laborers do not form a sizeable proportion of the agents. However, some ninety percent of the vasectomy clients were day laborers.

Most of the women agents were working women; they reported their tasks as housewife and worked in the fields. A little over twenty percent of female agents were widows, and many worked as female village organizers for the family planning program. In one district many of these women were formal members of the planning organization and were being paid to bring in women for intra-uterine contraceptive device insertion. This was difficult for them, so they brought in the husbands for vasectomy and thus improved their incomes.

Dr. Tietze wanted to know if Dr. Ratcliffe's sample was drawn from all over East Pakistan.

Dr. Ratcliffe said that this sample was limited to three districts and that he had a very detailed paper on methodology for anyone who was interested. Since there were three trends in the vasectomy rate, a district representing each trend was chosen. Of necessity, districts were kept close to Dacca: Dacca district was one part of the sample, and two other heavily rural districts were included.

Dr. Laurence wondered how effective female agents were in comparison to their male counterparts.

Dr. Ratcliffe replied that there was no sexual difference in effectiveness of the agents.

Dr. Phatak expressed worry about the incentive concept and the use of the term *incentive* in official communications. As a field worker she had always viewed the payment for vasectomy or tubectomy as a compensation for loss of wages or convenience, or a payment for baby sitters if they were required.

Dr. Phatak questioned Dr. Ratcliffe on the possibility that some patients considered the fee a compensation rather than an incentive. She was concerned with the possibility that certain patients might consider that they were being paid for a loop insertion or a tubectomy, and felt that no average person liked to think that he was being paid for something that was being done to him.

Dr. Ratcliffe said that he did not find that patients felt degraded because they were accepting money.

Dr. Tietze wanted to know if there had been any studies on the use of vasectomy by persons of upper or middle incomes and higher degrees of education. He inquired about the extent that vasectomy was employed as a method for the poor as opposed to those who can pick and choose.

Dr. Ratcliffe said that the clinics in his study were chosen at random and that there was a higher percentage of individuals from the lower socioeconomic groups. Other studies have shown the so-called Pakistani *elite,* the more established socioeconomic groups, use the pill, which they obtain from private physicians. This group does not use government clinics for anything.

Dr. Tietze expressed the expectation that these individuals would have private surgery.

Dr. Ratcliffe explained that private physicians were rather deeply involved with the government program. A doctor just has to register with the government and then he can perform as many vasectomies as he wishes; the government pays for this surgery. He said that he suspected that the agent system might have started when physicians sent agents out as *runners.*

Dr. Phatak said that she had known of some cases who had refused to accept the incentive payment.

Dr. Ratcliffe wanted to know if Dr. Phatak's patients were *elite* women.

Dr. Phatak replied that they were very poor women but the idea of an incentive payment just did not seem to suit them.

Dr. Taylor said he thought that in the United States the economically privileged had more sterilization surgery and more therapeutic abortions that the indigent. He felt that this was not due to economic reasons, but rather to the fact that wealthier persons had more immediate contact with physicians and so could obtain information on sterilization. He said that the situation in America was the reverse of that in the countries under discussion, and said he did not think that there was anything inherent in the situation except local circumstances, communication, availability of information, and knowledge of what possibilities exist.

Dr. Taylor asked Dr. Pai if psychological screening was done in India, for he was told more than 130 operations a day were done in Indian vasectomy camps and he doubted that screening could be accomplished with that case load.

Dr. Pai stated that the 130 cases Dr. Lee spoke of were not done in a single camp but rather at twenty different places operating for more than six hours daily. That means that 120 doctor hours are involved, and all the physicians operating in the program had postgraduate qualification. So there are 120 specialized hours for a hundred operations. That works out to be more than a hour a patient and if a physician cannot do a good job in that length of time he is not qualified.

Dr. Lee wanted to know if that meant that more than thirty minutes were needed for interviewing the patient.

Dr. Pai said that was so: three minutes for surgery and thirty minutes for before, during, and after routine. It does not always work out like that, for there is an occasional physician who does not do a proper job. For example, unmarried men have been known to appear at camps and lie about their marital status. The physician cannot always tell and the man may be sterilized. This causes trouble, for someone is needed to recanalize him.

Dr. Zinsser wanted to know if Dr. Lee agreed with Dr. Darbari's impression that persons who reported postvasectomy sexual capacity difficulties could be detected preoperatively because of some sexual problems.

Dr. Lee responded by saying that there were some psychoanalysts involved and that some findings were characteristic of postoperative complaints concerning sexual activity. He felt that the peak of male sexual activity in Korea was at 20 years of age, while females reached peak capacity at 30. Then sexual potency declined rapidly, especially in men. Since the average age of vasectomized men is 40 and that of their wives is 36, it is clear that male sexual activity is declining to a low point while female activity potential is still high. This results in a big disparity in sexual performance. Some decrease in sexual strength should be felt postvasectomy, but Dr. Lee said he did not have sufficient data to evaluate presurgical versus postsurgical sexual activity.

Dr. Bunge expressed concern with the effect of vasectomy. He felt that an unwarranted assumption concerning male hormone production had been made because males have performed in a

Discussion: Foreign Programs

sexually satisfactory manner after vasectomy. But does vasectomy have an effect on testicular hormone production. He measured serum testosterone in prevasectomized and postvasectomized males and found no difference. This is confirmation of the theory that testicular hormone production is unaltered. He said that he hopes to evaluate the effects of vasectomy on the physiology of the testes by measuring seminal plasma components both pre-vasectomy and post-vasectomy. He felt that this was an appropriate area of research which had been neglected.

Dr. Schmidt stated that one of the indices of satisfaction with vasectomy is the number of requests for fertility restoration through vasovasotomy. He wanted to know if Dr. Pai, Dr. Ratcliffe, or Dr. Lee had figures for their respective programs.

Dr. Lee said that in Seoul City about one in a thousand vasectomies requested recanalization; the most common reasons were remarriage or children's deaths.

Dr. Schmidt considered this an index of an excellent job in presurgical education and screening.

Dr. Pai said that he had 135 cases in about 100,000 who requested reanastomosis. One patient appeared for reversal because of sexual weakness, not because he wanted more children. Dr. Pai felt that this was an insufficient reason for recanalization, but Dr. Shikondi, who considered contentment a part of the family planing program, performed the surgery and the patient proceeded to use condoms.

Dr. Moon wanted to know the extent of the follow-up program.

Dr. Pai said that they were constantly following up some cases.

Dr. Moon wanted to know if Dr. Pai had been involved in follow-up.

Dr. Pai said that since about 80 percent of the cases do not even come for a postoperative check-up, and there are about fifty tests which could be performed, the possibility of organizing a good follow-up program is slight. The patients are told that they should return if there are complications.

Dr. Bunge wanted to know if this meant when their wives became pregnant.

Dr. Pai said that it did and that patients returned when their wives were pregnant.

Dr. Taylor cautioned against taking the small reported percentages of alleged increases or decreases in libido seriously, for he thought that if you took a hundred nonsurgical cases and questioned them after a year you would obtain the same sexual activity variations.

He compared the postvasectomy data on libido changes to those obtained by gynecologists from posthysterectomy patients. At one time there was considerable interest in whether a hysterectomy made a difference in libido, and whether a supra cervical hysterectomy differed from a total hysterectomy; it was found that eighty percent of the women reported no libidinal changes, eleven or twelve percent reported increases, and five or six percent reported decreases. He thought that a great mistake would be made in interpreting the postvasectomy changes in libido as real data and assuming that you could predict, on the basis of psychological examination, which cases would show improved sexual activity and which would show a decline in activity.

Dr. Tietze said that he was puzzled by the reported differences in self-evaluation between Dr. Lee's subsidized and private groups until he considered the age factor. The private group was younger, so that the adverse effects on libido reported by the subsidized group could possibly be attributable to the fact that they were older men and were married much longer.

Dr. Chez extended Dr. Pai's comments on the value and efficiency of spending time with individual patients before, during, and after surgery. He felt that this would have little effect on subjective learning or teaching, for the motivation for sterilization is the impetus that brings the patient to the physician and that impetus is subject to minimal modification. Therefore, this may not be an effective use of personnel and their time. One negative aspect of the procedure might be that the patient would wonder about the inordinate amount of time spent with him during this particular procedure, whereas he never had had such concentrated attention before. This is a pertinent factor in contraception clinics in the United States also.

Dr. Taylor asked if Dr. Chez thought that there might be difficulties with the surgery if too much time were spent analyzing it.

Dr. Chez said that this could be so, since the time spent is incompatible with time spent with patients for other procedures.

Dr. Pai said that a sample of 300 cases was compared: 115 were vasectomized in camps; 115 in hospitals. The hospitals spent a good deal of time on psychological preparation and the percentage of cases who reported postoperative sexual weakness was much higher among hospital patients than it was among camp patients. He considered this peculiar, for he did not know if spending time discussing the possibility of sexual weakness might not precipitate the condition.

Dr. Clyman noted that, in relation to Dr. Chez's remarks, there is a promotional aspect in the patient-physician relationship in sterilization programs. The patient is induced to come for vasectomy because of publicity emanating from the health ministry or local physicians. But some sort of patient-physician relationship should be established, or, at the very least, the patient should be informed about what might happen.

Dr. Tietze felt that the important thing in dealing with these patients was listening to them, rather than talking to them. He felt that this was often omitted in services given nonpaying patients. He also raised a question about the qualifications of physicians or surgeons for patient interviewing.

Dr. Taylor asked if Dr. Tietze thought that a psychiatrist would be better qualified.

Dr. Tietze said that perhaps he would prefer a psychiatrist or a well-trained social worker; the type of individual who was involved with, for example, marital counseling.

Dr. Prager pointed out that it was extremely difficult to find a formula for patient evaluation and instruction which would work for both private patients in San Francisco and patients in vasectomy clinics in Korea or Bombay. In private practice it is much easier to spend more time with and reach patients, but in nations with certain family planning goals and limited personnel for hundreds of thousands of vasectomies the problem is not only different, but also more difficult.

Dr. Schmidt agreed with this thesis, but pointed out that the animated cartoon was a communication medium to which everyone might respond. He felt that if such cartoons were made, explaining vasectomy and answering patient's questions, then personnel time would be released and hundreds of people could be informed at the same time and place.

Dr. Chez pointed out that this was a discussion of learning aids, and that he felt that there was a question of imposing middle class values. The problem with many teaching aids is that they are made by middle class people and are shown to populations who have visual literacy but not reading literacy. He stated that the previous discussion on patient interviews and education, applied criteria and standards which were used in relatively pure medical environments, and these were not applicable to mass government programs or camp situations.

He agreed that being a listener was an important part of patient preparation, but wanted to know what relevancy objective criteria (age, number of children, motivation) had to the right of a patient to be sterilized. He wanted to know if objective data existed that showed that a twenty-seven year old woman with four children should be sterilized, while a twenty-five year old woman with three children should not. He suggested that the established standards and criteria were false.

Dr. Taylor asked for an alternative suggestion.

Dr. Chez said that the alternative should be the motivation of the person who wanted sterilization.

Dr. Taylor wanted to know if he did not think that people with six children should be sterilized.

Dr. Chez said that if this meant compulsory versus voluntary, he would say yes.

Dr. Taylor expressed concern over the situation of rights.

Dr. Chez said that the right of the individual over the right of the society was one matter. But he wanted to know how criteria other than the single criterion of wanting sterilization could be applied to cases who volunteered.

Dr. Tietze thought that the restrictions existed for the political protection of family planning program administrators who exercise what might be interpreted as unjustified limitations on freedom of choice in order to protect the program against political attack.

Dr. Chez accepted the pragmatic value of political reality but still said he did not see how criteria could be applied on a professional level.

Dr. Taylor referred to a recurring topic in the papers that had been presented, i.e. the decline in the frequency with which vasectomy is being performed in the last three or four years. The peak period in Korea, India, and East Pakistan appeared to be in 1964 or 1965 and then diminished. He wondered if this was an artefact, a temporary thing, or whether it was something that happens inevitably.

Dr. Neuwirth suggested that a more optimistic interpretation of the decline in sterilization cases might be to regard it as the difference between the number of people ready for vasectomy and its prevalence over the years.

Dr. Shubeck rebutted the decline following peak theory by citing the intra-uterine device campaigns in both South Korea and Taiwan. In South Korea the target of fifty thousand insertions a year has been met whenever funds were made available by the government; there has been no diminution.

Dr. Neuwirth suggested that this could be a function of setting targets.

Dr. Tietze mentioned that the sterilization decline in East Pakistan occurred at a time when the family planning program was vulnerable because it was an activity of the central government, which was unpopular in East Pakistan at that time.

Dr. Pai stated that in the intra-uterine device insertion camps there was an insertion peak and then a decline, and the same thing occurred in vasectomy camps. The latter decline was slight and might not be significant.

He suggested the need for tubectomy camps for nonpuerperal women; but the possibility existed of declining acceptance with this group. Postpartum tubectomy is done on completely prepared women in a clinic setting, where the problems of complications are reduced to an absolute minimum. He suggested that, under controlled conditions with proper precautions, female sterilization might be the answer to birth control.

II PERMANENT STERILIZATION

Ralph M. Richart, *Moderator*

Chapter 7

A MODIFIED OPERATIVE TECHNIQUE FOR VASECTOMY

HEE YONG LEE

In recent years, male sterilization by bilateral partial vasectomy has become increasingly popular as a birth control method. Fundamental surgical techniques have not been changed, but there have been numerous minor modifications. Criteria of a satisfactory operative procedure are the following: technical simplicity; minimization of complications; and feasibility of future recanalization.

Vasectomy is indicated when economic factors force limitations on family size; child-bearing endangers maternal health and tubectomy is contraindicated, the parents have physical or mental handicaps; genetic factors suggest the possibility of congenital anomalies; fear of pregnancy disturbs marital life; and the couple does not wish to have any more children.

Eligibility criteria for free government service in Korea are a low family income and the existence of more than three living children.

The couple's reason for requesting vasectomy must be determined and both partners should consent to the procedure. Preoperative screening is of the utmost importance in the prevention of a postoperative sterilization neurosis. A vasectomy patient must be mentally competent, and hypersensitivity and neurotic tendencies are contraindications for vasectomy.

Insofar as possible, the vasectomy operation should be explained to the patient. Great care must be taken to avoid confusion between sterilization and castration. The possibility of restoration of fertility should be discussed; but the couple must be made to understand that this cannot be guaranteed.

Both marital partners should sign an adequate consent form.

The procedure described here was performed on more than two thousand patients. It involves such modifications as a single scrotal incision, double ligation of the folded end, and immediate sperm clearance. A new instrument (Lee's vasectomy hook) has been employed in these procedures.

On the evening prior to surgery, the patient should shave the skin, take a shower, and have sexual intercourse, if possible.

SURGICAL PROCEDURE

The patient is placed on the operating table in the supine position and is asked to keep both hands behind his head. To keep the penis and pubic hair away from the operating field, they are fixed to the suprapubic abdominal wall with a wide adhesive plaster. The scrotal skin is shaved, and both scrotum and inner thighs should be washed thoroughly. The operative field is draped so that only the scrotum is exposed.

The surgeon should stand to the right of the patient and palpate both vasa to determine the anticipated operative level; this may be slightly below the radix of the penis. The incision should be made sufficiently distant from the vaso-epididymal junction so that future reanastomosis may be performed.

About 5 cc of a 2% procaine solution is infiltrated into the scrotal skin at the median raphe and into the tissues surrounding the vasa.

The course of the superficial scrotal vasculature determines the direction of the incision. A longitudinal or transverse incision (½ cm) is made on the median raphe of the scrotum just below the penile radix.

The point of a closed mosquito forceps is inserted into the center of the tissues and then the blades are opened. This enables the surgeon to grasp the vas more easily with an Allis forceps.

An Allis tissue forceps is then introduced through the median incision; the forceps should be directed towards the left vas, which is grasped by the forceps and pulled out through the incision.

A longitudinal incision (0.5 cm) is used to dissect out the superficial tissue covering the vasal wall. The vas is then exposed. If necessary, an additional infiltration of procaine may be infused along the course of the vas.

A vasectomy hook* is inserted into the interspace between the vas and its covering. The hook should be passed through the interspace until the largest shaft circumference is reached. The exposed vas is bluntly separated from its covering tissues and held for the next procedure.

A 3–0 silk thread nipped in a pair of mosquito forceps is passed through the space, while the hook is removed. The silk is then divided. Both ends of the thread attached to the distal vas (seminal vesicle side) are pulled upward; the thread attached to the proximal vas (epididymal side) is pulled downward. This bluntly separates the vas from its coverings for about 1 cm.

A pair of mosquito forceps is applied to the middle section of the separated vas. For immediate sperm clearance, the distal portion of the vas is lifted and lavaged with a solution of 5 cc of 0.1% potassium permanganate spermicidal solution.

A single ligature of 3–0 silk thread is applied to the distal vas; an additional tie with the same thread is done to the same vas at a point just below the mosquito forceps; this forces the cut end back on itself. The long ends of the thread are not cut but are held in a pair of mosquito forceps.

Another ligature of 3–0 silk thread is used on the proximal vas 0.5 cm below the previous distal ligature; the long ends of this thread are held in the same forceps as the distal ligature threads. The vas is interrupted between the two ligatures, but no section is removed. The distal end of the vas has been folded back and tied; but the proximal end has been tied singly, preventing spontaneous recanalization.

Both ends of the left vas are dropped back into the scrotum, but the long ends of the silk sutures are kept outside of the scrotum.

The ligated and divided left vas is pulled through the incision by the long ends of the silk threads in order to search for bleed-

* The vasectomy hook employed by the author (Lee's vasectomy hook) is made of stainless steel and is pointed, tipped, and angular in shape. The entire hook length is 18 cm (handle, 11.5 cm; shaft, 7.5 cm; beak, 0.4 cm); the shaft circumference grades from 0.5 to 2.5 cm. Chung Whang Instrument Company, Seoul, Korea, manufactures this instrument.

ing or oozing points. If there is no bleeding, the long silk sutures are cut, and both ends of the vas are released by a pull on the scrotum; the cut ends fall back into their original positions.

The right vas is handled through the same scrotal incision and in the manner previously described.

Bleeding points in the subcutaneous tissue of the scrotal wound are clamped and tied, and a small amount of antiseptic powder is applied to prevent local infection.

The scrotal wound is closed with a single suture of chromic catgut, eliminating the need for suture removal. A simple dressing is applied and the scrotum is elevated with a suspensory or T-bandage.

POSTOPERATIVE CARE

Patients are given 400,000 units of penicillin plus 0.5 gm of streptomycin. This is followed by the use of sulfa drugs or oral penicillin for two to three postoperative days.

The patient is advised to do only light work for two days postoperatively and is cautioned to avoid hard labor for five days.

When the *washing out* method is not used, the patient is advised to use other methods to guard against conception until at least six postoperative ejaculations have occurred. The postoperative semen specimen is examined for sperm at this time.

All normal activities, including showers and sexual intercourse, may be resumed after seven days.

POSTOPERATIVE RESULTS

There is usually mild discomfort in the area of surgery and in the lower abdomen. A slight swelling in the ligated portion of the vas may persist for a few days; a small area of induration may persist for a longer period without pain or discomfort. The most common postoperative complaints found in this series of 2,250 cases were the following: decreased sexual drive (123 cases); deterioration of general health (90 cases) sperm granuloma (32 cases); and bacterial epididymitis (15 cases).

The technique of a single median scrotal incision proved to be satisfactory. No single vas was cut twice, and among the fifteen epididymitis cases, none was bilateral.

Various techniques have been suggested to avoid spontaneous recanalization: sealing the cut ends of the vas by fulgurating them, and closing the fascial sheath of the vas over one end; arranging the cut vasal ends so they overlap; and folding the cut vasal ends back on themselves. In this series, there were only two cases of spontaneous recanalization. This might be attributable to the technique of folding back the cut end of the distal vas and using a double silk ligature on the distal vas and a single ligature on the proximal one.

The immediate sperm clearance technique has been effective in preventing the presence of residual sperm in the ampullae. The rate of sperm exhaustion from the ampullae should be judged by the frequency of ejaculation; therefore, several semen specimens should be examined postoperatively. The *wash out* technique was tried on more than 250 cases and no pregnancy resulted from intercourse. The immediate sperm clearance technique of instillation of a spermicidal solution into the reservoirs at the time of surgery appears to be effective.

To permit reanastomosis, vasectomy should be performed at a sufficient distance from the vaso-epididymal junction and no section of the vasa should be excised. Among the sixty cases who required anastomosis, an average of three years elapsed between the vasectomy and the request for vasovasotomy; reversal was requested because of the death of children or remarriage. Of fifty cases who were reanastomosed, forty-three showed semen positive for sperm, but only eight cases successfully impregnated their wives. In nine cases of reanastomosis, the untoward effects of vasectomy were reversed.

Chapter 8

VAS REANASTOMOSIS PROCEDURES

STANWOOD S. SCHMIDT

PRINCIPLES

To understand the principles behind vas anastomosis, one must consider first the anatomy of the vas, the technique of the previous vasectomy, and the results of the vasectomy.

The vas is markedly convoluted as it arises from the epididymis. These convolutions are three-dimensional; the angles are acute, and the vas sometimes even turns back upon itself. This portion of the vas cannot be straightened without interfering with its blood supply. A probe in the lumen can be passed to the first angle, but not around it.

As the vas progresses, the convolutions become less acute and fewer until, at the top of the scrotum, the vas becomes straight. Any procedure to anastomose the vas will be more successful, and technically easier, if the previous vasectomy has been done in the straight portion of the vas.

The average vasectomy is poorly done. It is performed without a clear understanding of the optimum technique. Even worse, it is usually done without regard to future reanastomosis.

All too often, the vas is interrupted in the midscrotum, where it is easily accessible, but convoluted. Many physicians will resect lengths of the vas in the belief that this is necessary to insure success in sterilizing the man. Cases exist where the vas was resected from epididymis to above the external ring; obviously this makes anastomosis impossible. A vasectomy should be done at the top of the scrotum, and the vas should not be resected (Fig. 8–1).

Following vasectomy, the testicular (or proximal in terms of flow of sperm) side of the vas changes (Fig. 8–2). Along with the epididymal tubules, the vas dilates. This results not only in dilation of the lumen of the vas to four times its original di-

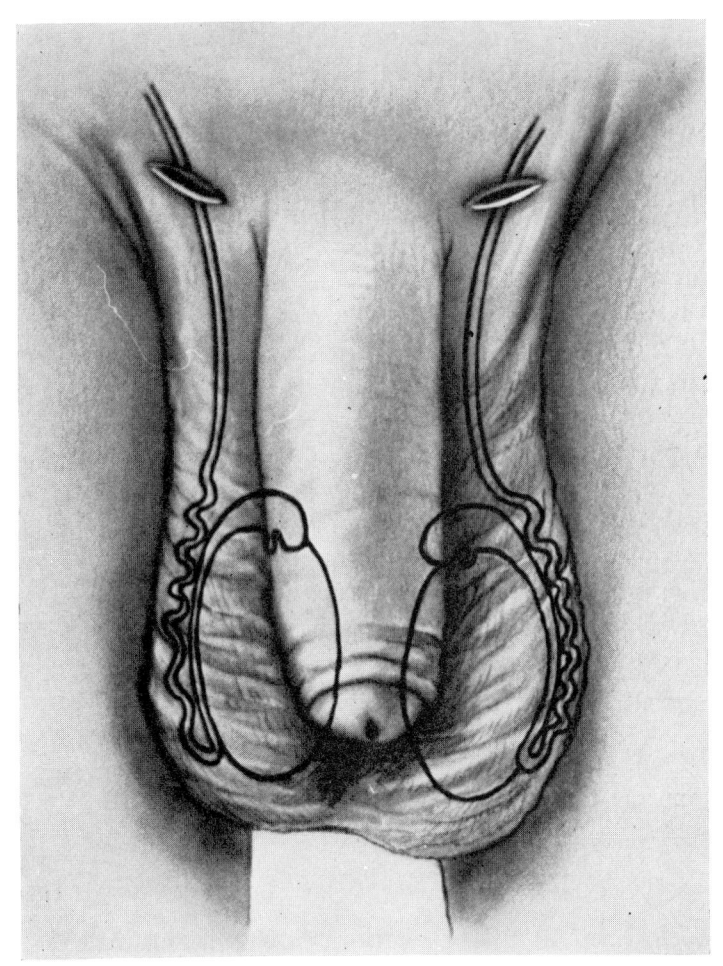

Figure 8-1. Diagram showing optimum location for vasectomy.

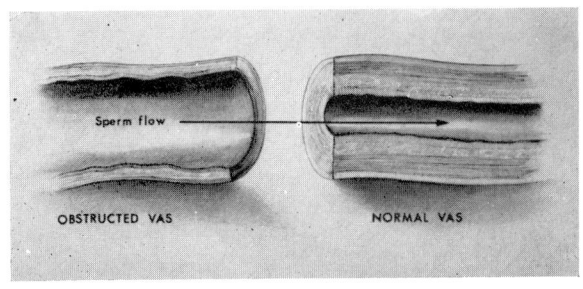

Figure 8-2. Diagram showing difference in lumina after vasectomy.

ameter, but also in a thinning of the wall of the vas. Vas anastomosis, therefore, calls for joining structures with lumens of different diameters.

In the epididymis, this dilation is pronounced and may cause temporary discomfort from engorgement. Rupture of such a tubule will result in the formation of a spermatic granuloma of the epididymis, followed by permanent obstruction at that point. This is a significant complication (in excess of 4%) of vasectomy. It explains not only the failure to secure sperm from the proximal vas at surgery, but also is the reason why vasectomy will never be reversible in all cases. This epididymis will show the typical acute granuloma initially. Later, it will merely show dilated, often patchy tubules in the head of the epididymis and collapsed tubules elsewhere in the epididymis. Here, success depends on an epididymovasostomy, sometimes with a simultaneous vasovasotomy. Success rates are poor in these cases.

An unproven belief exists that spermatic granuloma sometimes can result in auto-immunity to one's own sperm. This may explain cases where vasovasotomy is followed by a high count of nonmotile sperm.

Spermatic granuloma is a major cause of failure of vas anastomosis. Conversely, it is also the mechanism of spontaneous vas anastomosis following vasectomy.

TECHNIQUES

The location of the previous vasectomy determines the technique that can be used. If the vasectomy has been done so that the proximal end of the vas is convoluted, only one basic method is possible. If the proximal end is straight for 1 cm or more, a variety of operations may be employed. Often two different techniques are used on the same patient, one on each side.

Regardless of method, the surgery is best done in a hospital operating room with the patient under anesthesia. It should not be done as an office procedure. It is too painstaking a procedure to risk the distractions to the surgeon that will accompany the use of a local anesthetic. With present-day anesthetics, the patient may be released after he has fully awakened. If the scrotum is immobilized with a good suspensory, limited general activity is not harmful, and the patient usually has little postoperative pain.

The point of previous vasectomy can usually be palpated as a nodule or as a defect in the vas. The scrotum is incised over this area. The vas is grasped above and below this point with Allis clamps. The ends of the vas are freed from their overlying fascia for 1 cm and are then freshened with transverse cuts (Fig. 8–3).

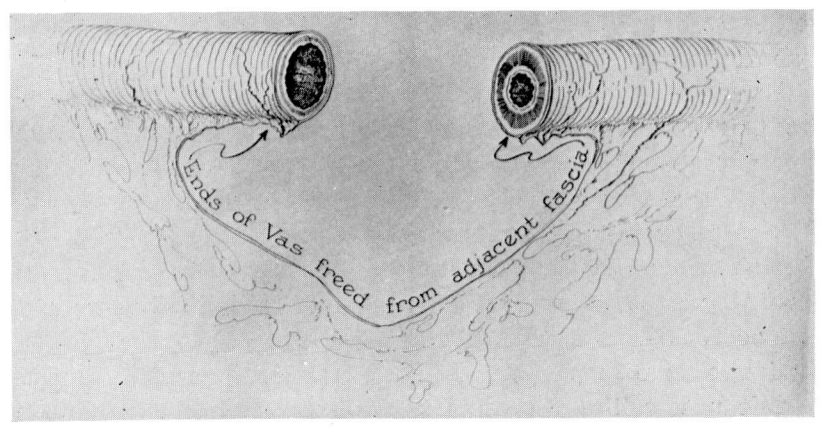

Figure 8–3. Ends of the vas are freshened with transverse cuts.

Patency of the distal arm is proven by injecting saline with a blunted hypodermic needle (#23). The patent vas accepts this readily and with little pressure. Should the needle not pass, the vas may be probed with a nylon suture.

Spermatic fluid is often seen upon freshening the proximal (testicular) end of the vas. This is examined for spermatozoa. If they are found, it is certain evidence that the duct is patent to that point. Sometimes macrophages are seen without sperm. Any amount of spermatic fluid is presumptive evidence of patency. If no fluid is immediately apparent, the vas may be milked to produce it. The epididymis should not be milked, for its tubules might be ruptured. Where epididymal obstruction has followed the vasectomy for weeks or longer, the vas may show a dilated lumen without spermatic fluid. If the lumen is not dilated, the testis may never have produced sperm and a testicular biopsy should be done.

After the patency of the vas has been determined, the testicular end is probed with a nylon suture (#00 or #000) to determine how far it is straight. If it is straight for 1 cm or more, an endosplint may be used. If not, as with a convoluted vas, a solid, removable splint must be used.

Regardless of the type of splint used, the ends of the vas are next brought together by placing one or more nonabsorbable sutures in the adjacent fascia. This should permit the ends to rest together even when mild traction is exerted to separate them. The anastomosis is performed end-to-end, never side-to-side.

Any of several techniques can be employed at this point. All construct the anastomosis over a splint, for this aligns the lumen and puts the anastomosis at rest. Vasovasotomy can be done without splinting the vas, but a splint seems to make healing better and success greater.

A simpler method, which must be used in a convoluted vas, involves placing a #00 nylon splint into the distal vas for a distance of 5–10 mm. Using #00 nylon swaged onto a blunted straight needle (Ethicon ×–0821) or threaded through a hypodermic needle, the other end of the splint is inserted into the proximal vas to either the first convolution or, if possible, for a distance of 2 cm. It is then stabbed through the wall of the vas and through the skin (Fig. 8–4). The splint is held in place by a skin suture crimped, along with the nylon, into a lead shot. A wire splint may be used, but it would be far less comfortable.

An exciting alternate method, which has resulted in pregnancies but which is not yet fully evaluated, uses a permanent internal cannula or an endosplint. This conducts the spermatic fluid across the anastomosis and prevents leakage, and thus granuloma, at the anastomosis.

This endosplint is tapered, with the larger diameter placed into the proximal (testicular) end of the vas. It is placed without external fixation (Fig. 8–5). Its larger diameter prevents it from moving immediately into the distal vas. It is made of Silastic, and thus is biologically inert. Polyethylene may be used similarly, but it is less flexible than the vas, which is a disadvantage.

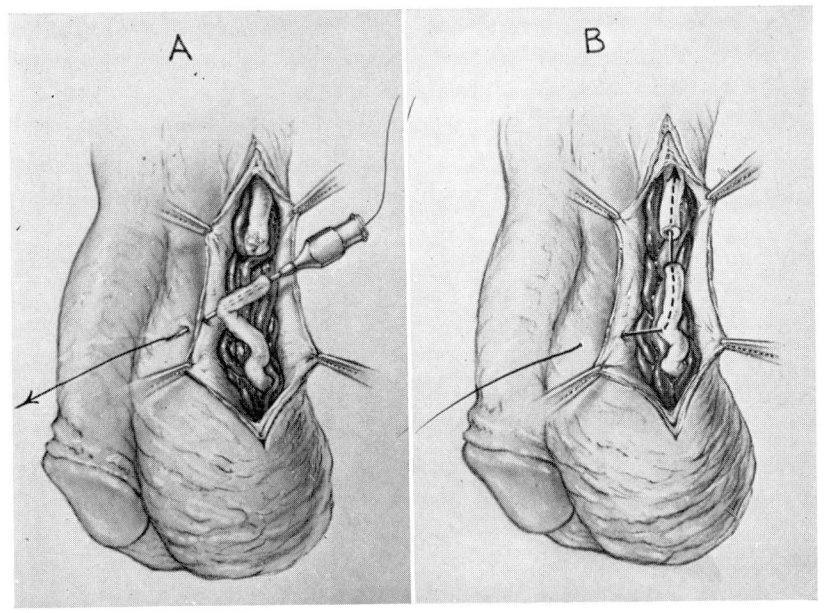

Figure 8-4A. The removable nylon splint may be placed by threading it through a hypodermic needle. B. After placement of the removable nylon splint.

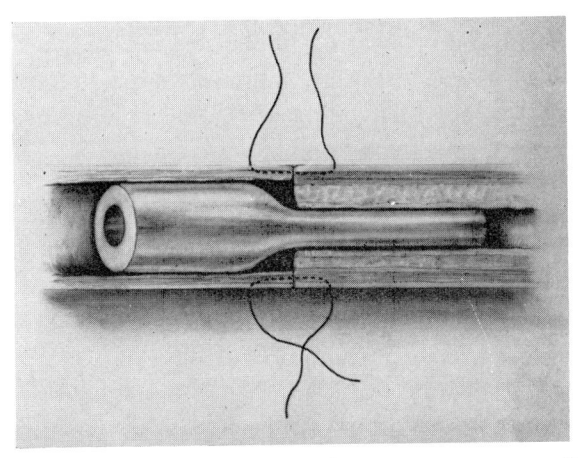

Figure 8-5. Diagram showing completed anastomosis using silastic endo-splint.

To date, these endosplints have been made by hand and vary in size. The lumen of the vas also varies in size and a splint must be chosen to fit the particular vas. The larger diameter of the splint should be at least 1 cm long and the smaller diameter may be 1½–2 cm long. The proximal, or testicular, arm is inserted easily, and thus sometimes is placed last. It is useful in placing the distal arm, to thread a 4–0 or 6–0 monofilament nylon suture through the endosplint. This suture is placed into the distal lumen, and the endosplint then is passed over the suture into place; after this the suture is withdrawn.

Occasionally, it is a simple matter to insert the endosplint into the distal vas. In this case, the proximal arm may be placed first. When this is done, the endosplint often starts to drip spermatic fluid. After it is placed into the distal vas, the fluid will continue to pass.

A previous technique involved a cannula which was brought through the wall of the distal vas to the outside, to drip spermatic fluid there. This avoided leakage at the anastomosis. However, it was almost impossible to keep the cannula in place in the proximal vas.

Any spillage of spermatic fluid must be wiped away or flushed away with saline irrigation. Sperm in the tissues results in a spermatic granuloma, which is a major reason for failure of the anastomosis. Theoretically, an endosplint will conduct spermatic fluid in spite of a granuloma, an added advantage.

Regardless of the splinting method, the actual anastomosis calls for precise suturing. Three or four interrupted sutures of #6–0 monofilament nylon or Prolene may be used around the circumference of the vas. The posterior suture is placed first, as it is the most difficult (Fig. 8–6). These sutures should be placed so that they do not enter the lumen of the vas.

From a practical standpoint, placing three sutures in a structure that averages 2 mm in diameter is difficult at best. A carelessly placed suture may cross the vas and obliterate the lumen. For this reason, the surgeon should use magnification in placing these sutures. He can use a visor-type of magnifier (which magnifies 2½x to 3x at a reasonable focal distance) or he can use an operating microscope (at 6, 10, or 16x). The visor can

Vas Reanastomosis Procedures

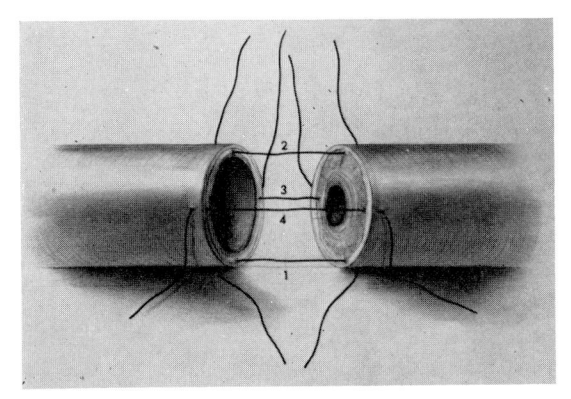

Figure 8-6. Order of placement of sutures.

be used with no prior experience. The microscope, however, requires considerable practice in use.

The sutures are swaged onto needles, minimizing the puncture hole. Sutures to #9-0 are available, but their needles are weak and bend easily.

These sutures are best placed in the wall of the vas before placing the splint and before tying the fascial sutures. When they are drawn up, it is important to make sure that the approximation is good and that the endosplint is not kinked. The wound is closed with subcutaneous and cutaneous sutures of plain gut. A suspensory always is applied.

Because of the thick walls of the vas, some of the techniques of fine vascular surgery do not seem applicable, e.g. tissue cements, staplers, and suturing by everting the walls.

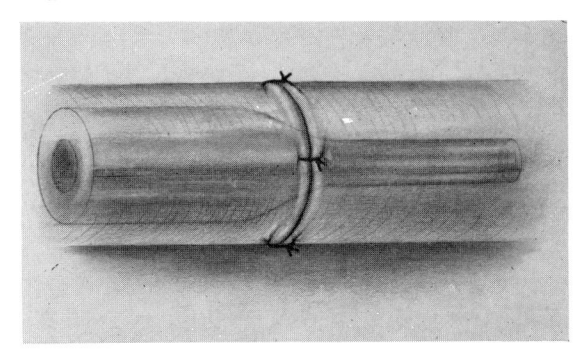

Figure 8-7. Completed anastomosis using endosplint.

The patient may resume bathing in two to three days, although the suspensory should be used for a week or more. When an endosplint is used, intercourse is permitted in one week. When a nylon splint is used, it is removed ten days postoperatively and intercourse is allowed two days later.

With a satisfactory anastomosis on one or both sides, a full count of sperm is often seen within several weeks. If the count is low, it may be due to a granuloma at the site(s) of anastomosis or possibly to a delay in the change from phagocytosis to transport of sperm. Reoperation should not be done within six months, for success may appear late.

Spontaneous anastomosis does occur through means of spermatic granuloma. This drains through the distal end of the vas. Eventually an epithelialized tract forms. This anastomosis usually occurs within a few weeks of vasectomy. An opposite effect, that of obstruction, seems to occur when a spermatic granuloma complicates vasovasostomy.

FAILURES

Since the opportunity to reoperate is infrequent, little is known about failures.

With such a small structure, misalignment can occur easily. Splinting will minimize this and will prevent kinking and overriding. The use of magnifying lenses while suturing also will aid in securing an exact alignment.

Unless particular care is taken, the anastomosis may pull apart. The wall of the vas is not strong. Sutures placed in the vas are for approximation, not for strength. The sutures in the adjacent fascia must provide the strength to hold the ends of the vas together. When a long segment of vas has been excised previously, these sutures must support the weight of the testis.

When the ends of the vas are not approximated well (e.g. sutures are not placed equally around the circumference, or a transverse face has been anastomosed to an oblique face of the vas) the anastomosis will not be watertight. Sperm may leak from the anastomosis into the surrounding tissues, forming a spermatic granuloma. The resulting inflammation and scarring may obstruct the anastomosis.

A spermatic granuloma of the epididymis is not unusual. It causes an obstruction in the epididymis which may prevent sperm from reaching the vas. This may occur following vasectomy, and is often, but not always, symptomatic. Vigorous attempts to milk the epididymis at the time of vasovasotomy may produce this. The anastomosis of the vas may succeed then, but the patient will remain sterile.

Evaluating the results of vasovasotomy is difficult; twenty-five percent of the patients do not return for evaluation or do not inform their physicians of the results. Many of these men have undergone surgery to please their wives, and often these are younger, second wives. Perhaps they think if sperm are not present in the seminal fluid they will have to undergo additional surgery, or perhaps, since they may have had children by a previous marriage, they are less anxious for children than their wives.

After six postoperative months, it is unlikely that the results will change, and surgery is indicated again. The anastomosis is exposed. A vasotomy is made in its testicular side, close to the anastomosis. A longitudinal incision is used, and the vas is probed distally with a nylon suture. If it is impassable, punching through with a probe may be attempted, and then a nylon splint or a Silastic endosplint may be placed. Often it is more certain to excise the old anastomosis and construct a new one.

Chapter 9

EVALUATION OF THE OPTIMAL TIME FOR TUBAL LIGATION

Lelia V. Phatak

Tubal ligation and/or minimal bilateral salpingectomy by a modified Pomeroy method are accepted contraceptive procedures for population control. Human sterilization by vasectomy or tubectomy is one of the most widely accepted methods of contraception in India.

The National Program of Family Planning of the Indian government has aided this program in a number of ways. Obstetrical and gynecological departments which do not have operating theaters are given aid in building them in order to make round-the-clock sterilization possible. Grants are also given to maintain extra beds especially for tubectomy cases; and tubectomy camps, staffed by teams of experienced surgeons, have been encouraged. Financial compensation is adequate for the medical and paramedical personnel involved in these programs.

The degree of acceptance of the program has been most encouraging.

Certain targets in family planning have been established in order to attain the desired level of population control. An attempt is made to sterilize as many women as possible who have a family of two, three, or more children. However, acceptance of any method is one of the main considerations in its evaluation. Since motivation for sterilization is greatest in the perinatal period, postpartum sterilizations have been encouraged and play an important part in the national program. In order to reach the desired target, twenty percent of all delivered women should be sterilized.

Before deciding on the optimal time to perform tubal ligation, it is necessary to have a comparative evaluation of the operation done during the following periods: early puerperium, less than forty-eight hours; from two to ten days postpartum; nonpuerperal periods; and incidental sterilization performed with other gynecological or surgical procedures.

The first two categories of patients are of great importance to the success of the government program, and it is important to obtain as much data as possible on the long-term and short-term effects of sterilization during these periods.

The data herein presented are drawn from two of the largest hospitals in Delhi; the experiences of one group of patients is studied, and a long-term follow-up of another series of women is presented. A total of 948 sterilizations were performed from 1963 through 1968.

Table 9–I presented the distribution of these cases. The ac-

TABLE 9-I
DISTRIBUTION OF STERILIZED CASES

Period of Sterilization	Number of Cases	Percent of Cases
Early Puerperium (less than 48 hours)	530	55.98 ⎫
Late Puerperium (48 hours-10 days)	267	28.10 ⎬ 84.08
Nonpuerperal	44	4.64
Incidental	107	11.28
TOTAL	948	100.00

ceptance of sterilizations is greatest in the puerperal period; this agrees with observations made by many other physicians.

The 797 cases of sterilization performed in the puerperal period were studied clinically in order to assess morbidity in relation to the time of surgery. Short-term studies were done on the puerperal cases, and a comparison was made between sterilization performed in early puerperium (under 48 hours) and late puerperium (48 hours to 10 days).

SHORT-TERM STUDIES

When the puerperal sterilization cases are considered alone, 64.9 percent and 65.4 percent in each hospital were done within forty-eight hours following labor; the remainder of the 797 cases were sterilized later than two days after delivery.

The mortality rate in all the cases was zero.

Morbidity data on the 797 cases are presented in Tables 9–II, 9–III, and 9–IV.

Morbidity as defined by the Joint Committee on Maternal Welfare is a temperature of 100.4° on any two of the first ten postpartum days, exclusive of the first twenty-four hours; temperature is taken by a standard technique at least four times a day.

TABLE 9-II
MORBIDITY IN RELATION TO STERILIZATION TIME

Period of Sterilization	Total Cases	Morbidity Cases	Morbidity Percentage
Early Puerperium (less than 48 hours)	530	79	14.9
Late Puerperium (48 hours-10 days)	267	34	12.7
TOTAL	797	113	14.1

TABLE 9-III
MORBIDITY IN RELATION TO STERILIZATION TIME IN NORMAL AND ABNORMAL LABOR

Period of Sterilization	Normal Labor Morbidity Cases	Normal Labor Morbidity Percentage	Abnormal Labor Morbidity Cases	Abnormal Labor Morbidity Percentage
Early Puerperium (less than 48 hours)	24	4.60	55	19.8
Late Puerperium (48 hours to 10 days)	15	2.88	19	6.85

TABLE 9-IV
MORBIDITY INCIDENCE IN RELATION TO HEMATOLOGICAL STATUS

Hemoglobin (in gm %)	Total Cases	Morbidity Cases	Morbidity Percentage
6.0 or less	11	5	45.00
6.5 to 10.0	486	68	14.20
10.5 or more	265	34	12.83

Table 9–II shows the incidence of morbidity in relation to the time of surgery. Table 9–III relates the morbidity to the type of labor. Both sets of data show that better results are obtained in cases operated on during the early puerperal period.

Of the 68 cases of morbidity in group B, 64.7 percent of the patients were involved with obstetrical surgery, and morbidity incidence was 14.2 percent. Of the total of 113 cases in this series exhibiting morbidity, 74 (65.5%) had obstetrical problems; the morbidity level here was 14.1 percent.

An estimation of the hemoglobin was done in 473 cases, and the influence on the morbidity patterns is very interesting (Table 9–IV).

Moderately low levels of hemoglobin do not appear to have an influence on morbidity, and variations in time of surgery may not be significant in cases with moderately slight anemia. Severe anemias, however, appear to be conducive to a very high morbidity rate.

Tubal sterilization is done under many different circumstances, and clinical outcome is influenced by the institutional environment and management, the type of patients, and the personnel involved with the patient. Special interest in any particular area also contributes to the success of the surgical procedure.

Table 9–V compares the incidence of abnormal labor in two

TABLE 9-V
ABNORMAL LABOR, PROPHYLACTIC ANTIBIOTIC USE, AND POSTOPERATIVE MORBIDITY
Comparative Study of Two Hospitals

Hospital	Total	Cases Abnormal Labor	Morbidity	Prophylactic Antibiotics
A	505	179 (33.3%)	92 (18.0%)	465 (92.0%)
B	292	99 (33.8%)	21 (9.1%)	192 (65.7%)

hospitals, and also shows the use of preoperative antibiotics and the incidence of postoperative morbidity. It is of great interest to note the extreme difference in the morbidity rates and in the administration of preoperative prophylactic antibiotics. Obviously, clinical results obtained at varying institutions are influenced by numerous factors; this is of the utmost importance in the implementation of a large-scale countrywide program.

LONG-TERM STUDIES

The late effects of puerperal sterilization has been an issue of great interest for a long while; there is need for follow-up studies in many aspects of the program. Available studies are not helpful in setting clear guidelines for the optimal time of tubal ligation.

A long-term follow-up study was done on a sample of 277 cases who had been sterilized; the postoperative study period ranged from six months to five years.

The relative proportion of puerperal, nonpuerperal, and incidental sterilizations was similar to that observed in the previous series of cases studied. In a series of 400 women, 256 (99%) had puerperal sterilizations; this is similar to the 84.17 percent of sterilizations done in the puerperal period in the initial sample of 799 cases.

A series of 277 women have been followed for the following time periods: up to six months, 125; six months to one year, 63; one to two years, 28; two to three years, 22; three to four years, 16; four to five years, 9; and five to twelve years, 19.

An endometrial biopsy was done on 254 of these cases; the remaining patients either declined the procedure or did not appear. In those patients who had started menstruating, the biopsy was taken three to four days before the menstrual period was expected. In the other patients, the biopsy was taken when the patient appeared for follow-up. Of the biopsies obtained from women who were seen postoperatively up to a maximum of five years (245 cases): 94 cases showed a proliferative phase; 157 showed a secretory phase; and 4 showed an inflammatory reaction. Three of the cases exhibiting inflammations were biopsied within the first three months after sterilization; the other case had a biopsy taken two years postoperatively.

Nine biopsies were obtained from women who were seen five years or more after sterilization. Five cases showed a secretory phase; one showed atropic changes; two revealed a hyperplastic nonsecretory phase; and one case had cystic glandular hyperplasia.

Pathological correlation of the clinical findings revealed that in two cases an inflammatory reaction had associated menorrhagia, while the third case with chronic endometritis had amenorrhea at the time of examination (three months postoperatively). The fourth case complained of no particular symptoms.

Histopathological examination of the fallopian tubes was done in 296 cases: 97 percent of the tubes were normal; 1.1 percent exhibited acute salpingitis; and 1.3 percent showed chronic salpingitis.

In the cases with acute salpingitis (five in all), two had had morbid pregnancies; one incomplete abortion and one ectopic pregnancy. Both of these women showed a mild hydrosalpinx three and six months postoperatively. The remaining three cases remained normal for nine months following sterilization.

Of the four cases with chronic salpingitis, two appeared to have no complaints for a year after surgery. One of the cases also had chronic endometritis and postoperative menorrhagia. The fourth case had chronic endometritis and developed a mild hydrosalpinx associated with menorrhagia three years after surgery.

Menstrual irregularities were reported by nearly 21 percent (40) of the 194 cases studied for this. While the number of patients who reported for follow-up decreased as time went by, the number who complained of menorrhagia increased. Definite conclusions concerning the incidence of menorrhagia as a complication of sterilization are difficult to make, for the incidence of the symptom in the population is not sufficiently documented. Authors reporting on menstrual irregularities have given widely different data. Many authors have concluded that if tubal ligation is delayed for more than forty-eight hours after delivery, it should not be undertaken until late in the postpartum period. The optimum time is considered to be beyond ten days; but this may be the longest period that a patient can be hospitalized in a well-financed institution in India. Many physicians think that tubal edema, bacterial contamination, risk of hemorrhage, technical problems, and morbidity increase in proportion to the delay in time of sterilization.

CONCLUSIONS

Bacteriological studies were not undertaken with this series, but an attempt was made, on the basis of available clinical data, to evaluate the two immediate postpartum periods in terms of morbidity patterns.

Patient response to sterilization while they are in the hospital is most favorable; and there appears to be no extra morbidity risk in tubal ligation at any time after delivery.

Prophylactic administration of antibiotics seems to be of secondary importance in an efficient obstetric service. However, it is necessary to assess the hematologic status of the patient and defer sterilization in poor-risk patients for fear of postoperative morbidity.

Long-term follow-up indicates that there is a definite hazard of potential infection of the apparently normal fallopian tube This topic needs further study on a larger scale.

Chapter 10

TUBAL STERILIZATION BY OPERATIVE CULDOSCOPY

Martin J. Clyman

Tubal sterilization in the United States is used widely, but is not an important part of current birth control programs. Most procedures are done abdominally and usually in the first twenty-four hours postpartum or at the time of cesarean section. In the developing countries, however, it is increasing in importance as a major effort to provide a more efficient means of population control.[1]

Transvaginal tubal ligation primarily using the Pomeroy technique has been advocated as an interim procedure. Boysen and McRae[2] used both the anterior and posterior colpotomy approach in 169 patients with one failure. Fort and Alexander[3] describe their techniques and the advantages of the vaginal Pomeroy sterilization in a hundred cases with a failure rate of two percent.

More recently, surgical sterilization by fimbriectomy has been reported to be a very effective means of sterilization. Kroener[4] reported over a thousand without any known pregnancies.

The purpose of this presentation is to introduce a rapid, simple transvaginal approach to tubal sterilization by the operative culdoscopic technique. Details of the culdoscope and operative culdoscopy have been presented previously.[5,6] The prime advantages of this technique are the following: ease of tubal visualization through the culdoscope; good exposure; rapidity of procedure; use of local anesthesia; no visible scar; and a short hospital stay.

METHODS

Preoperative preparation of the patient includes the following: an enema; miniperineal preparation (this need not include shaving of pubic hair); intramuscular administration of Pantopon®

20 mg, Scopolamine® 0.3 mg, and Compazine® 10 mg, one hour prior to procedure. Immediately prior to the procedure, the patient is given 50 mg of Demerol® intravenously.

The patient is placed in knee-chest position with the thighs perpendicular to the surface of the table. Shoulder braces hold the patient in this position adequately and prevent her from sliding forward. The buttocks, perineum, and vulvar area are wiped clean with Zephiran®, (benzalkonium chloride 1 : 750) or Betadine®. The patient is draped sterilely, and a specially designed fulcrum perineal retractor is used for good vaginal exposure (Fig. 10–1). The vagina is wiped clean with the same solution and then dried.

A 1% solution of lidocaine with Adrenalin 1:100,000 is used; 3 cc are injected into the parametrium and 2 cc into the mucosa at the maximum point of concavity of the posterior fornix. A #12G trocar is used to puncture the fornix at the maximum point of concavity. Air is then heard to hiss into the peritoneal cavity spontaneously.

The 7 mm trocar then is used to puncture the mucosa and

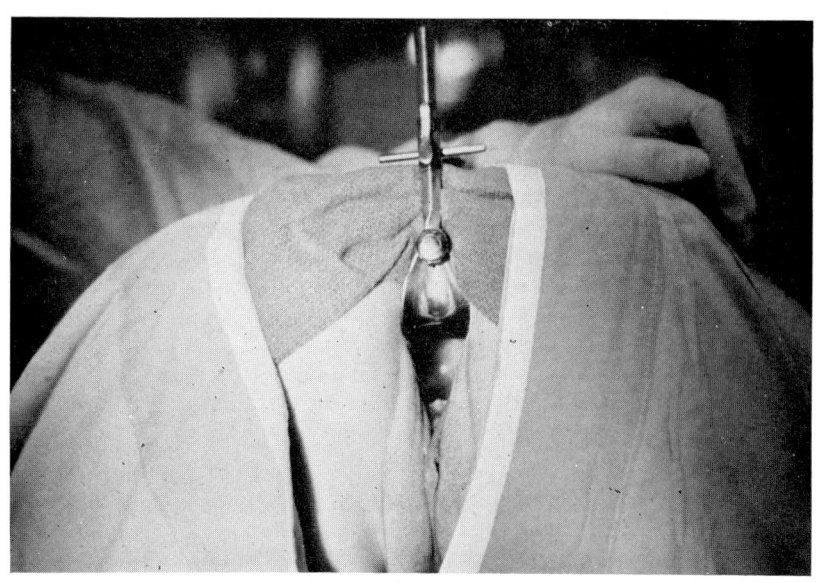

Figure 10–1. Vaginal exposure secured by fulcrum perineal retractor with variable pitch blade.

peritoneum in the same area. The pelvic organs are visualized when the intestines have fallen cephalad. An additional 0.5 cc of local anesthesia is placed in the mucosa (using a #23 gauge tonsillar needle) lateral to the cannula. The cannula is removed, and a nine-inch straight clamp is placed into the puncture hole and the opening is enlarged to 2 cm by spreading the tips of the clamp. The area is usually avascular, and any oozing from the vaginal mucosa is checked by additional injection of lidocaine plus Adrenalin. The culdoscope is introduced into the larger opening, and a specially designed mesosalpinx clamp* (11 inches long) is placed into the peritoneal cavity. Both culdoscope and clamp are moved forward until the edge of the clamp is at the superior pole of the ovary. Then the clamp is used to grasp the mesosalpinx ligament near its tubal insertion (Fig. 10–2). This ligament is firm and can be used to bring the tube into the vagina (Fig. 10–3). The culdoscope is removed. A Pomeroy sterilization is then performed. The midportion of the tube is grasped with a straight clamp, the top pulled forward and tied with plain $\overline{0}$ or $\overline{1}$ catgut (Fig. 10–4). The loop of the tube is then excised. This is repeated on the other side. The

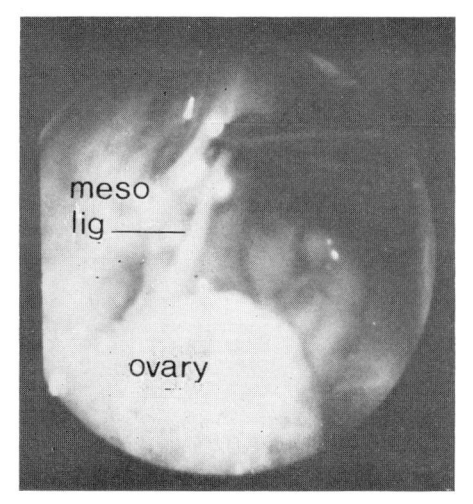

Figure 10–2. Culdoscopic photo showing mesosalpingeal ligament being grasped near end of fallopian tube.

* John Marco & Son, 601 Dow Avenue, Oakhurst, New Jersey 07755

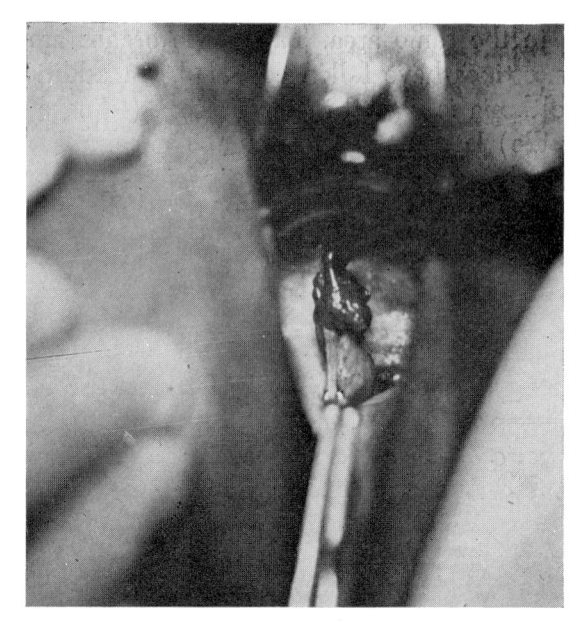

Figure 10-3. Fallopian tube brought into vagina.

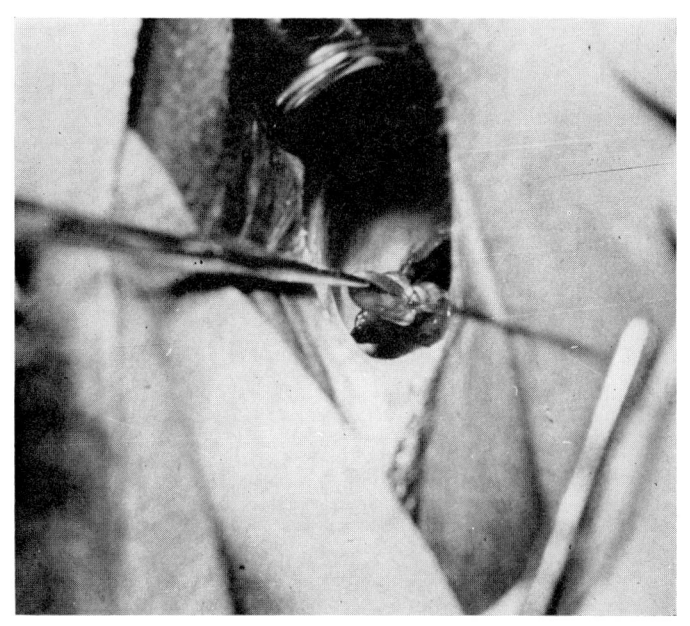

Figure 10-4. Ligating midportion of tube.

culdoscope is reintroduced to make sure that hemostasis is secure.

The posterior fornix is then closed with a figure-of-eight chromic $\overline{0}$ suture through both mucosa and peritoneum. Then the cannula is reintroduced, and the patient is placed into a prone position, with the operators hand on the suprapubic area of the abdomen. In this way, all of the intraperitoneal air is expressed. The cannula is removed, and a Sims perineal retractor is used to expose the posterior fornix. The suture is then tied. The patient returns directly to her room, and remains in the hospital for twenty-four hours or less.

The Kroener fimbriectomy sterilization is even more rapid and simple to do by culdoscopic technique. After the tube is brought into the vagina, the fimbriated end of the oviduct is grasped with a clamp and a silk suture is passed through the mesosalpinx and tied. The suture is passed around the tube and tied. The distal third of the tube then is excised.

OPERATIVE CULDOSCOPIC TUBAL STERILIZATION BY CAUTERY OR CRYOSURGERY

Using the operative culdoscopic technique described, the human fallopian tube can be coagulated and cut by cautery current as a means of sterilization. This can be accomplished intraperitoneally or intravaginally.

An intraperitoneal technique employs a Teflon coated clamp. This clamp is coated completely, except for the inner surface of the distal 1 cm; the distal 2 inches is angled at 45° and can reach the fallopian tube 1 cm from the cornual end. The distal end of the clamp has a 5 mm blade capable of crushing the fallopian tube. When this clamp is connected to the Bovie Cautery unit, it completely coagulates the tube for a distance of 1–2 cm, depending on the duration and intensity of the coagulating current. However, histologic examination of the coagulated tube reveals that the lumen is not obliterated with coagulation alone. It, therefore, is necessary to cut the tube and coagulate the proximal end. At present, long-term follow-up data are not available on this technique, and it is impossible to state what the rate of failure might be.

Coagulating and cutting the fallopian tube in monkeys and rabbits results in complete occlusion.

Better results in endosalpingeal destruction are obtained when the tube is brought out into the vagina and the cautery tip is inserted high into the lumen of the fallopian tube before coagulation. This destroys the endosalpingeal mucosa, and occlusion results.

Cryosurgical tubal sterilization with a cryoprobe at $-60°C$ has been attempted in monkeys and rabbits. At present, because of the expense of the equipment and the failure to obtain complete tissue destruction, this method of tubal closure does not appear promising.

OPERATIVE CULDOSCOPIC TUBAL STERILIZATION WITH TISSUE ADHESIVES

Tissue reaction to the injection of tissue adhesives such as isobutyl-2-cyanoacrylate monomer or n-octyl 2-cyanoacrylate monomer results in a local fibroblastic reaction.[7] Corfman et al. used methyl-2-cyanoacrylate in rabbits to obliterate the cornual ends of the fallopian tubes with the idea of transuterine cornual sterilization.

The technique of operative culdoscopy ideally lends itself to the trial use of these compounds to occlude the fimbriated ends of the tubes.

Four Macaque monkeys and four white New Zealand rabbits were used in an experiment to occlude the fimbriated ends of the tubes. The liquid monomer, isobutyl-2-cyanoacrylate,* polymerizes within a few seconds upon contact with the cations of the surface fluid of the endosalpingeal mucosa. The monomer was introduced by a sterile tuberculin syringe with a 25 gauge needle (a 1 cm length of Teflon tubing of appropriate size is placed over the needle). The Teflon tubing was introduced into the tubal ostium under binocular magnification (10x); 0.05 cc of the monomer was introduced by a special holder with a micrometer screw-thread advancement device. Great care was taken not to spill the liquid outside the desired area.

* Supplied in sterile containers by Ethicon Corporation, Somerville, New Jersey.

Gross examination of the ends of the fallopian tubes after three months and six months revealed that the polymerized plastic was still present in the lumen of the ends of the tubes. The tubes appeared to be occluded, and this was tested by introducing fluid above the obstructed ends. However, histologic examination revealed damaged endosalpingeal mucosa with scattered multi-nucleated giant cells and interspersed refractile nonstaining (H & E) granular polymer plastic. The same picture is seen in the human fallopian tube.

Studies are being conducted to determine if this is a functionally closed tube.

DISCUSSION

Where a similar result is required, the simplest, safest approach is best. The operative culdoscopic approach of tubal ligation by Pomeroy or the Kroener fimbriectomy technique is considered safe. It requires no recovery room; is performed under local anesthesia; the round ligament cannot be seen and mistaken for the tube; there is no postoperative pain and a short hospital stay. It can be done four to six weeks postpartum with no visible scar, direct visualization of the fallopian tubes, and therefore, no blind groping. One suture can be used to close the posterior fornix. It lends itself well to use in the developing countries where anesthesia and bed space are a problem—especially in India, where vaginal procedures are not considered as serious surgery by the populace.

Garb[8] reviewed tubal sterilization failures in 1957, and in a total of 29,496 cases, the failure rate was 0.71 percent. There were 0.40 percent failures in 5,477 Pomeroy operations; this was the current operation of choice.

If the lumen at the end of the fallopian tube can be completely occluded by tissue adhesives, Silastic, or other plastic material, the technique of operative culdoscopy could be used with great potential for reversibility.

REFERENCES

1. Ranganathan, K.V., and Hulka, J.F.: Tubal ligation as a part of family planning in India. *Amer J Obstet Gynec*, 105:434, 1969.

2. Boysen, H., and McRae, L.A.: Tubal sterilization through the vagina. *Amer J Obstet Gynec, 58:*488, 1949.
3. Fort, A.T., and Alexander, A.M.: Vaginal Pomeroy sterilization. *Obstet Gynec, 28:*421, 1966.
4. Kroener, W.F., Jr.: Surgical sterilization by fimbriectomy. *Amer J Obstet Gynec, 104:*247, 1969.
5. Clyman, M.J.: Operative culdoscopy. *Obstet Gynec, 38:*840, 1968.
6. Clyman, M.J.: A new panculdoscope, diagnostic, photographic and operative aspect. *Obstet Gynec, 21:*343, 1963.
7. Corfman, P.A., Richart, R.M., and Taylor, H.C., Jr.: Response of the rabbit oviduct to a tissue adhesive. *Science, 148:*1348, 1965.
8. Garb, A.E.: A review of tubal sterilization failures. *Obstet Gynec Surv, 12:*291, 1957.

Chapter 11

NONPUERPERAL STERILIZATION BY LAPAROSCOPY

Robert S. Neuwirth

Interest in applying laparoscopy for sterilization developed in the Bronx-Lebanon Hospital Center because of an acute shortage of beds, particularly obstetrical beds. Many of the patients in this series represent women who were delivered at the hospital and could not have their desired postpartum tubal ligation. They were followed up at discharge, and when a bed became available they were admitted and sterilized during the course of a one or two-day hospitalization period.

Tubal sterilization performed under laparoscopic control has gained wider interest in the United States and Western Europe during the past several years. The currently accepted approach was devised by Dr. Rauol Palmer of Paris; in 1962 he reported ten cases done during laparoscopy with a coagulation cautery.[3] Subsequently, Palmer designed a special biopsy forceps. This is a grasping as well as a coring or boring instrument, and it can also be electrified at its tip. Palmer's instrument, or modifications of it, is currently being used to coagulate and transect the fallopian tubes at laproscopy.

Tubal sterilization at laparoscopy was reported initially in 1941. Power and Barnes[4] attempted this procedure using the Ruddock peritoneoscope, an instrument designed in about 1935. Anderson also discussed this procedure in a paper in 1937.[1] The instrument had an incandescent lighting system; a good optical system; and an alligator type biopsy at its tip, which could be electrified. There were three major problems which made sterilization with this equipment unsatisfactory. The first was the incandescent light, which increased the risk of inadvertent intestinal burns. The second was the lack of an automatic constant pressure-flow gas system to maintain a good pneumoperitoneum and free the operator's hands for manipulation. The third, and most important problem, was the arrangement of the coagulation and cutting features of the instrument, which were located immediately below the optical system. Thus, as the instrument approached the target for coagulation, relationships were lost and only a close-up of the tissue could be seen. This clearly made the procedure a bold undertaking, as an error was possible when the tube was actually grasped. Nonetheless, tubal sterilization was feasible, though difficult, by laparoscopy.

Subsequent developments in laparoscopic equipment followed, and by 1960 fiberoptic, and quartz rod, cold light laparoscopes were available; and self-regulating pneumoperitoneum instruments were being refined. It also was becoming evident that the number of abdominal wall punctures did not add to the morbidity, and accessory instruments introduced at second and third sites significantly improved the operator's ability to see and manipulate tissues. With the accessory instruments introduced away from the optical instrument, the operator could continue to see relationships while performing various manipulations. The only minor problem remaining is monocular vision, for which correction can be made readily.

Dr. Patrick Steptoe modified Palmer's technique,[3,6] and began a large series of sterilizations in January, 1966. By December, 1967, he had performed 310 such procedures in Oldham, England. There were no serious complications. This is the largest sample of such cases to date and has been followed up for almost four years.

INDICATIONS

Women who fulfill the usual criteria for sterilization and who are beyond the puerperium are prospective candidates. Previous pelvic surgery is not necessarily a contraindication, but abdominal hernia, abdominal masses, and severe pulmonary disease are contraindications.

TECHNIQUE

The patient is admitted either the night before or the morning of surgery, having fasted since the previous midnight. A routine blood and urine study are made, and the abdomen and perineum are shaved and scrubbed. A rectal suppository is given. An enema generally is less satisfactory, for the restosigmoid often becomes distended, partially obscuring the view of the pelvis.

Nonpuerperal Sterilization by Laparoscopy

Anesthesia is either regional or nonexplosive gas administered by endotracheal tube. Palmer has used intravenous Pentothal,® and Barnes employed morphine with local anesthesia.

The position is dorsal lithotomy, with the hips at approximately 60 degrees and the table tilted to 20 degrees or 30 degrees Trendelenburgh. A negative electrode is placed under the patient. After an abdominal-perineal preparation, draping is applied so that the abdomen and perineum are in the same field. A bimanual examination is done. The patient is catheterized. A tenaculum is attached to the anterior lip of the cervix and a Jarcho cannula introduced into the cervical canal. This enables the surgeon to move the uterus readily from below.

Pneumoperitoneum is established by inserting a 16 gauge spring type needle (Fig. 11-1) with cannula into the abdomen at the midpoint of the lower margin of the umbilicus. Carbon dioxide is allowed to flow at no greater than 50 cm water pressure through the cannula to distend the abdomen. This may require about 4 liters of gas and take a few minutes.

Once the abdominal wall has been distended away from the intestines, the cannula is removed and a 1 cm transverse incision

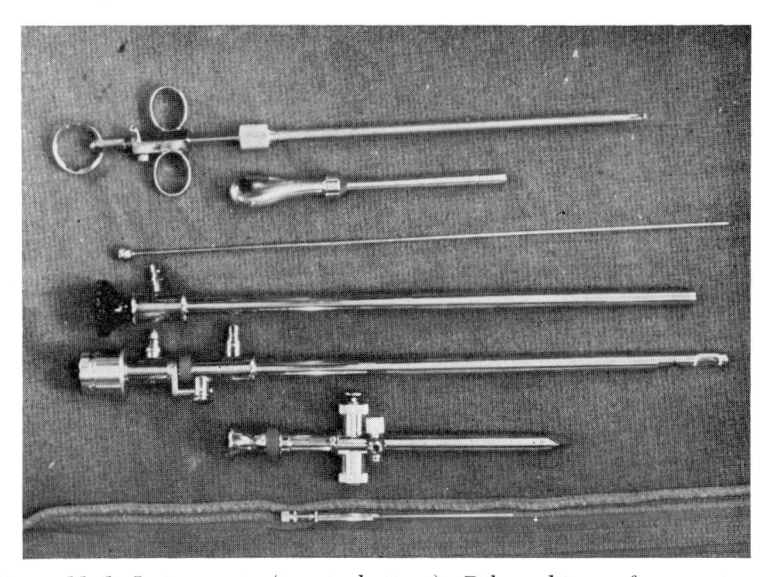

Figure 11-1. Instruments (top to bottom); Palmer biopsy forceps, trocar, probe, 180 degree laparoscope, photolaparoscope, trocar with cannula, insufflation needle.

is made at the lower margin of the umbilicus. An 8 mm sharp trocar and cannula are then introduced; the tip is aimed at the axis of the pelvic inlet. This avoids the risk of striking the great vessels at the sacral promontory.

With the large cannula in place, the gas tubing is attached to maintain the pneumoperitoneum by slow gas flow, and the laparoscope is inserted after removal of the trocar. Examination of the pelvic structures and lower abdominal parietal peritoneum is performed. A site is selected which is free of adhesions. Major abdominal wall vessels are visualized by transillumination of the right or left lower quadrants. The site should be at least 8 cm from the umbilicus. A 4 mm stab wound of the skin is made, and the trocar and cannula of the Palmer biopsy forceps is inserted. Next the biopsy forceps is introduced via the cannula.

Under visual control from the laparoscope, the biopsy forceps is used to mobilize the tube and identify it (Fig. 11-2). A point on the tube about 0.5 cm from the uterus is usually best for grasping. The area is lifted away from surrounding structures. Coagulating current is used to cauterize the tube slowly, in about 30 seconds (Figs. 11-3 and 11-4). Only the surgeon must control

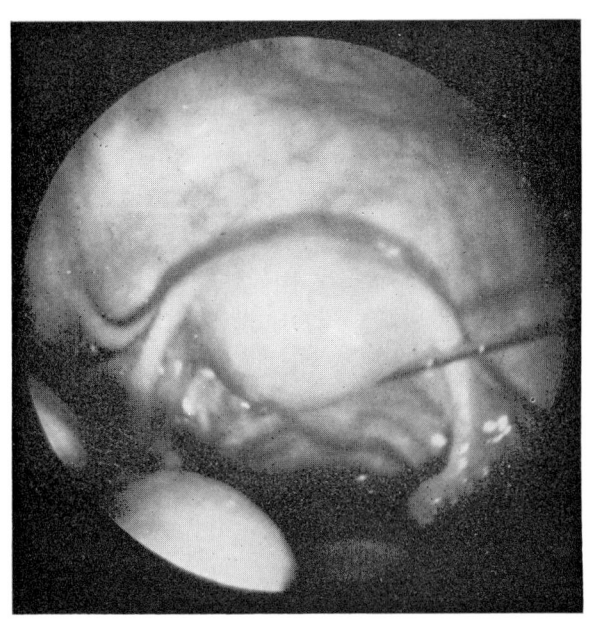

Figure 11-2. Identification of uterus, tubes, and round ligament.

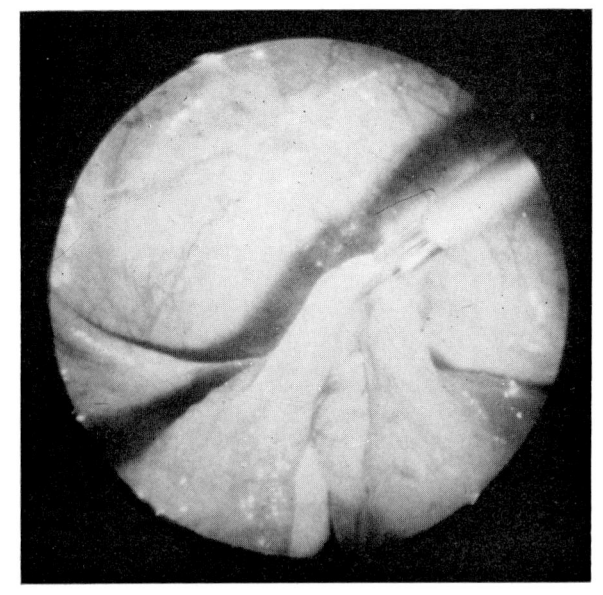

Figure 11-3. Pick-up of left tube.

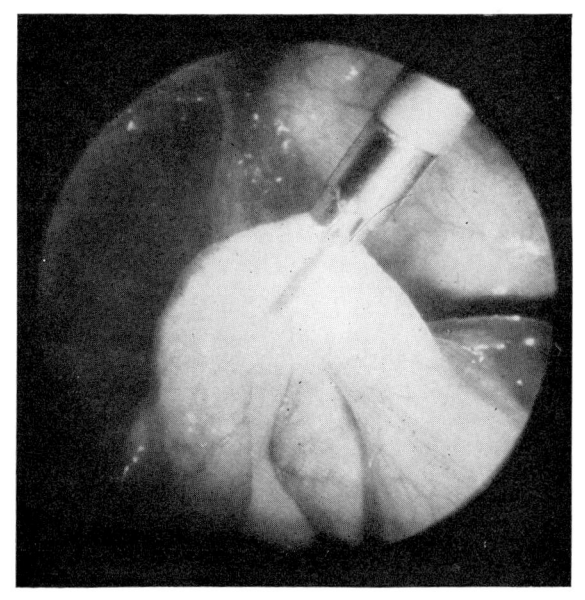

Figure 11-4. Close-up of coagulation.

the diathermy foot pedal. Once the area has turned white over a 2 cm length of tube, including the cornual position, coagulation is stopped. The tube is transected by unscrewing the boring cylinder of the Palmer biopsy forceps so that the sharp edges cut through the tube on either side of the place where it is being held by the teeth of the instrument (Fig. 11-5). The cuts should

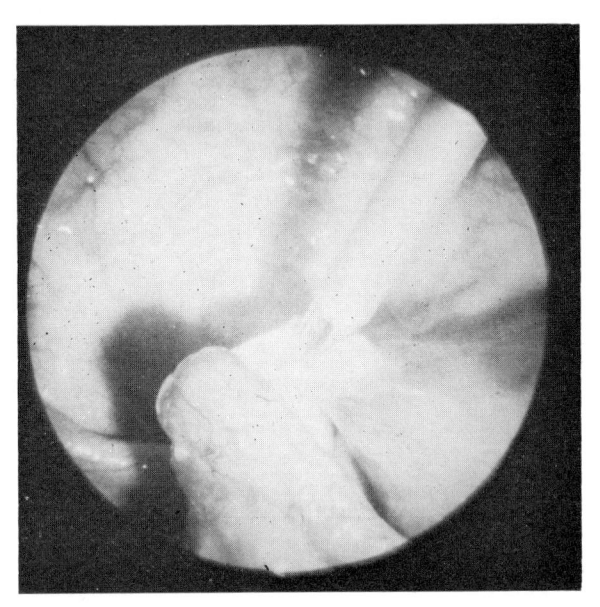

Figure 11-5. Close-up of transection left tube.

pass through the entire diameter of the tube at these points (Figs. 11-6 and 11-7). The boring cylinder is retracted by reversing rotation on the thread. The tube then can be released and recoagulated on each side of the transections. The isolated segment of tube can be removed by using cutting current. It is not advisable to pull it free; in practice it is rarely removed. The procedure is repeated on the contralateral side (Figs. 11-8,9 and 10). The instruments are then removed, and the gas allowed to escape. Clips or subcuticular catgut sutures can be used on the two small wounds. Strip adhesive dressings are applied.

Postoperatively, fluids or a soft diet may be given in the evening. Hospital discharge is usually on the following morning after

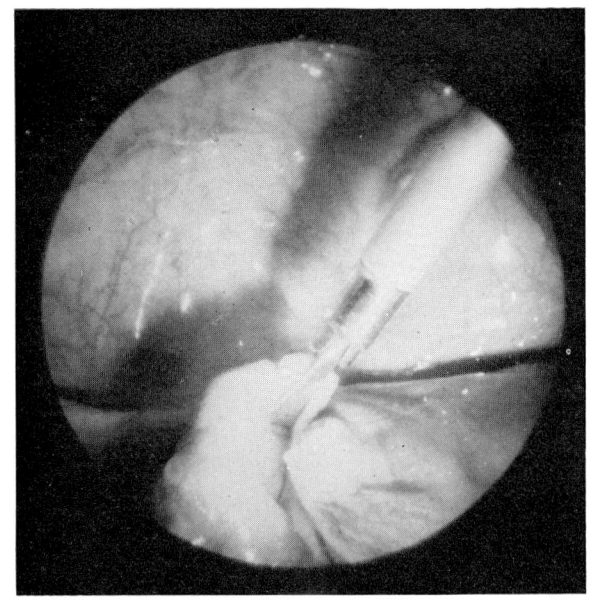

Figure 11-6. Tubal transection completed on left.

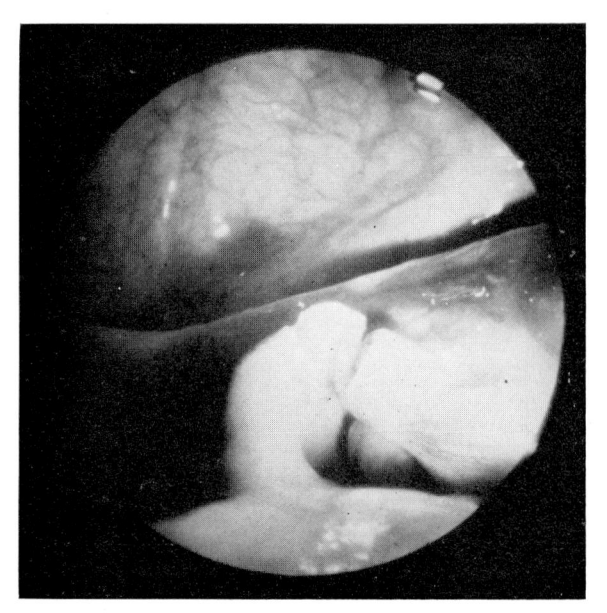

Figure 11-7. Removal of Palmer forceps from left tube.

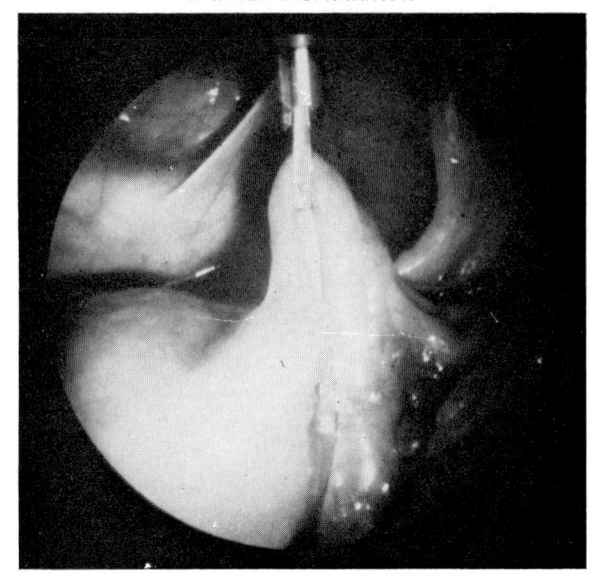

Figure 11-8. Pick-up right tube.

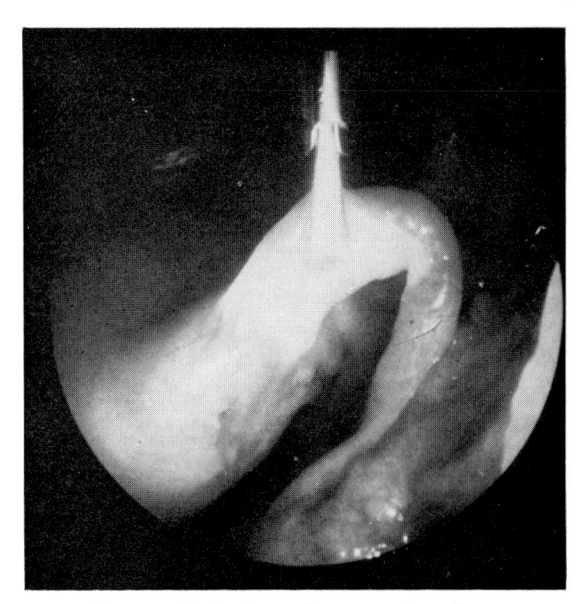

Figure 11-9. Coagulation right tube.

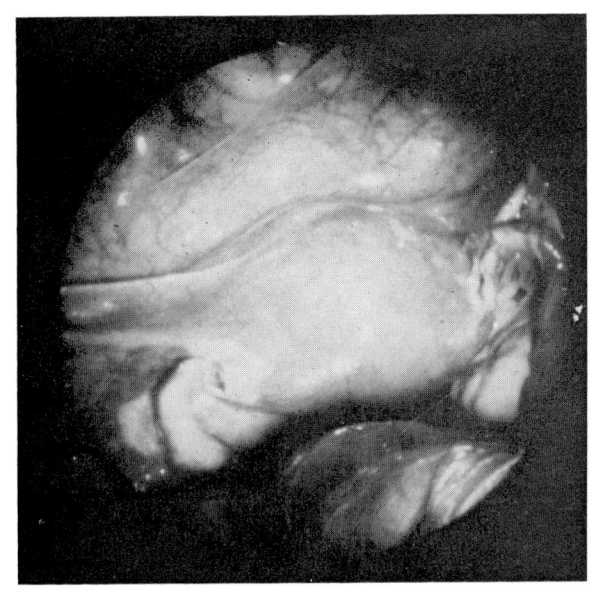

Figure 11-10. Uterus and both tubes following procedure.

breakfast. Darvon® or codeine might be required for the first twenty-four postoperative hours. All of the patients were back at their usual activities within one week or less. They have been followed up after six weeks, and a hysterogram was performed.

RESULTS

It is difficult to be certain, but there have probably been about 500 laparoscopic sterilizations done to date (Table 11-I). The largest group is Steptoe's 310 or more cases; he has had no serious

TABLE 11-I
COLLECTED EXPERIENCE WITH TUBAL STERILIZATION AT LAPAROSCOPY

	Cases	Pregnancy	Failure on Hysterogram
Behrman*	38	2 (cryosurgery)	0
Cohen*	60	0	1
Neuwirth	30	0	0
Palmer	50	0	0
Steptoe	310	1 ectopic 2 (cryosurgery)	0
Total	488	1	1

* Personal communication.

complications and reported one ectopic pregnancy in his group after about four years of follow-up. Palmer[2] reported about a year ago that he had done 50 cases since 1964 without failure or complications. Behrman reported 38 cases. He has used electrocautery as well as cryosurgery to produce tubal damage; there were two pregnancies in the cryosurgery group.

Other institutions using this technique include Michael Reese Hospital, Downstate Medical Center in New York, and the Johns Hopkins Hospital. Unfortunately, the exact results obtained by these groups is not available. Thus far, there appears to be only the one failure reported by Steptoe using the technique developed by Palmer and Steptoe.

The current sample consists of 30 cases and there have been neither complications nor failures in a period of just under two years. Two cases were done in connection with first trimester therapeutic abortion.

Operating time is usually about twenty minutes; postoperative hospital stays have not exceeded two nights, and are usually one night. Postoperative hysterograms have all shown tubal closure, with the exception of one case (Fig. 11–11). In this instance,

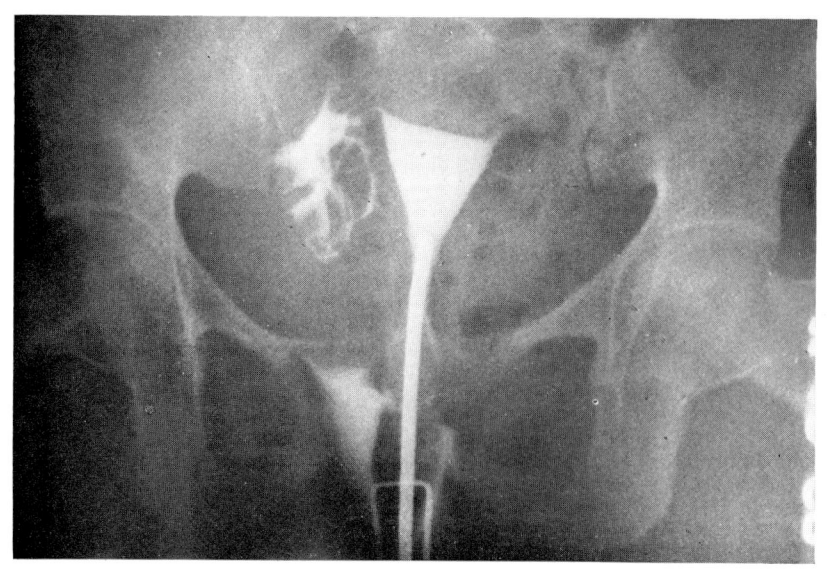

Figure 11–11. Tuboperitoneal fistula six weeks after procedure.

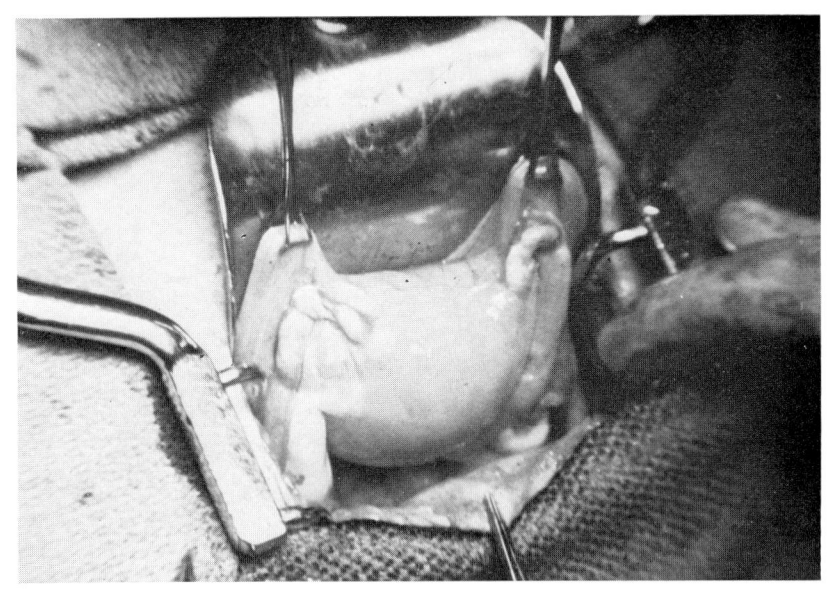

Figure 11-12. Gross appearance of the tubes six weeks after tubal coagulation and transection.

a tuboperitoneal fistula was demonstrated at the proximal stump of the tube; the fistula was confirmed at laparotomy and salpingectomy six weeks after sterilization (Fig. 11-12).

The pathologic data which have been collected show the initial microscopic findings are remarkably benign (Figs. 11-13 and 11-14). At six weeks there is necrosis and early fibrosis (Figs. 11-15 and 11-16). Steptoe has found complete fibrosis after three to six months.

CONCLUSIONS

The current data being accumulated from sterilizations at laparoscopy by electrocoagulation and transection indicate that it is a feasible procedure and not difficult to learn by an individual already trained in general surgery or gynecology. The cryosurgical variation of the technique does not seem to be as reliable, based on very limited data. This apparently is due to rapid recanalization. The equipment for cryosurgery is more expensive than electrocoagulation equipment.

The total experience is limited in numbers and in time. Not

112   *Human Sterilization*

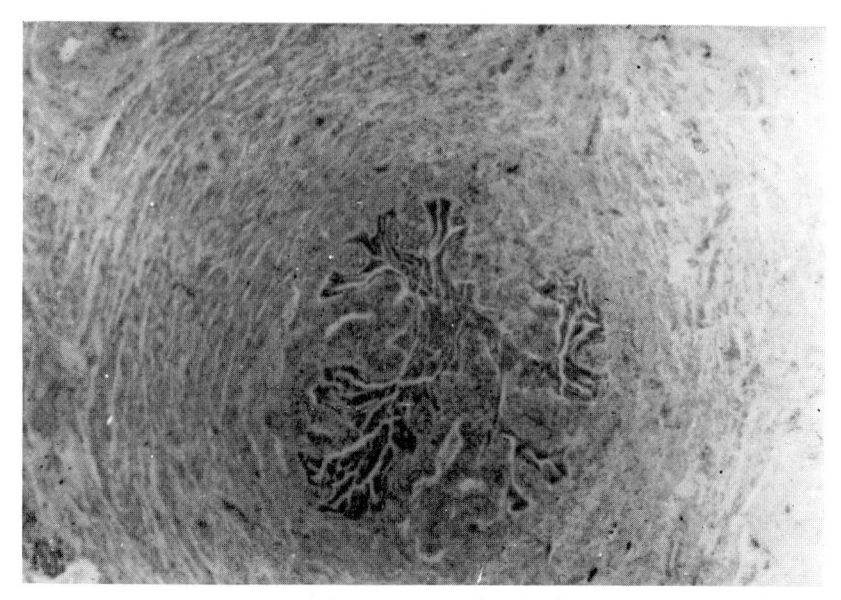

Figure 11-13. Low-power photomicrograph of tube removed immediately following coagulation and transection.

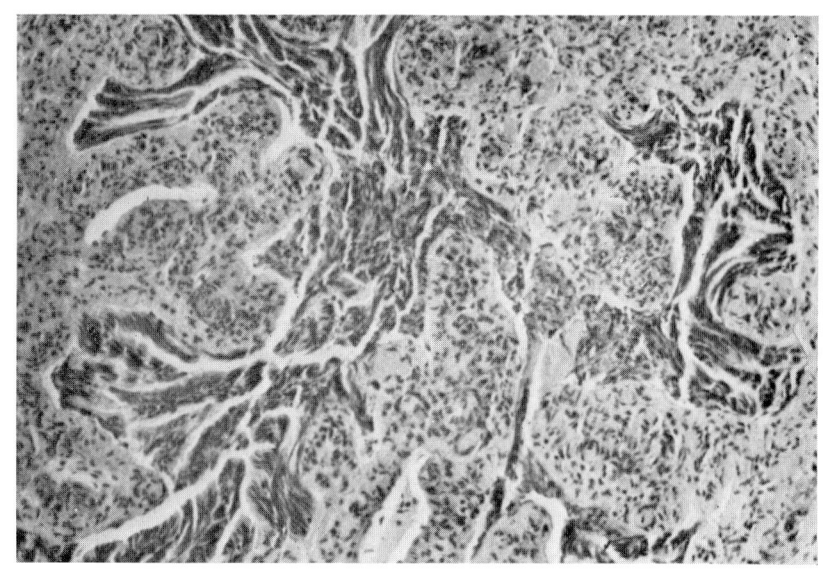

Figure 11-14. High-power view of specimen in Figure 11-13.

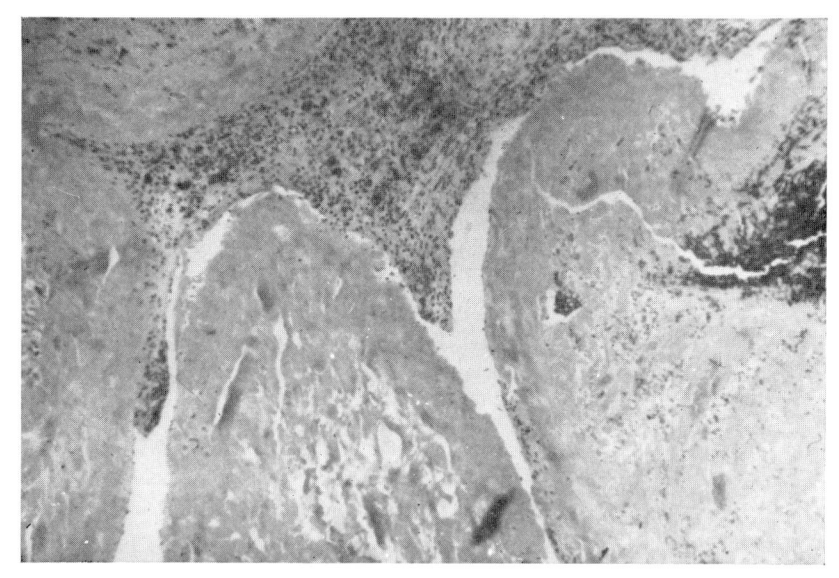

Figure 11-15. High-power photomicrograph of tube seen in Figure 11-12 showing necrosis and early fibrosis.

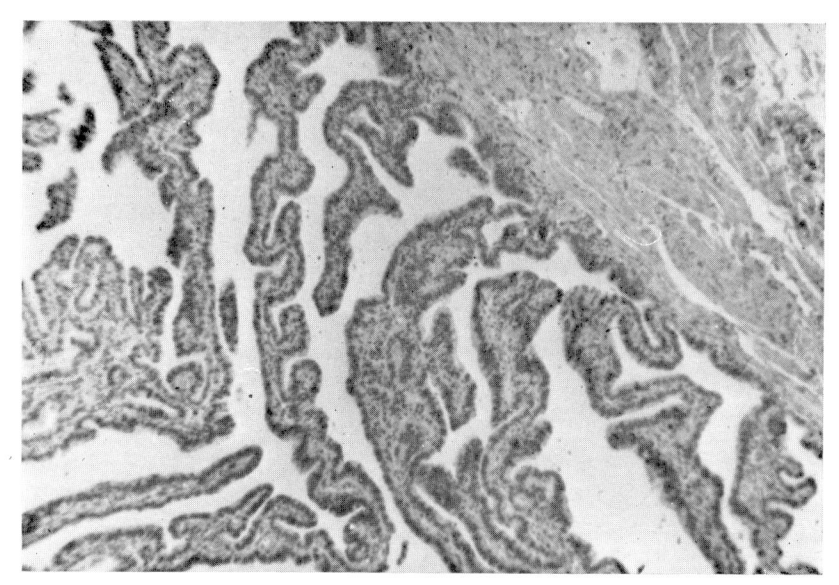

Figure 11-16. Appearance of adjacent normal tube seen in Figure 11-12.

more than eight years have passed since the first of this group of patients was sterilized. Yet the procedure holds distinct promise for certain situations where permanent sterilization is desired. It is relatively atraumatic usually permitting discharge from the hospital in twenty-four hours and return to activities in a week or less. It appears to be remarkably free of surgical complications and it seems to compare favorably in success rate to such procedures as the Pomeroy operation. If the success rate is truly comparable, then the advantage of a brief hospitalization time and rapid recovery for a nonpuerperal sterilization is clear. Furthermore, it is relatively easy to train personnel, especially after the technique of laparoscopy is accomplished.

The disadvantages are the cost of the equipment, approximately 1500 dollars minimum, and the need for an operating room. It is generally thought that the procedure should be done under general or regional anesthesia. However, Power and Barnes[4] performed the technique under sedation and local anesthesia in 1941. Virtually all groups currently employ general or regional anesthesia. It appears that the feasibility of using local anesthesia and heavy sedation for this procedure has not been really tested.

In the matter of large numbers of sterilizations, such a procedure is limited because of equipment costs, the need for an operating room and experienced, highly-trained personnel. Thus, as a mass technique it would be limited to situations where these factors are available. The ability to use sedation and local anesthesia, would make the procedure more widely applicable, however.

It is necessary to be cautious, although the results of this procedure are favorable in terms of low complication rates and apparently high success rates. However, these data have been obtained from medical centers with a particular interest in the operation. It is only lately that other hospitals are trying this technique; results of wider use may prove to be less encouraging. This, plus the relatively short-term experience with the procedure, forces a careful approach. At present, however, the operation appears to be used increasingly without difficulty, suggesting that its use may become even more widespread.

REFERENCES

1. Anderson, E.T.: Peritoneoscopy. *Amer J Surg, 35*:136, 1937.
2. Palmer, R.: Tubal Sterilization under Laparoscopy. Ford Foundation Meeting, Venice, May, 1966.
3. Palmer, R.: Essais de sterilisation tubaire coelioscopique par electro coagulation isthmique. *Bull Gynec et Obstet, 14*:298–301, 1962.
4. Power, F.H., and Barnes, H.C.: Sterilization by means of peritoneoscopic tubal fulguration. *Amer J Obstet Gynec, 41*:1038, 1941.
5. Steptoe, P.C.: Sterilization by Laparoscopic Techniques. Sixth World Congress on Fertility and Sterility, May, 1968.
6. Steptoe, P.C.: *Laparoscopy in Gynecology.* London, Livingston, 1968.

Chapter 12

OVIDUCT ANASTOMOSIS PROCEDURES

Celso-Ramon Garcia

It is understood that techniques considered are proposed to reverse the previously intended or desired sterility. It is also assumed that the patients' general health (which includes physical, mental, and social well-being) is such that a reversal of the sterile state is desirable. Moreover, it is essential that the ovulatory, endometrial, and insemination factors (including coital habits) are such as to permit a realistic prognostic view of fertility restoration.

Review of the adnexa by culdoscopy or laparoscopy is highly desirable to assess the extent of the previous sterilizing procedure and the condition of these structures, since an unconstrained adnexa is also an important factor in the prognosis of sterility restoration.

Tubal sterilization (Fig. 12-1) usually involves the resection of a small midsegment of the oviduct; some surgeons prefer to bury the excised fimbria beneath the peritoneum. On occasion, fimbrial burial between the leaves of the mesosalpinx or anteriorly in the bladder flap; fimbrial resection; and even total salpingectomy is encountered. Moreover, depending primarily on the care and skill of the surgeon, among other factors, periadnexal adhesions of varying degree can occur. These may contribute substantially to a decreased restorative prognosis and in some instances might reasonably deter the surgeon from attempting tubal reconstruction, for example, in cases of severe dense periadnexal[1] adhesions.

Reviews of the literature usually present any and all procedures carried out on the fallopian tubes without regard to either degree or type of pathology or to the site of obstruction, if any exists. The analyses usually present an overall pregnancy rate, without a breakdown of specific procedures, and without indicating the outcome of the pregnancy. Obviously, the oviduct damaged by

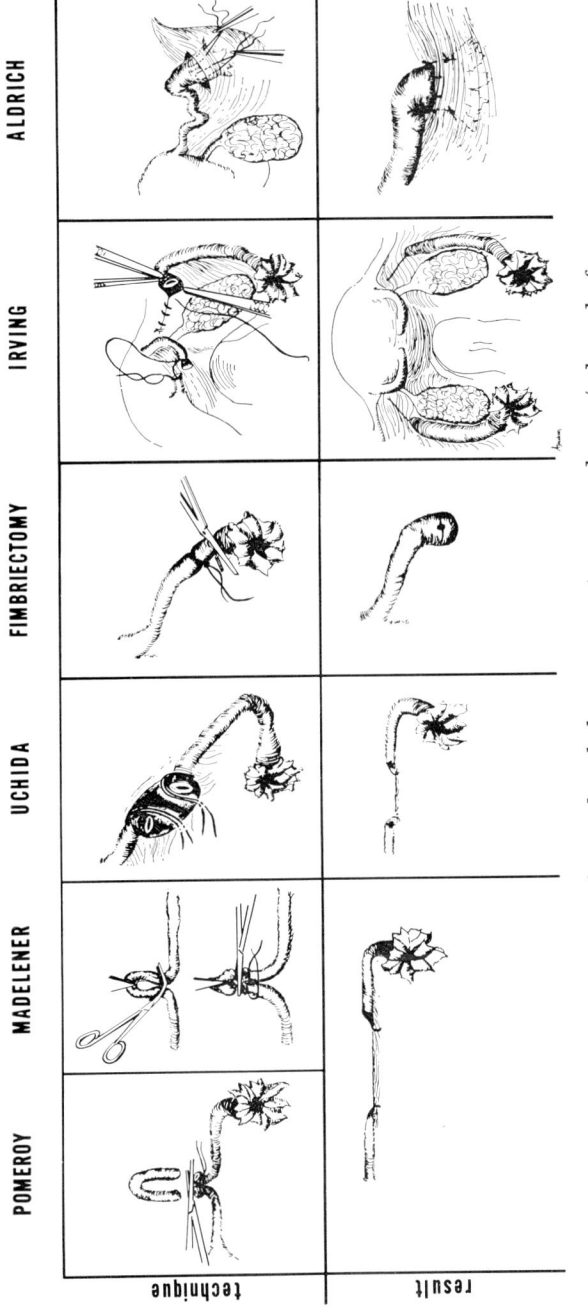

Figure 12-1. Surgical tubal contraceptive procedure (adapted from Kroener, W.F., Jr.: Surgical Sterilization by Fimbriectomy. *Amer J Obstet Gynec, 104:247*, 1969).

trauma will be affected less than that altered by severe infection. This is shown dramatically in the extreme case of the hydrosalpinx, where mucosal destruction produces alterations in secretory activity, and fibrous replacement of the muscularis produces potential derangement in tubal motility.[6] It is conceivable that patients could have suffered varying degrees of such pathology without tubal occlusion prior to, but more likely following, the tubal ligation. Nonetheless, most women seeking tubal ligation can be expected to have normal tubal function, since they are seeking a means to prevent further fertility.

The number of women who desire reversal of tubectomy in our society is usually small. They usually have remarried, lost children, or have religious or other regrets. When screened for the above contraindications, the number of ideal candidates is even smaller. In many cases the patients age or health contraindicate such procedures.

TECHNIQUES

Among the techniques proposed or used to reverse previously produced female sterility are the following: hydrotubation; end-to-end anastomosis; uterotubal implantation; the snorkel procedure; and substitute and bypass procedures.

HYDROTUBATION

Although hydrotubation has been recommended for tubal occlusion reversal, the potential hazards of its use and its general lack of success limit the usefulness of the procedure. This is particularly so when the proximal segment of the ligated tube is short and its wall is thick.

END-TO-END ANASTOMOSIS

Resection of the occluded ends and their anastomosis, with or without polyethylene splinting, have been advocated for restoring tubal patency. Table 12-I shows the results obtained from the literature of the past ten years. While the data are by no means complete, they show the paucity of reported experi-

TABLE 12-I
END-TO-END ANASTOMOSIS (1959–1969)

Author	Number of Cases	Number Patent	Number Pregnant	Percent Pregnant
Mutch (17)	4	4	4	100
Palmer (19)	31	—	0	0
Hanton (11)	2	2	1†	50
Hayashi (12)	6	—	4	66.7
Garcia (8)	4	3	0	0
Crane and Woodruff (3)	8	—	3	37.4
Siegler (25)	7	—	2	28.6
Total	62	—	14	22.5
	31*	—	14*	45*

* Based only on the smaller series, with Palmer's larger series eliminated.
† Aborted.

ences with this approach. Simple approximation and mucosal regeneration over polyethylene was carried out in the monkey by Castallo and Wainer.[2] In humans there is disparity of opinion regarding the need for splinting of the anastomosed area. If the lumina that are to be approximated are of similar diameter, patency restoration can be anticipated to a greater extent. However, if the resected segment is extensive, interference with muscular activity and possible secretory function may further complicate the successful fertility restoration, even though patency may have been restored. Of course, when a longer segment of oviduct is resected, the disparity in diameters and the wall thicknesses of the segments to be reunited will vary considerably, (Fig. 12–2).

Attempts to reunite oviducts by side-to-side approximation of small windows opened in the lateral walls of both segments are generally unsuccessful. When there is a disparity between the distal, larger segment and the thicker proximal segment with a smaller lumen, the following procedure is recommended. Excise the scarred end sharply at right angles to the lumen of the distal segment; excise the scarred, occluded end of the proximal oviduct with an oblique incision to develop scar-free luminal openings compatible in diameter.

Most descriptions of reanastomoses describe the use of several simple interrupted approximating sutures penetrating all layers of the wall of each segment of the tube. It probably is better to utilize an everting stitch, which eliminates the need for poly-

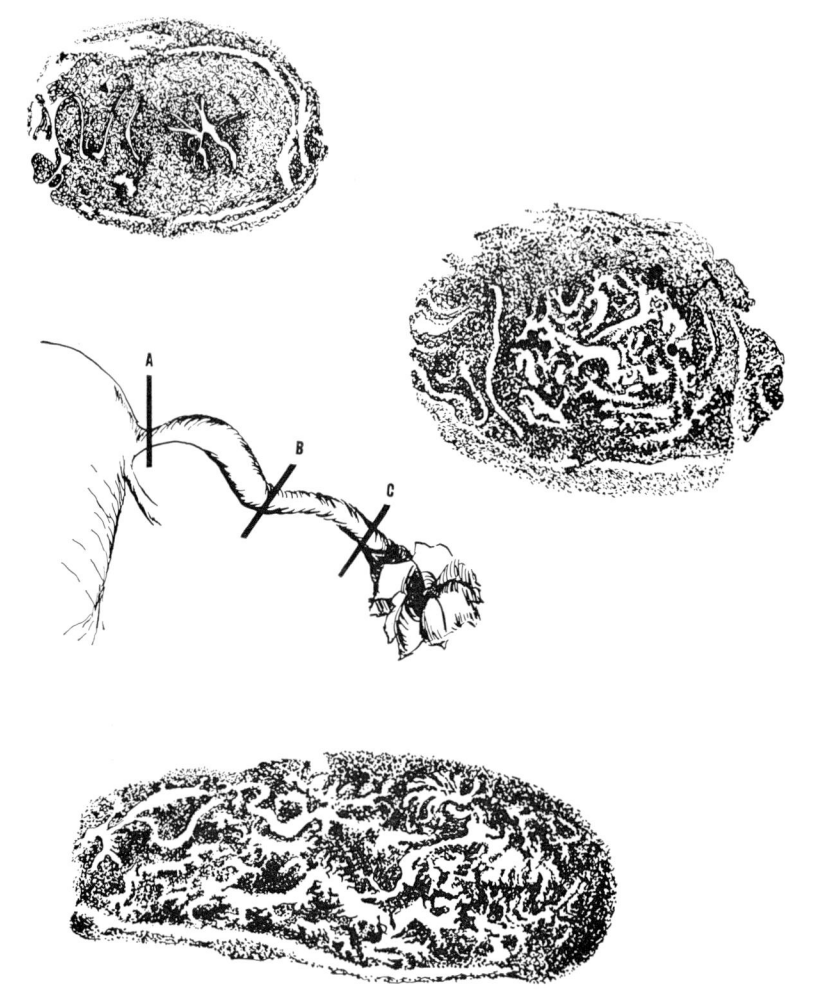

Figure 12–2. Cross-sections of the fallopian tube (adapted from Behrman, S.J., and Gosling, J.R.: *Fundamentals of Gynecology*, 2nd ed. New York, Oxford, 1960, p. 27).

ethylene splinting. Absorbable and silk sutures should be avoided. Nonabsorbable synethetic fibers of narrow caliber (e.g. #8–0 nylon) are most desirable. Certainly, if a splint is used, there is no justification in threading it through the uterotubal junction into the uterine cavity. Not only is the intramural lumen exceedingly narrow, but it is convoluted and kinked.[13] It is this narrow tortuosity which prevents luminal passage of a probe. The superimposed luminal shadow at the time of radiographic evaluation appears straighter and wider than is actually the case. The use of intrauterine installation of indigocarmine saline, either transcervically or, preferably, transfundally, while occluding the cervical uterine junction with the aid of the Buxton or the Dartique clamp better delineates the lumen.

Following the reported use of a microsurgical reconstructive technique in a patient by Platt,[21] the author and his colleagues acquired experience in the rabbit,[4,5] and subsequently applied these techniques to four women over the past twenty months. The results of these anastomoses are not included in Table 12-I. However, the first of these microsurgical procedures was succesful; a bilateral reanastomosis restored fertility and the women had a term, live female infant. The second patient has not become pregnant, but restoration of patency was demonstrated by hysterosalpingography six months postoperatively. The other two cases have not had a long enough follow-up to justify radiographic evaluation.

The microsurgical approach permits easier identification of the mucosa, the muscularis, and the visceral peritoneal layers. After approximation of the mesosalpinx with a holding suture, the scarred portions are excised and the luminal diameters made approximately equal in size. The endosalpinx is everted with four interrupted everting #6–0 nylon (monofilament) sutures placed in the muscularis (Fig. 12–3). The visceral peritoneal edges are inverted for peritonization. Once the sutures are placed, the probe is removed and the sutures tied. Placement of each suture is done under direct visualization with the operating microscope. The sustained patency with continuity across the line of anastomosis is tested with indigocarmine instilled transfundally while the cervicouterine junction is occluded with a Buxton clamp. It is too soon to assess the advisibility of this approach, but the meticulous layer-to-layer approximation has theoretical appeal and may eliminate the need for a residual splint.

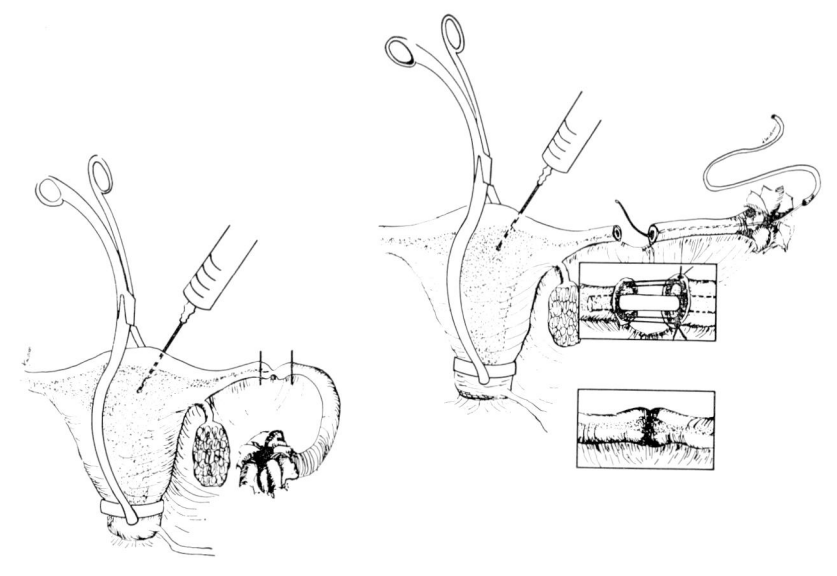

Figure 12-3. Tubal reanastomosis.

UTEROTUBAL IMPLANTATION

Uterotubal implantation techniques have been used to reanastomose the distal segment of the previously ligated oviduct to the uterine cavity. Unfortunately, it is not clear from the literature which of the cases reported were carried out following ligation or for occlusion secondary to congenital, traumatic, infectious, or spasmotic etiology. Table 12-II lists representative results reported during the past ten years. Moreover, it does not appear particularly pertinent whether cornual resection and implantation is carried out with direct approximation of endosalpinx to endometrium (Figs. 12-4 and 12-6a) or whether the Corkborer technique (Fig. 12-5) is used and the oviduct implanted blindly (Fig. 12-6b). Further, there is controversy regarding the use of a splint after implantation.[120] It seems odd that there are so little differences in end-results with so many variations in technique. It should also be pointed out that the pregnancy results include relatively high abortion and ectopic rates. In some experiences, the only conceptions reported were tubal pregnancies!

TABLE 12-II
IMPLANTATIONS (1959–1969)

Author	Number of Cases	Percent Patent	Number Pregnant	Percent Pregnant
Gallegos (7)	22	45.5	2	10.0
Mazziotta-Maribal (15)	6	—	1	16.7
Vara (27)				
(With Polyethylene)	33	—	6	18.0
(Without Polyethylene)	27	—	7	26.0
Green-Armytage (9)	50	—	23	46.0
Guerrero (10)	48	—	6	12.5
Moore-White (16)	16	41.2	9	56.3
Palmer (19)	108	—	39	36.0
Pous-Puigmacia (22)	726	—	196	27.0
Shirodkar (24)	140	90.0	49	35.0
Snaith (26)	30	—	3	10.0
Hanton (11)	22	45.4	10	45.5
Peel (20)	27	—	6	22.0
Botella-Llusia (1)	33	—	4	12.0
Hayashi (11)	45	—	7	15.6
Garcia (8)	14	57.1	2	14.3
Crane & Woodruff (3)	18	—	4	22.2
Siegler (25)	12	—	10	83.3
O'Brien, et al. (18)	36	88.8	16	43.3
Total	1,433	—	402	28.0

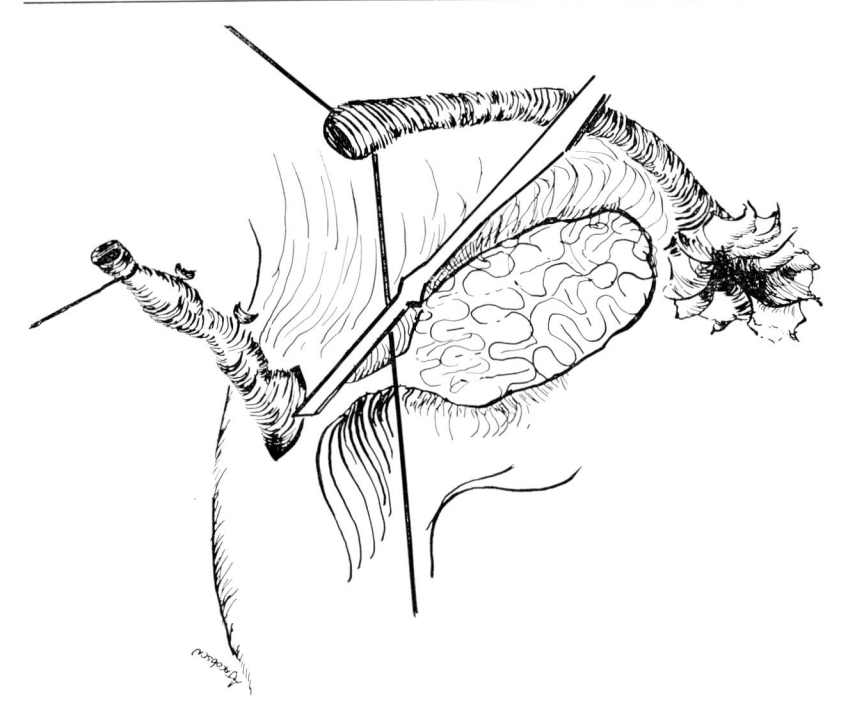

Figure 12–4. Uterotubal implantation: Scalpel resection technique.

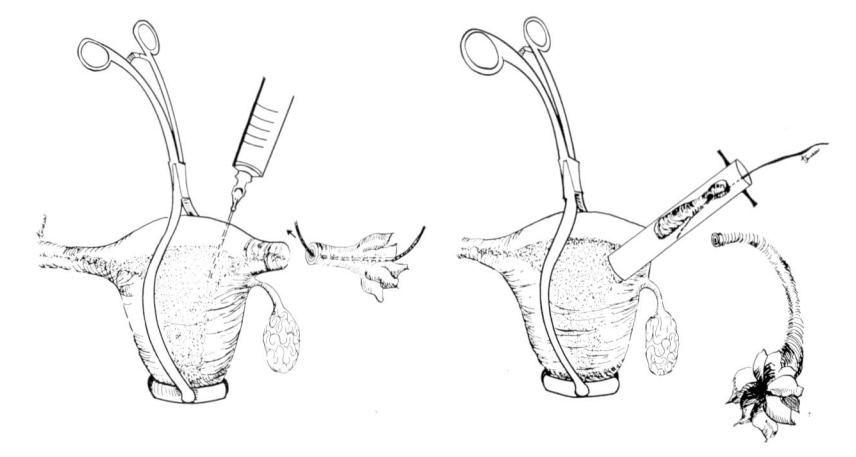

Figure 12–5. Uterotubal implantation: Cork-borer resection technique.

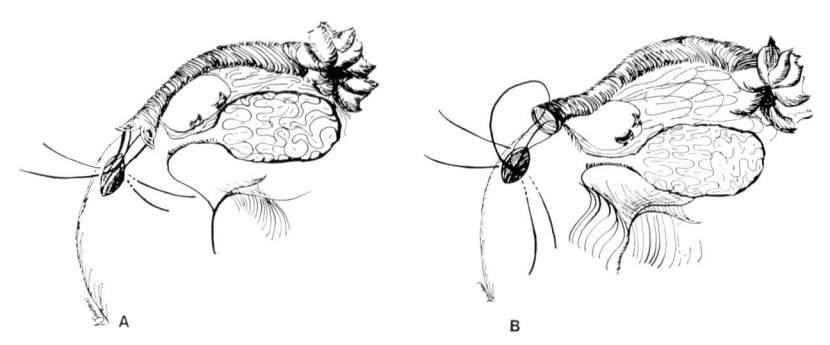

Figure 12–6. Uterotubal implantation: a) bivalve of oviduct with endosalpinx to endometrium; b) simple direct implantation of oviduct.

SNORKEL PROCEDURE

This technique is used when the distal segment of the oviduct has been resected. The visceral peritoneum is dissected off the distal 2 cm of the oviduct, which is then opened and folded back on the raw surface; this should permit the flap to adhere better after its edges are sutured to the peritoneal edge. Maintenance of patency is less than satisfactory, and pregnancy outlook is even less impressive. It seems that once the distal end of the oviduct is excised, there is little chance of restoring fertility.

SUBSTITUTE AND BYPASS PROCEDURES

Substitutes of ileal grafts, peritoneal tubes, vermiform appendices, blood vessels, plastic ovisacs, and intra-uterine relocation of the ovary (Fig. 12-7) have been so singularly unsatisfying, that their use cannot be justified. Transplantation of the human oviduct has been unsuccessful.[23] It is unlikely that these approaches will be utilized in the immediate future, since much needs to be done to improve microsurgical as well as immunosuppressive techniques.

COMMENTS AND CONCLUSIONS

At this time it seems that end-to-end anastomosis holds the greatest promise of restoring fertility in women who have had prior tubal ligation. Yet at times it is difficult to decide whether it is wise to accept the challenge to reverse the tubal occlusion that was previously meant to be permanent. One of our colleagues[14] performed a reanastomosis on a woman who had had a tubal ligation because of severe mitral stenosis. Following a successful commissurotomy, the patient's cardiac function was apparently restored to normal. The woman then sought fertility restoration. This was reestablished, and she was delivered of one live normal infant at term. She subsequently became pregnant again, went into congestive heart failure at seven months and died.

A happier note is struck in the case of a forty year old woman who had a tubal ligation for social reasons after her fifth pregnancy. She remarried and found it emotionally important to have a restoration of her fertility. This patient was the first to volunteer to have the microsurgical techniques applied at the Hospital of the University of Pennsylvania. She was delivered of a normal term infant some fifteen months postreanastomosis.

Recently we have been asked to consider reestablishing tubal patency in a forty-five year old woman who finds it emotionally important not to end her potentially reproductive years in an infertile state. She had a tubal ligation following her sixth pregnancy about fourteen years ago. The justification for attempting a reanastomosis procedure under such circumstances is less than

126 *Human Sterilization*

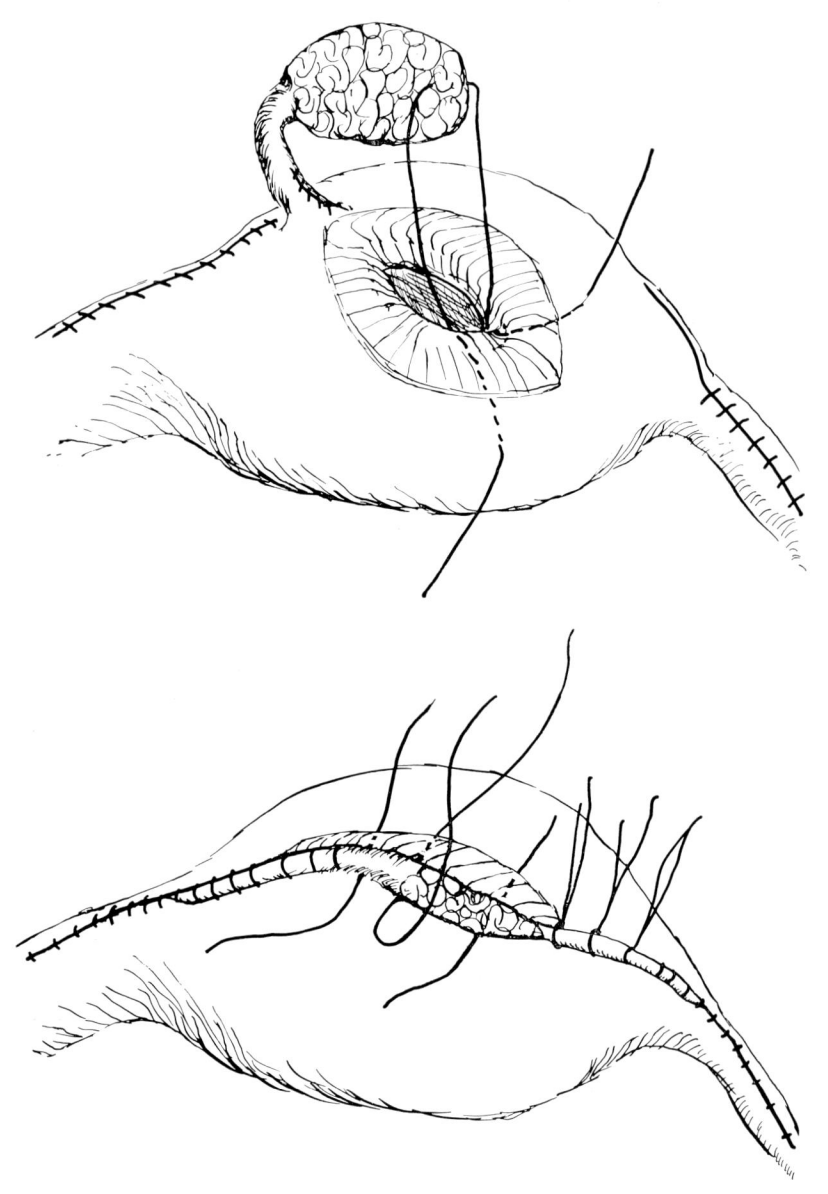

Figure 12–7. Intra-uterine relocation of ovary (the so-called *Estes* procedure).

compelling. While the surgical exercise may be acceptable to the patient, the enthusiasm of the surgeon should be tempered by his evaluation of the total circumstances surrounding the case. Special attention should be paid to the general health and the supportive potential fertility of the woman.

It must be reemphasized that the experience of individual surgeons is limited and the proposed techniques are quite variable. More meticulous and delicate approaches to tissue handling, fine sutures and their placement, as well as the careful selection of subjects without periadnexal involvement and with minimal tubal resection, theoretically should yield better results. In performing a tubal ligation the surgeon should use a technique which would interrupt the oviduct and resect a *minimal segment* of the fallopian tube. Certainly, this, and the preservation of the distal or fimbrial end of the tube are essential, if tubal ligation is to be considered reversible.

REFERENCES

1. Botella-Lluisia, J. In Botello-Llusia, J., Caballero-Gardo, J.A., Clavero-Nunez, S.A., and Vilar-Dominquez, E. (Eds.): *Esterilidad y Infertilidad Humana.* Barcelona, Editorial Ceintifico-Medica, 1967, pp. 401–403.
2. Castallo, M.A., Stack, J.M., and Wainer, A.: Experimental recanalization of the fallopian tubes in the Macacus rhesus monkey. *Fertil Steril,* 1:435–442, 1950.
3. Crane, M., and Woodruff, J.D.: Factors influencing the success of tuboplastic procedures. *Fertil Steril,* 19:810–820, 1968.
4. David, A., Brackett, B.G., and Garcia, C.R.: Effects of microsurgical removal of the rabbit uterotubal junction. *Fertil Steril,* 20:250–257, 1969.
5. David, A., Brackett, B.G., Garcia, C.R., and Mastroianni, L.: Composition of rabbit oviduct fluid in ligated segments of the fallopian tube. *J Reprod Fertil,* 19:285–289, 1969.
6. David, A., Garcia, C.R., and Czernobilsky, B.: Human hydrosalpinx. *Amer J Obstet Gynec,* 105:400–411, 1969.
7. Gallegos, D.A.: Cirugia conservadora de las trompas de fallopia. *Rev Esp Obstet Ginec,* 19:193, 1959.
8. Garcia, C.R.: Surgical reconstruction of the oviduct in the infertile patient. In Behrman, S.J., and Kister, R.W. (Eds.): *Progress in Infertility.* Boston, Little, Brown, 1969, pp. 255–272.

9. Green-Armytage, V.B.: Discussion on the etiology and treatment of cornual occlusion of the tubes. *Proc R Soc Med, 48*:87, 1960.
10. Guerrero, C.D.: in Pous-Puigmacia, L.: Estudio y criticia de la cirugia tubarica. Neuva revision mundial del problema. *Rev Esp Obstet Ginec, 19*:310, 1960.
11. Hanton, E.M., Pratt, J.H., and Banner, E.A.: Tubal plastic surgery at the Mayo Clinic. *Amer J Obstet Gynec, 89*:934, 1964.
12. Hayashi, M.: Tubal factor in sterility. Proceedings of the Third Asiatic Congress of Obstetrics and Gynecology, Manilla, Phillipines, *Assoc Fed of Obs & Gyn,* January, 1965, p. 361, 1965.
13. Harnstein, A., and Neustadt, B.: Uber den Intranuralen tubenteil. *Z Geburstch Gynal, 88*:431, 1924.
14. Kroener, W.F., Jr.: Surgical sterilization by fimbriectomy. *Amer J Obstet Gynec, 104*:247, 1969.
15. Mastrioanni, L.M.: Personal communication.
16. Mazziotta-Mirbal, R.L.: Tratomicuto quirurgico de la esterilidad par obstruccion tubarica. *Rev Esp Obstet Ginec, 19*:215, 1959.
17. Moore-White, M.: Evaluation of tubal plastic operations. *Int J Fertil, 5*:237, 1960.
18. Mutch, M.G.J.: Sterility and tuboplasties: Critical analysis of 42 cases. *Fertil Steril, 10*:240, 1959.
19. O'Brien, J.R., Arronet, G., and Eduljee, S.Y.: Operative treatment of fallopian tube pathology in human fertility. *Amer J Obstet Gynec, 103*:520, 1969.
20. Palmer, R.: Salpingostomy—a critical study of 396 personal cases operated upon without polyethylene tubing. *Proc Roy Soc Med, 53*: 357, 1960.
21. Peel, J.: Uterotubal implantation. *Proc Roy Soc Med, 57*:710, 1964.
22. Platt, M.: in Smith, J.W.: Microsurgery: review of the literature and discussion of microtechniques. *Plast Reconst Surg, 37*:240, 1966.
23. Pous-Puigmacia, L.: Estudio y critica de la cirurgie tubarica, neuva revision mudial del problema. *Rev Esp Obstet Ginec, 19*:299, 1960.
24. Ritala, A.M.: Tubentransplantation bei sterilitat in der frau verursacht druch occlusia tubae. *Acta Obstet Gynec Scand, 25*:493, 1946.
25. Shirodkar, V.N.: *Contributions to Obstetrics and Gynecology.* London, Livingston, 1960, p. 65.
26. Siegler, A.M.: Salpingoplasty: Classification and report of 115 operations. *Ostet Gynec, 34*:339–344, 1969.
27. Snaith, L.M.: in Chiara, A. (Ed.): *Studi Sulla Sterilita.* Turin, Minerva Medica, Torino, Italy, 1961, p. 53.
28. Vara, P.: Ergebnisse und erfahrunger bei operatives behandlung der sterilitat. *Gynecologia (Basel), 147*:445, 1959.

DISCUSSION: PERMANENT STERILIZATION

Ralph M. Richart, *Moderator*

Dr. Richart asked for discussion of Dr. Lee's presentation on an improved vasectomy technique.

Dr. Garcia inquired if it were possible to try a second reanastomosis if the first one failed.

Dr. Lee said that he had done this three times in the same case.

Dr. Garcia wanted to know if all three attempts failed, while Dr. Richart wanted to know the degree of success with the new reanastomosis.

Dr. Lee replied that he could remember procedures which had failed, but after reoperation, success was achieved and pregnancy followed.

Dr. Schmidt suggested that one reason for the failure of a second procedure was the fact that the epididymis might have been massaged vigorously at the time of the first operation. This is done in hope of expressing fluid-containing sperm; unfortunately, the tubules of the epididymis break very easily. He said that in some cases he had performed unsuccessful surgery when seminal fluid with sperm was in the vas. Then, upon a second attempt, he had found a dry vas with no sperm. He also has opened the tunica vaginalis and has seen dilated tubules in the epididymal head with empty tubules below it. It was his opinion that there was no reason that a second attempt should not work even if this were not done.

Dr. Moon inquired if there were any pus or inflammation with the use of 5 cc of 0.1% spermicidal solution.

Dr. Lee explained that a very dilute solution of potassium permanganate was used as the spermicide. There was some difficulty when the solution was used, for a small number of patients complained of some sort of discomfort. He saw no inflammation or complications with his lavage technique, but could not speculate on the possibility of chemical inflammation.

Dr. Moon objected to the possibility of tissue damage with the potassium permanganate solution. He agreed that lavage was a good technique, but he would not do it with that solution for fear of the side effects. He said it was possible to get inflammation in the seminal vesicles or in the prostate.

Dr. Chez wanted to know how many ejaculations were required to exhaust the sperm reservoir.

Dr. Lee said that after six ejaculations no precautions to prevent conception should be necessary. He had seen many cases where the reservoirs were almost empty after three ejaculations, and that after five ejaculations, except in two cases, there were almost no sperm in the ampulla.

Dr. Chez speculated that if there were a hundred million sperm per cubic centimeter of seminal fluid, he wondered how many ejaculations it would take to reduce the sperm count to low levels. He wanted to know if the percentage of sperm dropped with successive ejaculations.

Dr. Lee conceded that there was an abrupt drop, and then the sperm count continued to be small. But he emphasized that the remaining sperm could still be responsible for impregnation.

Dr. Pai agreed that the semen did not show sperm after six ejaculations.

To return to a discussion of the midline technique, he had heard both positive and negative opinions concerning the procedure. Opposition to the midline incision is based on the following: it is effectively a blind procedure; the septum is a possible site of tumor origin, and trouble may arise if the surgeon is not extremely skillful; also, the midline incision may be in such a position in relation to the vas that future reanastomosis may be impossible. A bilateral incision, where the straight ends of the vas are definitely caught, may be a much better procedure if reanastomosis is being considered. He is of the opinion that in a mass procedure, either tubal ligation or vasectomy, a simple technique which is implementable on a large scale, is desirable. The midline incision is not as simple as the bilateral technique. Therefore, in a mass program, where surgeons may not always be trained in urology, the simpler technique is the more desirable one. It was his opinion that complications arising from vasectomy were more frequent with the midline technique than they were with the bilateral technique. He requested Dr. Lee's opinion on this matter.

Dr. Lee said that he preferred the midline technique because a simple procedure minimized complications, a single incision was better than two, and it was better for a patient to have the smaller incision of the midline technique. In Korea, about two-thirds of the vasectomies done since 1965 have been performed with the midline technique.

Dr. Richart presented Dr. Schmidt's paper on vas reanastomosis procedures for discussion.

Dr. Hulka wanted to know the fate of the endosplint: did it remain *in situ* or did it migrate eventually?

Dr. Schmidt explained that polyethylene endosplints migrated sometimes, but the Silastic splints apparently remained in position. He felt that migration did not matter as long as the lumen remained open, but explained that the procedure is new and chances to reoperate have been few.

Dr. Hulka inquired over what period the endosplints had been observed for migration.

Dr. Schmidt explained that he had followed up for about two years.

Dr. Tietze wanted to know how one could differentiate between a successful vasectomy in which the sperm had not disappeared from the semen as yet and an unsuccessful surgical procedure.

Dr. Schmidt explained that in the spontaneous reanastomosis cases he had seen, the sperm count in the ejaculate decreased sharply, until only a few were left. The next semen sample showed a higher sperm count, and finally the sperm count returned to normal.

Dr. Schmidt said that he thought a major mistake in vasectomy was that the average technique involved ligating the vas. Surgeons are trained to ligate blood vessels, and blood vessels will thrombose back to the nearest branch; the vas, however, remains patent up to the point of the obstruction. He suggested that the vas should be fulgurized with an electric needle rather than being ligated. The needle electrode should be inserted into the vas for about 2–3 mm; it should destroy the mucosa and the submucosa; and then it should be drawn out to destroy the cut end of the vas. This technique results in fewer spermatic granulomas than the ligature technique. The next point in manipulation is to close the fascial sheath of the vas over one end and put a physical barrier over the cut end of the vas. Spermatic granulomata will not cross a fascial barrier. The suture should be placed fairly closely to the end of the vas.

Dr. Richart opened the discussion on culdoscopy and laparoscopy.

Dr. Neuwirth thought that local anesthesia might be an aid to laparoscopy.

Dr. Cohen said that such procedures could be done with local anesthesia plus Innovar®. Innovar is a combination of a morphine-like substance and a major tranquilizer; it has been used chiefly for otolaryngology. He said he did not think that Innovar itself had to be used, but that any narcotic-tranquilizer could be employed in addition to the local anesthetic. This also depends on the patient, for all patients are not receptive to local anesthesia.

Dr. Hulka said that they had been trying to introduce larparoscopy into the residency program in North Carolina, but that the resident staff had recently discovered vaginal tubal ligation. He asked about a comparison of vaginal tubal ligation through a posterior colpotomy with laparoscopy in terms of time, equipment, and procedure.

Dr. Neuwirth admitted that laparoscopic equipment costs are higher, but felt that the patient's hospital stay is shorter. Tubal ligation patients usually are not discharged from the hospital after one day—perhaps this is due to tradition—but tubal ligation patients do not seem to be as energetic postoperatively as laparoscopy patients. The key to a comparison of the two techniques is how well the surgeon can perform, and how little trauma the patient must undergo for the purpose of the surgery to be achieved. He stated that a larparoscopic approach produced more diagnostic knowledge and permitted more therapeutic attainment than did either culdoscopy or colpotomy. It was his opinion, however, that physicians had to do what they could do

Discussion: Permanent Sterilization

well, and that the procedures really should be complementary, not competitive, in their use.

Dr. Richart wanted to know if any of the gynecologists present had used both techniques.

Dr. Garcia commented that in Puerto Rico they used to do tubal ligations that took ten minutes, skin-to-skin.

These were interval tubal ligations performed transabdominally. He noted that the experience with laparoscopy was very recent and many problems had arisen from inexperience. A large amount of team work is needed; it is important to have the uterus handled for maximum visualization, and experience is needed for this procedure. There is no comparison possible insofar as time is concerned, for the contrast is too great. With a small transabdominal incision, a tubal ligation patient can be discharged from the hospital on the second day.

Dr. Cohen reiterated that the experience of the operator was of the utmost importance; there are some surgeons who do better with a vaginal approach and others who do much better with an abdominal approach. There is no equating the two physicians, but both techniques have a great deal of merit.

Dr. Cohen then admitted that he had never attempted Dr. Clyman's technique, He said he had become disenchanted with posterior colpotomy and felt much more at home with abdominal procedures.

Dr. Neuwirth noted that if you know how to stab a patient in the abdomen, you know how to use a laparoscope. Recognition is really not a problem, for laparoscopy has an optical advantage over the vaginal approach; you can get a panoramic view. In the initial phases of the procedure, and in the later phases, the whole pelvis can be surveyed; indeed, it can be seen in one view. This is of importance in training residents. One reason that the residents learn so rapidly is that once they learn how to use the laparoscope and how to insert it, they are more at home anatomically.

Dr. Richart inquired if these techniques had been applied to mass programs.

Dr. Cohen said Dr. Neuwirth reported on five hundred cases, but he would not call that a mass procedure.

doing. He admitted that visualization of the organs was a useful adjunct; but all they did in Puerto Rico was make an incision, get the tubes out, and employ the Pomeroy technique.

Dr. Clyman said he thought that where a similar result is concerned, the simplest and safest approach is best. He likes the transvaginal approach to culdoscopy because it does not require general anesthesia, does not require a major surgical procedure, and can be done on a mass basis. In many places it does not make much difference in the manner in which the procedure is performed. But for a large program, the suggested technique under local anesthesia is simple, efficient, and fast. In India and Pakistan beds and anesthesia are not available for large-scale programs.

Dr. Garcia asked Dr. Clyman if he used antibiotics.

Dr. Clyman said they were not necessary but that he had used them.

Dr. Garcia wanted to know if he advocated them.

Dr. Clyman replied that he did not.

Dr. Richart asked if the total procedure took ten minutes with local anesthesia and if the patient could then go home immediately.

Dr. Garcia explained that the patient was actually asleep during the procedure.

Dr. Richart said that the anesthesia was not local.

Dr. Garcia replied that the technical procedure took ten minutes, the patient was discharged on the following day, but the technique was not done under local anesthesia.

Dr. Hernandez explained that most of the interval sterilizations in Puerto Rico were performed by private practicioners with one-bed offices. They do a saddle block, perform tubal ligation, and permit the patient to return home on the following day. The surgery costs about sixty to one hundred dollars.

Dr. Richart brought Dr. Garcia's paper on oviduct reanastomosis up for discussion and asked him when patency was tested.

Dr. Garcia said the patency he had referred to was tested six months postoperatively. Immediately after the operation patency is tested by passing a needle into the fundus, indigocarmine saline is flushed through the needle into the uterine cavity and it can be observed flowing out of the oviduct.

Dr. Hernandez wanted to know if anovulatory drugs were used in the first two or three postoperative months because of the possibility of ectopic pregnancy.

Dr. Garcia said that there was some justification in maintaining a patient amenorrheic for a period after uterotubal implantation; he had heard of such practices, although he did not use them himself. He had had patient complaints suggestive of a reflux type of menstruation into the peritoneal cavity; this was associated with a mild peritonitis and discomfort that persisted through two or three menstrual cycles. He did not know what this represented, because the peritoneum of these patients had never been visualized.

Dr. Clyman explained that he had examined these peritoneal cavities postoperatively at stages of one, two, or three months, and then after a year. After one month there is a great deal of edema, but this is generally of the fluid type. He uses birth control pills that produce amenorrhea in cornual implantation, because the flow in the first and second cycles are usually very heavy after reimplantation. It takes from three to six months to get good healing in the peritoneal cavity, although the patient feels very well and there is no clinical evidence of inflammation.

Dr. Tietze wanted to know about ectopic pregnancies following oviduct reanastomosis.

Dr. Garcia elucidated the fact that the forty-five and fifty percent pregnancy rates following reanastomosis sometimes represented almost all abortions or ectopic pregnancies; the ectopic pregnancy rate varies from a minimum of ten percent to a maximum of from thirty to forty percent. These are very high rates of abnormal pregnancies.

Dr. Hernandez asked how soon after surgery the ectopic pregnancy appeared.

Dr. Garcia thought that this varied with the promptness of restoration of tubal function. With splints, pregnancy is less likely to occur; in fact he had never observed a pregnancy with a splint in place. Once the splints are removed, however, pregnancies have been observed in the first succeeding menstrual cycle.

Dr. Garcia noted that in order to match the diameter of the

tubal lumens, he cuts one tube in an oblique diagonal and the resulting tube size is more compatible. When the lumen size is compatible on both sides, reanastomosis can be performed more readily. Side-to-side approximations are terrible and have proved to be totally unsatisfactory.

Dr. Richart requested discussion of Dr. Phatak's paper on the optimal time for tubal ligation.

Dr. Tietze inquired if there were any studies comparable to her longterm studies on women who did not have tubal surgery. He wanted to know what would be expected when women were examined several months or years after their last pregnancies.

Dr. Phatak explained that since comparable studies of women of similar ages were not available she could not state with accuracy that twenty percent of the women would exhibit menstrual irregularities.

Dr. Neuwirth recalled that the failure rate with the Pomeroy procedure seemed to be higher when it is done in the puerperal state rather than in the nonpuerperal state. In some of the reports there were failure rates of one or two percent; but, in the interval series, the failures were about one or two in three hundred.

Dr. Clyman mentioned a study done by Dr. Michelle; he took oviducts removed one to eight days postpuerperally, ground them and cultured them; all cultures were negative. This contradicts the results obtained by Hellman in 1941, in which he demonstrated an infiltration of leukocytes in the lumen. It was assumed to be an indication of infection and to show that performing tubal ligation twenty-four to forty-eight hours after delivery was not wise. Dr. Michelle's work and Dr. Phatak's work open this up for questioning.

Dr. Phatak thought that the results were troublesome when there was a question of a tube which manifested a chronic inflammatory state; the late effects of this are not known. But in the patients ligated after the first forty-eight hours, no differences were found. Surgery at this point was preferred because the patient was properly relaxed and motivated towards sterilization.

Dr. Tietze gave his opinion that both vasectomy and tubal sterilizations should be considered as procedures that are normally nonreversible; patients should not accept these procedures unless they are reasonably certain, at least at the moment, that they do not expect or want additional offspring. He thought it would be correct to say that not many reversals had been done because most people do not request them. The results of these procedures, although they have improved in recent years, are not certain. Insofar as women are concerned, the prospects for pregnancy following sterilization reversal are very, very small. He agreed with Dr. Phatak that it did not make any difference if the procedure were performed after forty-eight hours or during the following week.

Dr. Taylor agreed in essence with what Dr. Tietze had said. But he said there had been good tubal reversal procedures. He raised the question of how often a tubal sterilization reversal is indicated and whether this should be taken into account when surgery is undertaken. Years ago, procedures were described where, instead of ligating or sectioning the oviducts, the fimbria was sutured under the reflection of the bladder peritoneum; the percentage of failures was higher than that under tubal ligation, but the techniques of the procedure were not pushed very far. Another procedure involved splitting the broad ligament and placing the fimbria either inside the broad ligament or the inguinal canal. He felt that if a temporary tubal ligation were required, reversal could be obtained in a very high percentage of cases if a technique were adopted which also had a slightly higher failure rate. It is necessary that these procedures be placed on record; they exist and their reversibility is very high.

Dr. Tietze asked Dr. Garcia if he would discourage a person, male or female, from undergoing sterilization with the afterthought that he could return and have it reversed.

Dr. Garcia agreed that if you wanted to be perfectly sure, this would be the only way to do it with the data available at the moment. But the available data are difficult to analyze because there are so many factors involved and it is difficult to come to any conclusions. He felt that patency and restoration of the conduit could be assessed. Function is another matter; there are so many things, e.g. a new mate, that have to be considered that it is extremely difficult to predict a possible pregnancy.

Dr. Hulka requested that Dr. Tietze summarize his impressions on the indications for sterilization in terms of age, parity, and program limits.

Dr. Tietze thought that this would depend to a great extent on the local situation. He believes that individuals should be permitted to make their own mistakes, and it is not the purpose of the state or the physician to do anything but advise them. If this principle is accepted, persons who do not wish to have children should be sterilized for no reason at all; he did not think this was practical on political grounds, however.

III BIOENGINEERING TECHNOLOGY (A)

Denis J. Prager, *Moderator*

Chapter 13

VISUALIZATION OF SOFT TISSUE STRUCTURES: PRINCIPLES AND LIMITATIONS

F.C. McLeod

Ultrasound has found increasing acceptance during the past thirty years as an energy source for the visualization and imaging of soft tissue structures. Ultrasonic imaging is now a common technique for the examination of the brain, heart, breast, and circulatory system. Considerations such as the relative transparency of soft tissue to this form of energy, the reflectivity of soft tissue to this form of energy, the reflectivity at soft tissue interfaces, and the convenience of the propagation velocities involved, have led to the development of several imaging techniques. Sonic imaging systems present single image planes or cross-sections, analogous to the x-ray tomogram. Three-dimensional images are attainable by stacking or superimposing several adjacent cross-sections. The more recently developed holographic techniques promise direct visualization of three-dimensional tissue structures. As with optical imaging, the resolution or clarity of sonic images is determined by the wavelength of the sonic energy and the transducer aperture.

The principle advantage of ultrasonic energy is that images of objects completely transparent to x-rays can be produced. This is made possible by the differing absorption and reflectivity of the two energy forms, as determined by different physical properties of the materials. Ultrasonic images are formed by reflection at tissue interfaces, whereas radiographic images are formed by different amounts of absorption within the structure. In general, the image obtained by ultrasonic techniques is of inferior resolution to those obtained by visible light or x-rays, because convenient sonic wavelengths are much longer.

IMAGING TECHNIQUES

Short-range, pulsed sonar techniques are most commonly employed for imaging soft tissue structures. In these techniques, short bursts of high-frequency sound are coupled into the tissue structure through an electromechanical transducer consisting of a piezoelectric crystal such as barium titanate. Such a crystal gives off pressure waves when excited electrically; conversely, it produces a voltage when pressure stimulated. The sonic pulse can be thought of as a combination pressure-vibration disturbance moving through the tissue at approximately fifteen hundred meters per second. This is in contrast to light waves, which are electromagnetic in nature and travel at three hundred million meters per second. The comparatively slow propagation velocity of the sonic wave makes it possible to determine the depth of a tissue interface. Echoes reflected from underlying tissue structures are recorded on an oscilloscope screen; the time delay between the transmitted pulse and the return echo is proportional to the depth of the reflecting interface. Most tissue structures of interest contain many interfaces at different depths; thus, the oscilloscope trace consists of a series of peaks, one for each interface. This most basic system, the *A scan,* is analogous to a core sample in that only tissue structures along the narrow transducer beam are visualized. This trace is useful for measuring distances between interfaces, and thus the size and position of a structure. Instruments using the simple *A scan* system have proved very useful in determing brain midline displacement and in observing motion of heart valves. (Fig. 13–1).

Only a small fraction of the ultrasonic energy can be reflected by each underlying tissue layer. While it is important that enough energy be reflected to provide a detectable echo, it is also important that not all the energy be reflected. Complete reflection would not leave any energy to be reflected off successive tissue layers. The result of complete reflection is a shadowing of all underlying tissue structures. Interfaces between tissue and bone, and/or tissue and air, reflect most of the sonic energy. Such interfaces are avoided, if possible, in ultrasonic imaging. Although complete reflection prevents or limits visualization of structures behind bone and gas spaces (e.g. lungs), it provides a useful tool for the detection of gas in the gastrointestinal tract, or bubbles accidently introduced into the bloodstream during surgery. Similarly, the absence of reflecting surfaces makes fluid-filled spaces readily identifiable. Cysts and the bladder are outlined easily because of their reflectionless content.

A two-dimensional image can be obtained by moving laterally over the surface to assemble a series of core samples. Such a scanning procedure is generally referred to as a *B scan*. Instead of displaying the return echoes as a series of peaks, the echoes

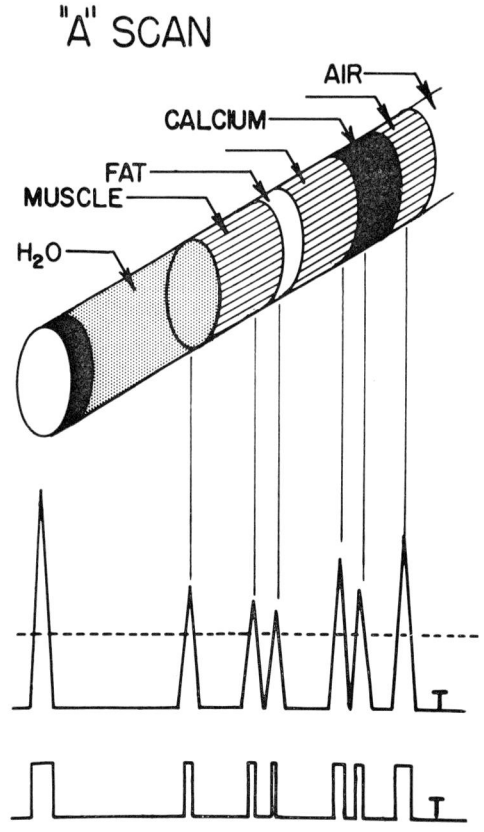

Figure 13–1. Echoes returned from interfaces between tissue structures. Echoes displayed on a time base corresponding to range are referred to as *A scan*.

are represented as a series of dots along a horizontal line. The position of the dot along the line corresponds to the depth of the reflection. The vertical deflection of the oscilloscope is synchronized with the lateral displacement of the transducer as it is moved over the tissue structure. A line of *points* or echoes is formed for each position of the transducer. Each line is retained by the memory property of the oscilloscope screen, thereby creating a two-dimensional image (Fig. 13-2).

'B' SCAN

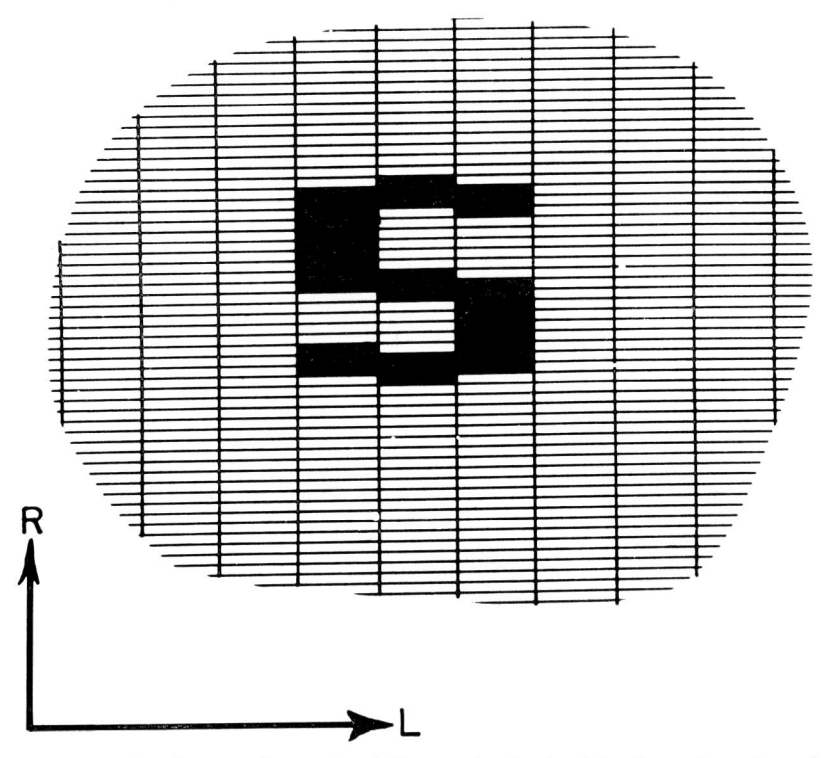

Figure 13-2. The two-dimensional *B scan* is obtained by lateral motion of the transducer over the tissue structure. Depth resolution is generally much better than lateral resolution; typical resolutions are depth, 50 points/cm, and lateral, 5 points/cm.

A variety of scanning techniques have been used for visualizing different biological structures. These range from slow hand movement of the transducer to rapidly rotating acoustic mirrors, which quickly cover a large area. The method chosen reflects the mobility of the organ. The scanning rate is limited by the mechanism and typically is less than ten frames per second. Use of these scanning systems thus is limited to stationary and slow-moving structures. There is little prospect for dramatic improvements in the future.

PULSE ECHO PRINCIPLE

The pulse echo principle is basic to all sonic imaging techniques except the recently developed holographic methods. The echo reflected back to a transducer by a simple point source target is an attenuated reproduction of the transmitted pulse. It has been delayed, in time, by an amount corresponding to the range delay, shifted in frequency by the Doppler effect resulting from the target's motion, and reduced in amplitude by the reflectivity and shape of the tissue interface. Reflection of sonic energy occurs at boundaries between tissues of differing acoustic impedances; this physical property is determined by the density and elasticity of the biological material through which the pulse is traveling. A portion of the pulse energy is reflected when a wave traveling through normal tissue enters a different tissue medium. Thus, a reflection will occur when a wave traveling through normal tissue encounters a cyst or other anomaly. A similar reflection will occur as the wave emerges from the cyst into normal tissue. The reflections are similar because a tissue-cyst interface is identical to a cyst-tissue interface. If the transmitted signal consists of a series of rectangular pulses on a sinusoidal carrier, the reflected echo will appear as a corresponding series of pulses. The time or range delay (T_r) between the transmitted and return signals indicates the distance (R) to the reflecting interface according to the relationship: $T_r = \frac{2R}{C}$. C is the velocity of sound in tissue ($\sim$ 1500 m/sec).

The frequency of the reflected pulse will be Doppler shifted from the transmitted frequency (F_t) by an amount: $F = \frac{2 F_t}{c} \frac{dR}{dt}$,

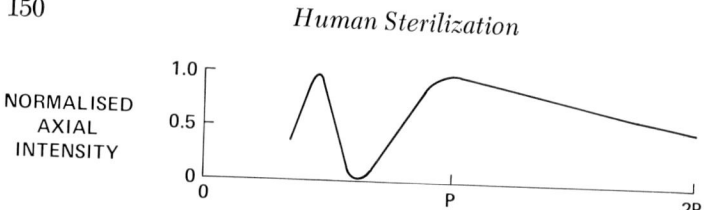

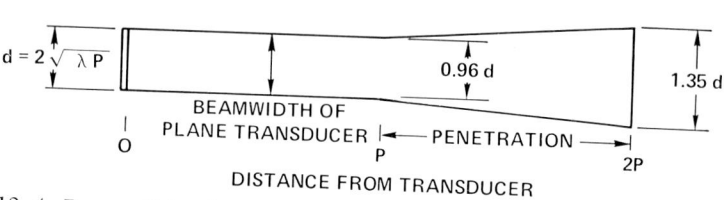

Figure 13-4. Beamwidth of a plane transducer spreads as penetration increases, limiting lateral resolution. Field of observation is generally limited from P to 2P to avoid nonuniformity near field of transducer.

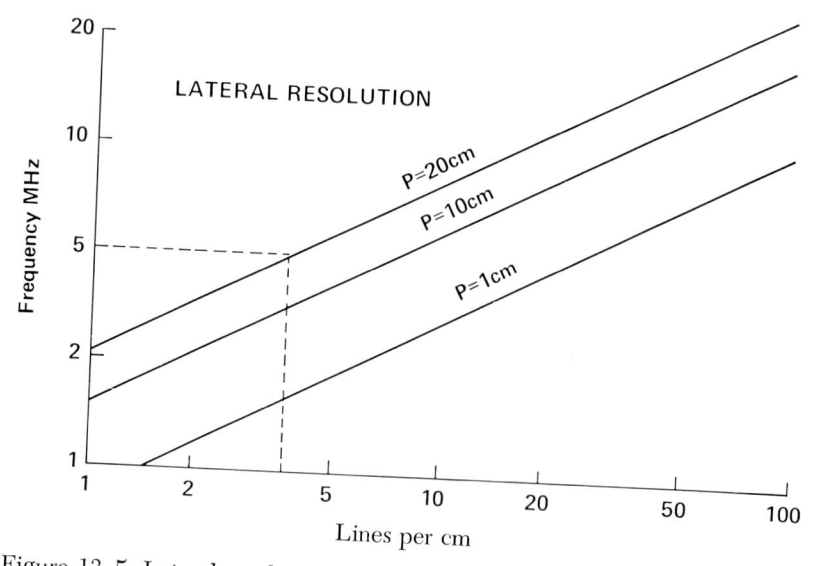

Figure 13-5. Lateral resolution is determined by both frequency and penetration.

wave as it passes through the material being imaged. Pulses, or short bursts of energy, comprise a broad band of frequencies. The rate of attenuation of sonic energy in tissue is a function of the center frequency (Fig. 13–6). Attenuation in average tissue is approximately zero to five decibel/MHz/cm. (The decibel here is defined as $10 \log \frac{P_{out}}{P_{in}}$). For example, the attenuation of a pulse having a center frequency of 5 MHz is 2.5 db/cm. After traveling only 8 cm, this pulse is attenuated 20 db, or reduced to 1% of its original power. A 10 MHz wave is re-

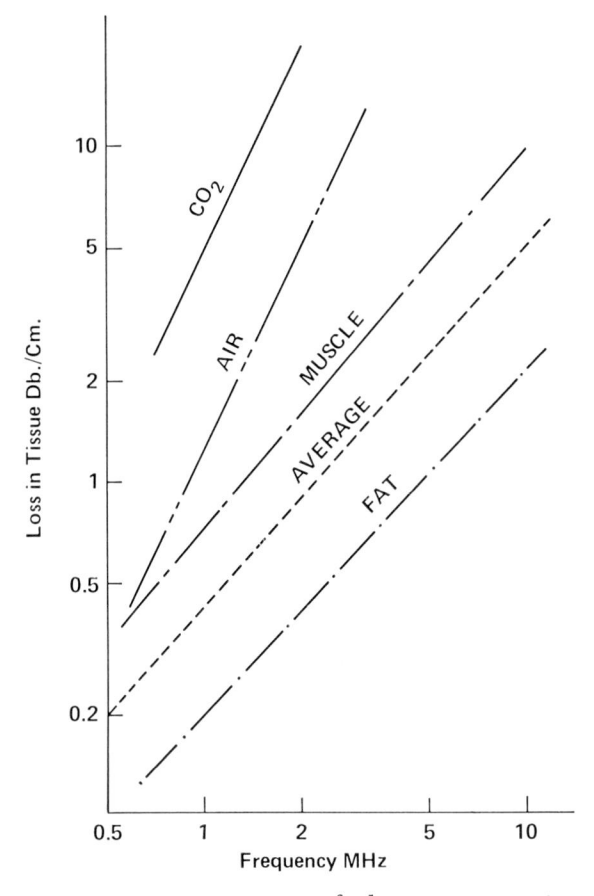

Figure 13–6. Approximate attenuation of ultrasonic waves in various biological media as a function of frequency. Average attenuation in soft tissue is 0.5 Db/MHz/cm.

duced to 1% in only 4 cm of travel. Thus, the resolution and range of an ultrasonic image obviously is limited by this severe attenuation of the ultrasonic wave. Assuming a maximum input power of 1 watt/cm^2 applied to the tissue structure, the maximum depth and resolution of an image can be computed (Fig. 13–7). Resolution can be obtained only at the expense of image depth. Frequencies in the two to five MHZ range generally are used for most ultrasonic imaging, and represent a practical compromise between range and resolution. Corresponding resolutions are in the order of thirty lines per centimeter.

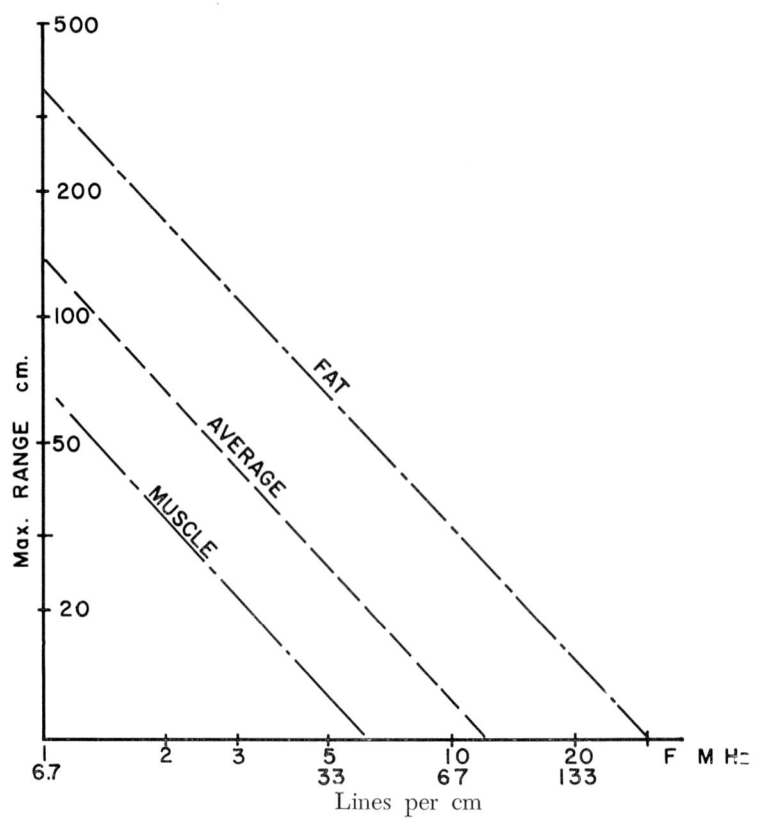

Figure 13–7. Maximum penetration is limited by the maximum energy that can be safely applied to the tissue, background noise, and frequency. Image resolution is gained at the expense of penetration. Values shown represent maximums attainable. Typically, maximum ranges are approximately one-half those shown.

SUMMARY

Ultrasound can be used to produce images of tissue structures that ordinarily would be transparent to radiographic techniques. The images are formed by reflection of sonic waves at the interfaces of different tissue media. Resolution generally is inferior to that attained with x-rays; however, ultrasound does not present the damaging side-effects of ionizing radiation.

Using simple pulse-echo techniques, structures several centimeters thick can be visualized. The echoes (shifted in time, frequency, and amplitude from the original) provide an image of the reflecting interface.

Current techniques include the one-dimensional *A scan* and the *two*-dimensional *B scan*. Holography offers the possibility of three-dimensional images in the near future.

REFERENCES

1. Howry, D.H.: Techniques used in ultrasonic visualization of soft tissues. In Kelly, E. (Ed.): *Ultrasound in Biology and Medicine*. Washington, D.C., American Institute of Biological Sciences, 1957, pp. 49–64.
2. Howry, D.H., Scott, D.A., and Bliss, R.W.: Ultrasonic visualization of carcinoma of the breast and other soft tissue structures. *Cancer, 4:* 354, 1954.
3. Reid, J.M.: Diagnostic applications of ultrasound. *Proceedings of IRE,* New York, November, 1959, pp. 963–967.
4. Baum, G., and Greenwood, I.: The application of ultrasonic locating techniques to ophthalmology: theoretical considerations and acoustic properties of ocular media. *Amer J Ophthal, 43:*319, 1958.
5. Joyner, C.R.: Diagnostic Ultrasound in the study of cardiac disease. In *Diagnostic Ultrasound,* University of Colorado Press, Denver, 1966.
6. Thompson, H.E.: Applications of ultrasound to obstetrics and gynecology. In *Diagnostic Ultrasound,* University of Colorado Press, Denver, 1966.
7. Ambrose, J.: Pulsed ultrasound: Illustrations of clinical applications. *Brit J Radiol, 37:*435, 1964.
8. Mason, W.P.: *Physical Acoustics*. New York, Academic Press, 1964, Vol. I, Methods and devices.
9. Kossoff, G., Robinson, D.E., and Garrett, J.J.: Ultrasonic two-dimensional visualization techniques. *Proc IEEE, SU-12,* 31, 1965.

10. Jabocs, J.E.: Ultrasound image converter systems. *Proc IEEE:* SU-15: 146, 1968.
11. Massey, G.A.: Acoustic imaging by holography. *Proc IEEE,* SU-15, 141, 1968.
12. Lobdell, D.D.: A nonlinearly processed array for enhanced resolution. *Proc IEEE,* SU-15:202, 1968.

Chapter 14

POLYMER IMPLANTS

FRED LEONARD

The wide range of mechanical properties of polymers make them attractive candidates for implants. These properties result from the structural characteristics of the polymer at the molecular level.

The main feature of synthetic organic macromolecules is a backbone chain composed of covalently-bound carbon atoms. Because of the tetrahedal geometry of the saturated carbon atom and the possibility of rotation about carbon-to-carbon bonds, a multiplicity of spatial configurations is possible.

Many macromolecular chains may include, in addition, atoms other than carbon, e.g. nitrogen, oxygen, or sulfur. Also, the chain backbone may be part of a more complex structure such as a branched molecule or a three-dimensional network.

The physical properties of a particular macromolecular species depend on the nature of its repeating units and the topology of its chain structure. By varying these parameters, it is possible to prepare polymers whose mechanical properties range from soft elastomers to hard, rigid materials. It is also possible to combine polymers with low-molecular weight substances to achieve specific mechanical and temperature-resistant properties or enhanced environmental stability. Thus, plasticizers may be added to achieve flexibility, reinforcing agents to enhance strength, and antioxidants to protect against oxidative degradation.

For a surgical implant, not only are mechanical properties of importance, but tissue compatibility is a principal requisite for long-term utilization. Tissue compatibility involves the interaction between the host and the implant: the effect of the tissues and body fluids on the implant and the effect of the implant on the tissues.

An implantable material may initiate a tissue response in

three general ways: by the release of low molecular weight toxic materials as a result of the biodegradation of the polymer; by simply occupying space in the internal milieu; or by the diffusion of low molecular weight materials from the polymer.

POLYMER STABILITY

Polymers for surgical implants may be either biostable or biodegradable. With biostable polymers, the effect of the host on the implant is minimal so that the implant can be expected to maintain its integrity for a lifetime. Biodegradable polymers are expected to degrade at a desirable rate; degradation products are eliminated through normal excretory routes, and none of the products are stored in tissues or organs.

The stability or instability of the polymers is dependent upon the structure of the polymer and the biochemical nature of the environment in which it is implanted.

Chemical reactions of significance in the organism are the following:

1. Formation and cleavage of macromolecules.
2. Dehydrogenation and hydrogenation of alcohols to carbonyl groups, of saturated to unsaturated compounds, of aldehydes to carbon acids, and of amines to imines.
3. Formation and cleavage of carbon-to-carbon bonds by decarboxylation and carboxylation; condensation of activated carboxylic acids to β-keto esters, reactions analogous to aldol condensation; and additions to double bonds.
4. Loss of water, leaving a double bond; and addition of water to a double bond.

It is interesting that the well-known *in vitro* degradation mechanisms, both hydrolytic and oxidative types for polymer molecules, are possible in biological systems.

Examples of the stability of some *stable* commercial polymers in the organism are shown in the subsequent tables and figures. Table 14–I demonstrates the changes in the tensile strength of plastics after implantation. Harrison tested the tensile strength of fabric grafts implanted in dogs to replace portions of the

TABLE 14-I
CHANGES IN TENSILE STRENGTH OF PLASTICS AFTER IMPLANTATION

Materials	Days Implanted	Loss of Tensile Strength (%)
Nylon	1073	80.7
Dacron	780	11.4
Orlon	735	23.8
	670	1.0
Teflon	677	5.3
	675	7.0

descending thoracic aorta; tests were performed prior to implantation and for as long as three years following implantation. The nylon graft lost most of its strength over this period.

Mirkovitch measured the tensile strength of a polyurethane sample implanted intramuscularly in dogs as a function of time (Table 14–II). Table 14–III summarizes the results of the intramuscular implantation of various plastics in dogs.

Unfortunately, most of the studies reported in the literature on the effects of polymer implantations are of a practical nature. However, a few studies have attempted to elucidate the mechanism of polymer degradation after *in vivo* and *in vitro* use as surgical implants. Examples of such studies are those made of

TABLE 14-II
CHANGES IN POLYURETHANE PROPERTIES WITH IMPLANTATION

Time (Months)	Tensile Strength, PSI
0	8150
8	1846
16	Disintegrated

TABLE 14-III
CHANGES IN PROPERTIES OF PLASTIC FILMS AFTER IMPLANTATIONS OF SEVENTEEN MONTHS

Material	Tensile Strength	Elongation
Polyethylene	2700	780%
Control	1930	
Teflon	2950	320%
Control	3720	250
Mylar	18,300	100%
Control	18,440	100
Nylon	9,300	550%
Control	5,200	140
Elastic	950	800%
Control	930	290

the degradation of the poly-cyanoacrylates and the degradation of poly L (+) (lactic acid). The cyanoacrylates are liquid monomers which polymerize in the presence of a moist environment to form high-polymer molecules. They are utilized as tissue adhesives and hemostasis-inducing compounds in nonsuture closure of wounds. By simply spraying such compounds on bleeding livers or kidneys, particularly friable organs not easily amenable to suture closure, the cyanoacrylates spread and polymerize to form films which achieve almost instantaneous hemostasis.

In vitro studies of the degradation of the homologous series of poly-cyanoacrylates have indicated that these polymers may degrade by chain scission, and/or by hydrolysis of the ester group and solubilization and diffusion of the polymer away from the site of implantation. In the chain scission reaction, formaldehyde is formed. *In vivo* degradation studies, made by implanting radioactive polymer subcutaneous give similar results. In the *in vivo* studies, degradation products are not found in the internal organs, but appear to be eliminated through the feces and urine.

Poly L (+) (lactic acid), a polymer of lactic acid, has been synthesized at this laboratory in order to develop a biodegradable surgical repair material which would undergo hydrolytic de-esterification to lactic acid, a normal intermediate in the lactic acid cycle of carbohydrate metabolism. Implantation of the radioactive polymer indicates that the rate of degradation of the L (+) polymer was approximately five percent per month. The data indicate that the polymer is degraded and eliminated as carbon dioxide in the breath. *In vitro* work indicates that random chain scission occurs, resulting in de-esterification. Poly L (+) (lactic acid) may be fabricated into films, sutures, and rods. Preliminary evaluation has indicated that this material may be useful in soft and hard tissue repair.

COMPOUNDING INGREDIENTS

Most commercially available plastics contain low molecular weight compounding ingredients which have been added to enhance specific properties. If such plastics are implanted, the compounding ingredients may diffuse out of the plastics into the surrounding tissues at a rate sufficiently high to elicit a local or systemic toxic response. Typical examples of such low molecular weight ingredients are plasticizers, which usually consist of high-boiling esetrs; stabilizers, which are organometallic compounds; and antioxidants, which are phenolic derivatives.

For materials which are to be implanted, it is preferable either to eliminate the necessity for the addition of such compounds or to develop nondiffusible compounding ingredients.

MATERIALS RESEARCH AND INTRAUTERINE CONTRACEPTIVE DEVICES

IUDs presently used generally are made of stainless steel or polyethylene. These materials usually are well-tolerated by the body and elicit minimal tissue response.

However, as the result of studies which indicate that chronic inflammation of the endometrium is associated with the intrauterine device, it has been suggested that such a reaction is essential to the anti-fertility effect. Similar reactions probably can be achieved through the use of a biodegradable polymer with a known controllable degradation rate. Therefore, it is suggested that a systematic study of the anti-fertility effects of biostable and biodegradable polymers be undertaken.

REFERENCES

1. Harrison, J.H.: Synthetic materials as vascular prostheses. *Amer J Surg,* 95:3–15, 16–24, 1958.
2. Mirkovitch, V., *et al.*: Polyurethane aortas in dogs, three year results. *Trans Amer Soc Art Int Organs,* 8:79, 1962.
3. Leininger, R.I.: Plastics in surgical implants. *ASTM, STP 386,* Nov., 1964.
4. Leonard, F., *et al.*: *Annals NY Acad Sci, 146:*203–213, 1968.

Chapter 15

ULTRASONIC SURGICAL TECHNIQUES

Francis J. Fry

Ultrasound interacts with the soft tissue structures of the human or experimental animal in a number of interesting ways. It provides direct structural visualization if the acoustic properties of the tissue are appropriate, and it provides a spectrum of selective interactions with tissue.[1-11] Unlike mechanical probes or chemical additives, ultrasonic methods can be completely noninvasive. The mechanisms of interaction between ultrasound and tissue, although not completely understood, appear to be quite different from ionizing radiation interactions, and the problems of cumulative long-term effects apparently are eliminated in most applications. In cases in which ultrasound has been used to produce tissue lesions in the experimental animal and man, the acoustically generated lesion can be detected immediately by acoustic means. It is possible in a number of circumstances to combine the tissue visualization possibilities of ultrasound with the production of selective tissue lesions so that some surgical procedures can be performed under direct visual control in a nonmechanical or chemical invasive mode.

In general, the interface between fluid-filled space and soft tissue is most readily visualized with ultrasound, but many other structural features can also be detected. The use of intense focused ultrasound to produce selective lesions in the experimental animal brain is well documented in the literature and has been used on approximately two thousand adult animals at the University of Illinois (cat, rhesus monkey, squirrel monkey, and rat). In addition, approximately two thousand one-day-old mice have been irradiated in a study of the physical parameters of the sound field responsible for the interaction with embryonic nerve tissue.

Approximately a hundred human patients have been irradiated

Ultrasonic Surgical Techniques 161

for the treatment of various hyperkinetic disorders.[12,13] In addition, we have initiated studies on a small series of human subjects, in which, for the first time, acoustic visualization and lesion-producing capabilities are being combined. Since the skull bone is a difficult barrier to ultrasound as it is presently applied, a section of skull is removed and replaced by a rigid acoustic transparent device. The visualization and modification are performed transcutaneously.

An example of the kind of selective lesion which ultrasound can produce is shown in Fig. 15-1 (adult human brain).

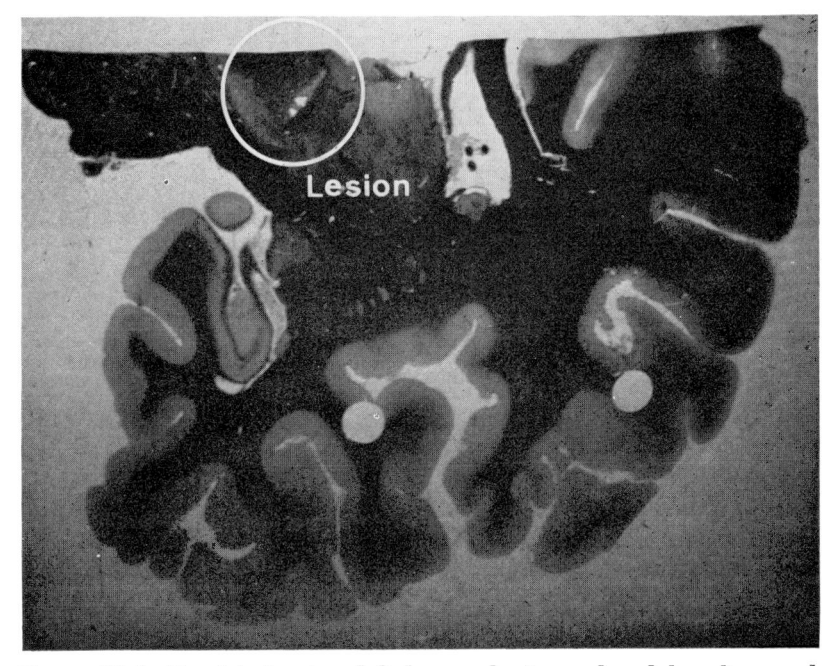

Figure 15-1. Focal lesion in adult human brain produced by ultrasound.

Figure 15-2, a partial coronal section of a human brain, shows the details of ventricular structures and demonstrates that the soft tissue, fluid-filled space interface can be seen readily. For more structural detail such as gray-white matter interfaces, an increased overall sensitivity is necessary (Fig. 15-3); the internal capsule can be outlined quite well.

Figure 15-4 exhibits a partial coronal section of a human

162   *Human Sterilization*

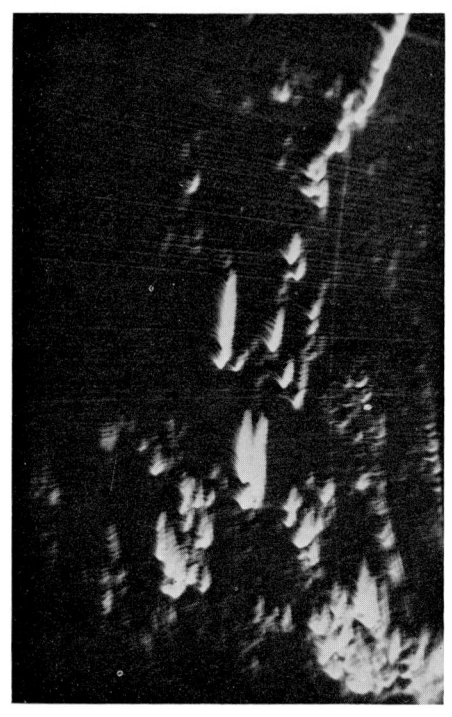

Figure 15-2. Coronal section of human brain showing details of ventricular structures.

brain in which there is evidence of considerable abnormal tissue growth; Figure 15-5 shows the same brain immediately following the generation of a lesion by means of ultrasound. Study of the acoustic echoes received from this brain shows that the acoustically generated lesion can be observed differentially with respect to other local brain features.

It is necessary when considering the use of ultrasound as a visualizing and tissue-modifying modality that each region be thoroughly investigated with regard to the problems associated with that area. If the structures of interest can be delineated acoustically, then such structures can be considered for potential modification by acoustic means. Only a study of the specific tissue of interest will determine if selective effects of ultrasound on different structures can be elicited. Although, at the present time, it is not possible to predict what type of interaction will

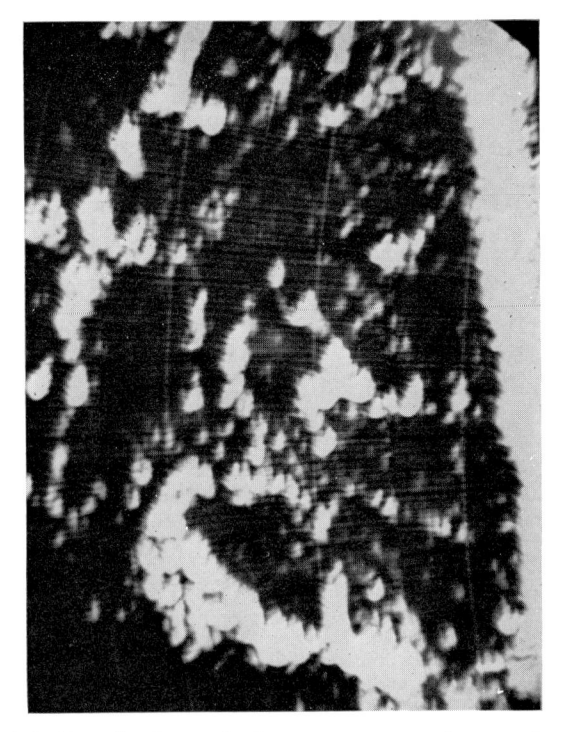

Figure 15-3. Detail of ventricular structures at increased sensitivity.

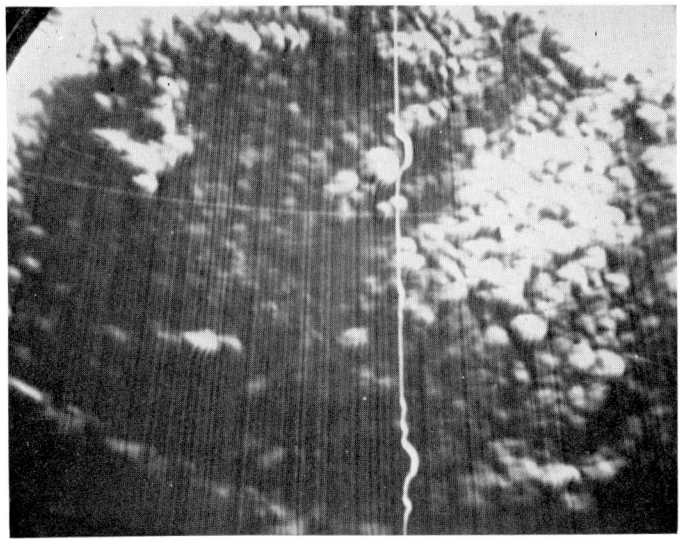

Figure 15-4. Partial coronal section just before ultrasonically generated lesion. Scan shows evidence of considerable abnormal tissue growth.

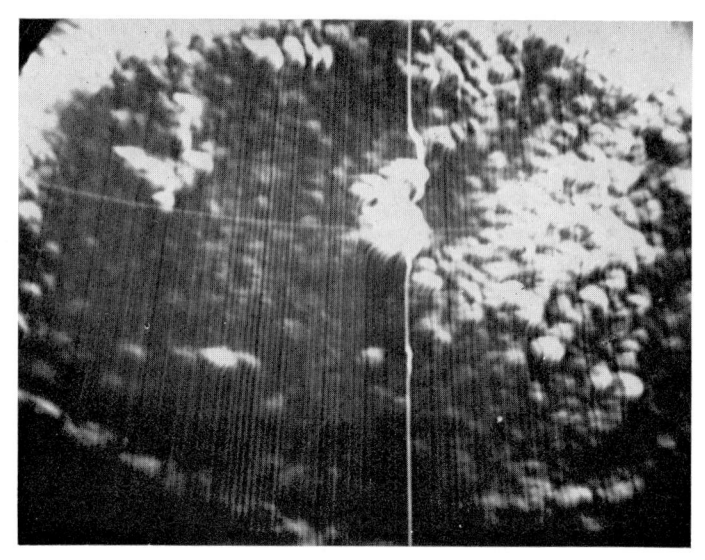

Figure 15-5. Immediate postultrasonically generated lesion scan of same brain as in Figure 15-4.

occur in various tissues, there are several possible ways of approaching tissue components not previously studied and the background information on neural tissue should be quite helpful.

Ultrasonic visualization of the human and animal brain, and ultrasonic lesioning methods are highly developed technologies. No equipment is commercially available for the full utilization of the methods; however, excellent commercial equipment is available for visualization of soft tissue structures.[14,15]

REFERENCES

1. Fry, W.J., Tucker, D., Fry, F.J., and Wulff, V.J.: Physical factors involved in ultrasonically induced changes in living systems: II. Amplitude-duration relations and the effect of hydrostatic pressure on nerve tissue. *J Acoust Soc Amer, 23*:364, 1951.
2. Wulff, V.J., Fry, W.J., Tucker, D., Fry, F.J., and Melton, C.: Effects of ultrasonic vibrations on nerve tissues. *Proc Soc Exp Biol Med, 76*: 361, 1951.
3. Wall, P.D., Fry, W.J., Stephens, R., Tucker, D., and Lettvin, J.Y.: Changes produced in the central nervous system by ultrasound. *Science, 114*:686, 1951.

4. Fry, W.J.: Action of ultrasound on nerve tissue—a review. *J Acoust Soc Amer, 25:*1, 1953.
5. Fry, W.J., and Fry, R.B.: Temperature changes produced in tissue during ultrasonic irradiation. *J Acoust Soc Amer, 25:*6, 1953.
6. Fry, W.J., Mosberg, W.H., Jr., Barnard, J.W., and Fry, F.J.: Production of focal destructive lesions in the central nervous system with ultrasound. *J Neurosurg, 11:*471, 1954.
7. Fry, W.J., and Barnard, J.W.: Selective action of ultrasound on nerve tissue. Convention Record, IRE, 102–106, 1954.
8. Fry, W.J., Barnard, J.W., Fry, F.J., and Brennan, J.F.: Ultrasonically produced localized selective lesions in the central nervous system. *Amer J Phys Med, 34:*413, 1955.
9. Fry, W.J., Barnard, J.W., Fry, F.J., Krumins, R.F., and Brennan, J.F.: Ultrasonic lesions in the mammalian central nervous system. *Science, 122:*517, 1955.
10. Barnard, J.W., Fry, W.J., Fry, F.J., and Brennan, J.F.: Small localized ultrasonic lesions in the white and gray matter of the cat brain. *Arch Neurol Psychiat, 75:*15, 1956.
11. Fry, W.J., Brennan, J.F., and Barnard, J.W.: Histological study of changes produced by ultrasound in the gray and white matter of the central nervous system. In Kelly, E. (Ed.): *Ultrasound in Biology and Medicine,* Washington, D.C., American Institute of Biological Sciences, 1957, pp. 110–130.
12. Meyers, R., Fry, F.J., Fry, W.J., Eggleton, R.C., and Schultz, D.F.: Determination of topological human brain representations and modifications of signs and symptoms of some neurological disorders by the use of high level ultrasound. *Neurology, 10:*271, 1960.
13. Fry, W.J., and Fry, F.J.: Fundamental neurological research and human neurosurgery using intense ultrasound. IRE Transactions on Medical Electronics, Vol. ME 7, pp. 166–181, 1960.
14. Fry, W.J., Leichner, G.H., Okuyama, D., Fry, F.J., and Fry, E. Kelly: Ultrasonic visualization system employing new scanning and presentation methods. *J Acoust Soc Amer, 44:*1324, 1968.
15. Fry, William J.: Intracranial anatomy visualized *in vivo* by ultrasound. *Invest Radiol, 3:*242, 1968.

Chapter 16

APPLICATIONS OF ULTRASONICS IN THE STUDY AND CONTROL OF POPULATION PROCESSES

Donald W. Baker

Effective population control depends on the development of techniques which are effective and which can be administered quickly, at low cost, and without serious side effects. Reproductive processes can be interrupted by either biochemical or mechanical means.

Biochemical techniques appear to have great promise for controlling population on a widespread basis. However, these techniques are not without their problems. Currently available chemical contraceptives produce undesired side effects, have temporary effectiveness, their cost is relatively high, and they are only available for the female. It also seems that the use of chemical agents is a method most readily used by a sophisticated society. If biochemical agents could be introduced in a more convenient, or even automatic manner, their effectiveness would not depend upon habit or memory, and more widespread usage might be possible.

Mechanical techniques, on the other hand, lend themselves easily to the less sophisticated classes. These methods can be absolutely effective (sometimes to the detriment of the individual who desires to be restored to full reproductive capability), have essentially no side effects (although emotional side effects are possible), and in the long term, the cost is extremely low.

What factors then prevent the more widespread application of mechanical techniques to sterilization of men and women? Although vasectomy is a simple and safe procedure which can be performed in minutes, it requires penetration of the skin. A better method would permit interruption of the spermatic passages without skin penetration. The ultimate technique would be a one-step process, producing little or no trauma to the individual, and necessitating no postoperative follow-up.

Mechanical sterilization techniques used on the female are considerably more involved because of the inaccessibility of the female reproductive organs. Techniques which take advantage of the vaginal approach have not yet been developed completely.

Clearly, there are opportunities to explore new methods and new approaches to mechanical sterilization in both sexes. Noninvasive techniques generally involve the interaction of some energy form with the organ or structure under study. Of the energy forms employed, light and ultrasound are the most controllable and have the greatest potential for use as sterilization tools. Unfortunately, because of the wavelength of light and its relatively high absorption by tissue, it is not possible to introduce enough energy through the skin and intervening tissues to map or alter biological structures. In contrast, because ultrasonic energy penetrates tissue relatively easily, it can be used to map tissue structure, and intense beams can be focused on a particular site to produce damage. This is feasible because the wavelength of ultrasound in tissue (for the commonly used frequencies 1–10 MHz) is 0.15–1.5mm. In this range, selective absorption and scattering caused by tissue interface becomes detectable. Ultrasound is generated with ceramic transducers and the resulting sound field can be shaped and focused into a narrow beam to facilitate directing the energy.

ULTRASONIC VISUALIZATION

Ultrasound should be a useful tool for mapping soft tissue structures and studying their geometric and dynamic properties. This knowledge could be applied clinically to develop devices for locating and producing lesions in particular ducts for permanent and nontraumatic sterilization. The first problem is to determine the effectiveness of ultrasound in mapping and visualizing soft tissue structures involved.

Ultrasonic mapping is based on the interaction of ultrasonic wavelengths with tissue structures. Generally, ultrasonic energy in the form of very short pulses, is introduced into the tissue with a suitable transducer; the same transducer detects the echo signal which is reflected from a tissue interface. The *round-trip* transit time of this pulse through the tissue is dependent on the velocity of sound in the tissue and the distance to the tissue interface. If the *round-trip* transit time and the relative intensity of the echoes from different interfaces are known, information concerning the geometry or structure of the tissue in the path of the sound beam can be derived. When the sound field is shaped into a very narrow beam and scanned through the region of interest, it is possible to map the position of echo-producing interfaces. The interfaces can be imaged on a cathode ray tube by modulating the oscilloscope trace with the reflected signal. Two types of displays are commonly used in ultrasonic tissue visualization. The simplest is called an *A-scan*. In this display, the echo intensity is plotted versus the *round-trip* transit time. Figure 16–1 (bottom) shows a typical *A-scan* taken through a section of the eye. This type of display can be interpreted easily if very simple structures are involved and if the boundaries between the structure and surrounding

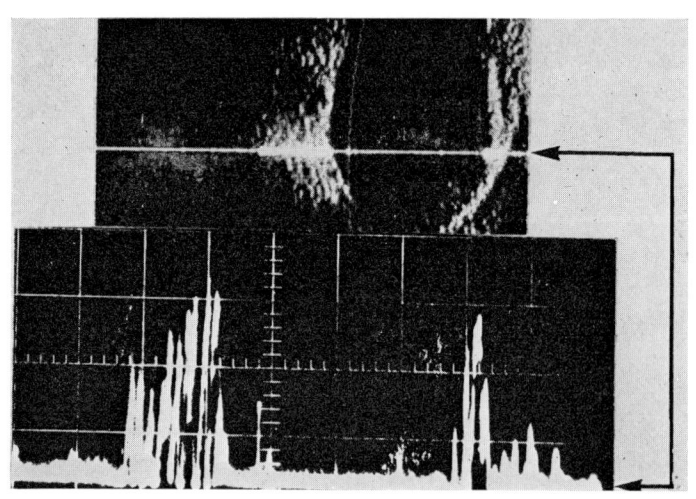

Figure 16–1. *A-scan* display of ultrasonic echoes from Ocular Section. Adapted from: Baum, Gilbert: A comparison of the merits of scanned intensity modulated ultrasonography versus unscanned *A-scan* ultrasonography. In Grossman, C. (Ed.): *Diagnostic Ultrasound*, New York, Plenum Press, 1966.

media are quite clear and distinct. The sharpness of the image of the tissue boundaries depends on the relative acoustic properties of the adjacent media. If the product of the density times the velocity of sound in one media is quite different than that in the adjacent media, there will be an interface which will produce strong echoes. Because this type of display is limited to showing echo intensity versus depth, it is sometimes difficult to identify and study complex structures. The upper half of Figure 16–1 illustrates *B-scan* display. Here, the reflected echoes are displayed in a two-dimensional array with coordinates of range and angle so as to show a one-to-one correspondence between the actual tissue structure and the displayed pattern representing the sound field interaction. This illustration shows a cross-sectional scan of an eye which the observer can identify easily. If the structure of interest has no regular pattern, then it becomes difficult to identify structures with a *B-scan* also.

A better understanding of the physics of ultrasonic scanning provides better appreciation of the potential usefulness and limitations of the method. The beam produced by the ultrasonic transducer is similar to the light beam emitted by lasers. They are spatially coherent in the far field, and usually are represented by plane sound waves perpendicular to the beam axis progressing through space. The angle between the sound-beam axis and a reflecting surface has a definite effect on the echo shape and amplitude because of the coherent nature of the impinging waves. When the surface is smooth and acoustically different from the coupling medium, echoes will be received only when the beam is normal to the surface. At other angles, the sound is reflected in another direction, depending on the shape of the surface. This is called the specular reflection properties of interfaces. If sound impinges upon a roughened surface at an angle slightly off normal, more of the energy will be reflected back in the direction of the receiving transducer. The reflection from nonsmooth surfaces is a scattering phenomenon in which the ultrasound is sent in many directions. Tissue, depending on its structure, sometimes acts as a reflector, other times as a scatterer. If a transducer is placed on the surface of the skin and moved back and forth in a sector-scan motion,

170 *Human Sterilization*

only those interfaces which are nearly at a normal angle to the beam will return echoes; interfaces at other angles will scatter sound in other directions and will not be detected. The result is an incomplete imaging of the region. The difficulties arising from the specular reflecting properties of tissue can be overcome partially by special scanning techniques.

 The type of scanning motion used depends on the nature of the tissue structure to be mapped. These special scans are called compound scans because the transducer is sector-scanned while it is translated simultaneously to the left, the right, or in an arc. The cross-sectional shape of the fetal head taken at various times during the course of pregnancy is shown in Figure 16–2 by a *B-mode scan* display. The images shown cor-

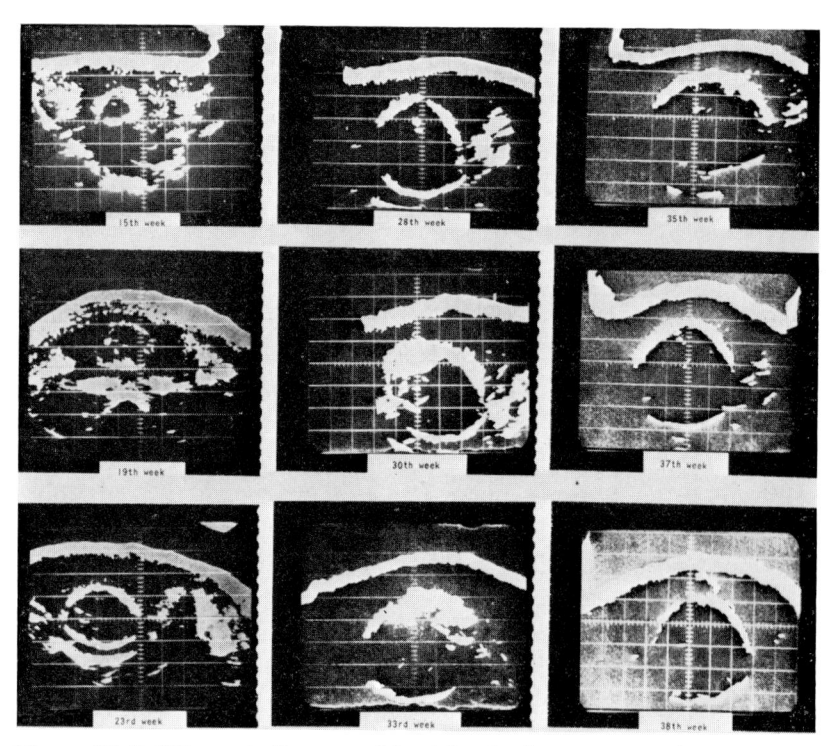

Figure 16–2. Ultrasonic *B-scans* of fetal head taken at intervals from 15 to 38 weeks. Adapted from: Thompson, Horace E.: Studies of fetal growth by ultrasound. In Grossman, C. (Ed.): *Diagnostic Ultrasound,* New York, Plenum Press, 1966.

respond to plane sections passing through the head of the fetus. It is easy to identify the round structure of the head in this cross-section, because the observer has a preconceived concept of its shape. This illustration provides an indication of the resolution capability of ultrasound for target identification in a rather typical application. As the structure becomes smaller and more complicated, it becomes increasingly difficult to identify particular structures within the body.

Ultrasonic techniques appear to have potential capability for mapping and visualizing sections of the female pelvis. However, more sophisticated techniques have to be developed before localization and identification of the oviduct will be possible. The overall resolution must be improved and better displays developed in order to permit differentiation of echoes from different interfaces. The actual echo information from the pelvis extends over a dynamic range of nearly a thousand-to-one. It is technically difficult to exhibit this wide range of information on a black and white display. A more sophisticated display using color to show this wide range of intensities would permit the identification and relation of the acoustic reflections to specific tissue interfaces.

Ultrasonic mapping of appropriate structures of the male reproductive system poses a different set of problems. Here the need is for a very high-resolution scanning system which can function within 2–3 cm of the surface of the skin. A conventional hand-operated *B-mode scan* display probably could not map the vas deferens with sufficient resolution, since hand scanning does not provide a reproducible scan over the region to be mapped.

A high-speed rotating scan transducer is being developed for cardiovascular applications.[*] This could demonstrate the feasibility and usefulness of high-speed scanning for the purpose of mapping the cross-section of the vas deferens. The principal feature of this type of scanning is not speed, but the exact repetition of each scan is along the same path. Figure 16–3 shows the functional block diagram of a rotating high-speed scanner. Three ultrasonic transducers are located on the periphery of a rotating

[*] This work was supported in part by NIH Grant 07293.

BLOCK DIAGRAM

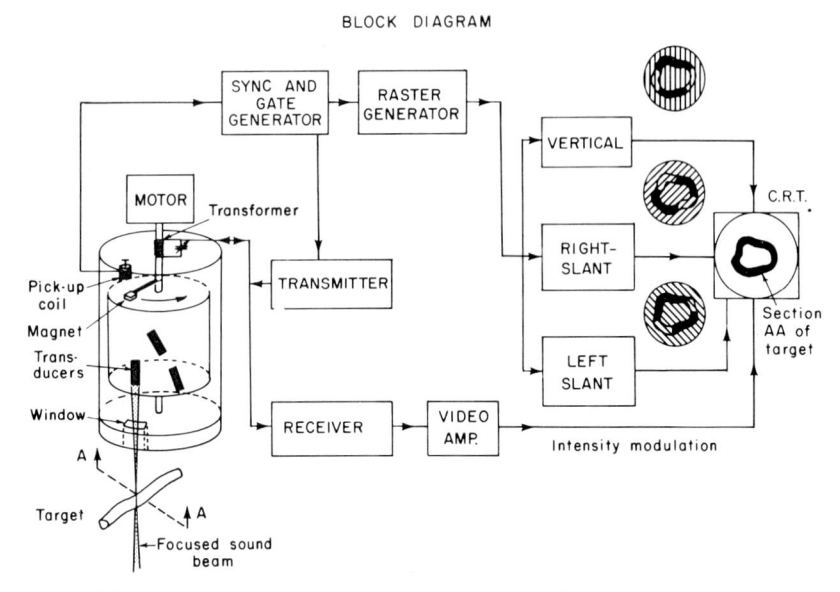

Figure 16–3. High-speed rotating compound scan for mapping blood vessel cross-section.

drum. As each transducer passes a pick-up coil, a trigger is produced to generate a raster on a cathode ray tube display. The orientation of the raster corresponds exactly to the alignment and orientation of the transducer on the rotating scan. The rasters are intensity modulated by the returning ultrasonic echoes from each transducer as it passes over the vessel or duct. Three modulated rasters, generated in sequence as they are triggered by the moving transducers, are superimposed on the cathode ray tube in proper registration to give a full two-dimensional image of the cross-section of the tube. This method has been used to obtain, transcutaneously, cross-sectional scans of the cephalic vein of a human subject.

Resolution is increased by using shorter transmitted pulse widths and higher ultrasonic frequencies. However, because of increased absorption at higher frequencies, it is not possible to increase the frequency or shorten the transmitted pulse indefinitely. An example of very high resolution scanning is shown in Figure 16–4; this is a compound sector scan of the eye taken with a fifteen megahertz echo ranging apparatus. Here the resolution

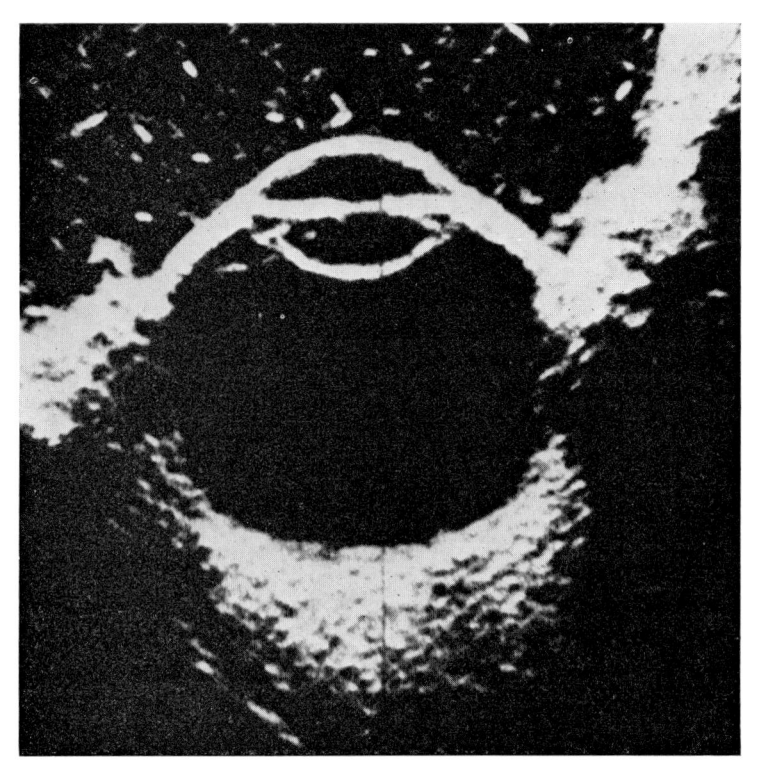

Figure 16–4. Intensity-modulated sector scan of eye taken with 15 MHz transducer. Adapted from: Baum, Gilber, *op. cit.*

is on the order of a fraction of a millimeter. Such a system might easily map the cross-sectional shape of the vas deferens.

It seems quite feasible to consider the development of a scanning apparatus which would have sufficient resolution to map the cross-section of the vas at a point of ligation. Then it would be possible to follow changes that occur after surgery. This device could be used for basic investigations of changes in tissue properties, and possibly, to follow the extent of recanalization following ligation.

LOCALIZATION AND LESIONING BY ULTRASOUND

The successful use of ultrasound to produce lesions in the vas or the oviducts depends to a large extent on the ability to localize these tissue structures and to aim suitably focused, high-power transducers upon them. At the present time, the vas seems to be the only duct which might be localized and identified transcutaneously without the use of an elaborate ultrasonic scanning system.

The oviducts, on the other hand, pose quite a different problem. High resolution ultrasonic scanning systems would have to be used to identify and localize them. An aiming control system would be needed to position the lesioning transducers so that energy could be directed properly to the specific site. This is a rather sophisticated objective that would involve the development of suitable coordinate systems whereby the scanning transducer could specify the exact location of the interface of interest. The lesioning transducer would be programed to focus at a particular site and then introduce the ultrasonic energy. Such techniques are being used by Fry to do destructive lesioning within the human brain. In this application, the sequence is one of scanning, mapping, aiming, and directing energy into a specific location. This is far less difficult than attempting to produce a lesion in the oviduct.

CONCLUSION

The prospect of mapping the tissue structures of the reproductive systems seems feasible. The examples presented here indicate technical progress. Application or reapplication of these techniques to particular scanning objectives depends on the development of methods which have higher resolution and improved displays to permit the identification of tissue properties and structures of interest. The possibility of using ultrasound for research is reasonable; however, its use as a clinical tool is limited by the extreme difficulty of implementing the methods.

DISCUSSION: BIOENGINEERING TECHNOLOGY A

Denis J. Prager, *Moderator*

Dr. Prager opened the discussion by asking for questions on ultrasonic technology.

Dr. Chez commented that ultrasound was a very exciting diagnostic, and potentially therapeutic, device. It can be applied to both obstetrical and gynecological problems. But he felt that the ultrasonic images presented were frustrating to him in that he could not visually comprehend what was apparently obvious to experts in the field. He wanted to know the requirements for competence in the interpretation of ultrasonic images: learning time as well as requisite intellectual competency.

Dr. Fry replied in terms of neurosurgery. Neurosurgeons and neurologists think in terms of the structural detail of the brain as they visualize atlases and stained sections. In an instrument employing ultrasonic techniques, the type of material that one is accustomed to seeing in a brain atlas would be presented on a monitor in either coronal or horizontal section as required. A color overlay would relate the two so that direct structural identification could be made between the atlas and the patient. A third color overlay could be used to focus on the lesion. Thus, the neurosurgical approach would involve a direct comparison between the structural detail with which the neurologist is familiar and the structural detail in the ultrasonic images.

Perhaps some image processing would be required to outline details further.

It was Dr. Fry's opinion that the brain did not present any great problem, since it was a highly structured system. Although he was involved with liver and kidney scans, for example, he could not state how long it would take to achieve complete familiarity with the subject matter. This is more complicated than the interpretation of x-ray pictures, for in these, the image is flattened into two dimensions. With ultrasonic imagery, a 1 mm brain cross-section is being observed. The problem of learning is at least as complicated as roentgenogram interpretation, possibly even more difficult. In neurosurgery, the attempt has been to present the neurologists with the type of structural detail with which he is familiar.

Dr. Chez said that he understood a theoretical application of the technique to human sterilization would involve the creation of a permanent acoustic lesion of the vas; this would be done transcutaneously without anesthesia. He wanted to know how long it would take from the time the patient presented himself to complete the procedure.

Dr. Fry speculated that it would take a few minutes.

Dr. Chez wanted to know if it is possible to achieve that.

Dr. Fry explained that it takes only a half a second to generate the image of a full cross-section of the brain. After that it is up to the operator to interpret and decide on a course of action. He said that this was pure speculation, for he had no experience in the area of sterilization. But the generation of both the image and the lesion is extremely rapid. How extensive this is to be, is of course a different matter.

Dr. Prager requested comments on the visualization of blood vessels or heart valves.

Dr. Baker commented that a great deal of work remained to be done; he did agree that the problems of visualization and display were important. The ability of access depends on the ability to visualize in three dimensions; any training would have to be directed toward enhancing three-dimensional visualization capabilities. By computer processing, the display can be enhanced to providing access to more visualization methods; all the data can be taken over a region and be displayed as they are taken, then can be followed through mentally.

He agreed that the problem for sterilization was what Dr. Chez had indicated; the interface of interest must be identified and the apparatus must be directed to produce a lesion at that point. The economics of the situation may be more of a problem than the engineering feasibility; for a given number of dollars in a given period of time the practicability of this could be shown. But to design a device that would be applicable in a vasectomy camp is quite another question. He expressed doubt that male sterilization was necessarily the place in which the technique should be applied. From an engineering standpoint, tubal sterilization appeared to be more complicated. If apparatus could be developed so that one woman could be sterilized every five minutes, transcutaneous techniques would be more useful. Certainly the individual would not be hospitalized for a day. He considered this a major factor in the economic aspects of the program.

Dr. Prager emphasized that very complicated systems, applicable to research, were being discussed. He wanted to know if there was any way that a simple system could be utilized, not necessarily for lesion production, but simply as an aid in visualization.

Dr. Baker expressed certainty that a small device capable of some visualization could be developed, but he felt that even that involves some speculation at the present time. He felt that the implementation of ultrasonic techniques would have to go through a series of stages; the first stage is the establishment of feasibility through research. Once the problem has been identified in the real engineering and clinical sense, the apparatus for the field of operation should be designed. He felt that statements of *what ought to be* were useless.

Dr. Tietze wanted to know if the lumen of a hollow organ could be identified. In other words, is it possible to use ultrasonic devices to verify the success of a sterilization procedure.

Dr. Baker thought it was quite possible, certainly in a research stage, to follow the cross-sectional area in either male or female tubes; the oviduct would present the more difficult problem.

Dr. Tietze explained that the vas was quite narrow and wanted to know if visualization could be done at a fraction of a meter.

Dr. Baker said that the vas is close to the surface and between fifteen to twenty megacycles should be sufficient to provide adequate resolution to see the lumen.

Dr. Prager emphasized that the technique had been used with

in the vas in the field, and would such a lesion block the vas or permit recanalization.

Dr. Fry said he could not answer the question, but he did not think that the instrument required to produce a vasal lesion could be small.

Dr. Southam wanted to know if lesions can be produced in other tubes with smooth muscle walls, like arteries; she inquired whether arteries can be occluded ultrasonically.

Dr. Fry explained that if you wished to produce a sonic level in the brain that was high enough to produce a hemorrhage, an artery could be occluded if the hemorrhage occurred in that area. Work has been done in the occlusion of smaller vessels, but not larger vessels of the brain. He could not say whether or not it would work in other systems.

Dr. Southam questioned the use of the term *irradiation* when ultrasound was spoken of, and wanted to know how irradiation as applied to x-ray was differentiated from irradiation as applied to ultrasound.

Dr. Fry said that the difference existed only in the sense that one is a mechanical vibratory phenomenon, (ultrasound), the other electromagnetic radiation.

Dr. Southam explained that she was speaking of the clinical differentiation, admitting that ultrasound irradiation and ionizing irradiation should be discussed.

Dr. Baker suggested that the use of the term *sonification* might be more appropriate in this usage.

Dr. Zinsser mentioned an experiment in which mice were kept and bred in a *sonifying* tank for a period of ten generations. Even when the body of the weanling rats were subjected to sound levels high enough to produce skin burns (perhaps six to ten watts per square centimeter), the breeding rates were not affected. This indicated that even immature testes are not susceptible to damage by ultrasonic energies of this level. He suggested that, if the vas were irradiated with a focused beam, it was very unlikely that spermatogenesis would be halted or the testes would be damaged by heat effects.

Dr. Fry agreed that the entire area of toxicity had not been explored definitively; there are areas which are unexplored in certain ways, and there are data scattered through the literature that demonstrate that there are no basic problems. But he emphasized that definitive data involving organ-specific irradiation, ultrasound, and toxicity levels were not existent.

Dr. Prager opened the paper by Dr. Woodward on tissue response to cyanoacrylates for discussion.*

Dr. Richart wanted to know which of the different polymeric compounds could be purchased and which had to be synthesized by the researchers.

Dr. Woodward explained that the materials he discussed were either synthesized at Dr. Leonard's laboratory or were supplied by Ethicon, or American Cyanamid. He continued by saying the synthesis of alkyl cyanoacrylates is not particularly difficult for organic chemists; the technique is fairly well known, and for experimental purposes, it might well be possible to custom synthesize cyanoacrylates. There are over four hundred publications or abstracts dealing with cyanoacrylates; many of these are studies of methyl cyanoacrylate, a very toxic material which possibly could be particularly useful for human sterilization. It is not really possible to compare results with various cyanoacrylates in a particular use setting, since the results might not be truly comparable.

Dr. Shubeck wanted to know if the variation in the adhesive qualities of the higher order of cyanoacrylates differed between methyl and hexyl, for example.

Dr. Woodward said that, in his experience most of the pure, properly stabilized cyanoacrylates were good adhesives. There are some exceptions, for neither the methoxy-ethyl nor the cyclopentyl cyanoacrylates are good adhesives; this is unusual. Pure, properly stabilized cyanoacrylates are good adhesives.

Dr. Richart inquired about species specificity and species response. Dr. Woodward's paper was concerned with hydroxyproline in a subcutaneous site; there may not be the striking species differences that are found with epithelial responses. He wanted to know if different species had been studied and if there were interspecific differences in responsivity to cyanoacrylates.

* See Dr. Woodward's paper, chapter 24, page 264.

Dr. Woodward said that there was not much interspecific difference in inflammatory response. A cyanoacrylate that produced a foreign-body response and a bland transient inflammatory response in rats or mice was likely liable to produce the same effects in monkeys or human; this appeared to carry over from species to species. When interspecific responses to epithelium regeneration are considered, they seem to be very similar. In addition, gastrointestinal anastomosis or mucosa regeneration does not appear to vary greatly between species.

Dr. Segal asked if there were a direct relationship between the resorption of cyanoacrylates and the toxicity or foreign-body reactions they elicit. Is the compound which is absorbed to a larger degree going to be associated with a more extensixe foreign-body reaction.

Dr. Woodward said that the cyanoacrylates which were resorbed rapidly were inflammatory and elicited very little foreign-body response. The polymers which were resorbed poorly elicited transient and mild inflammatory and foreign-body responses, and did not interfere with wound repair.

Dr. Segal pursued the matter further by asking if one were searching for a compound to form adhesions in a tube, would one attempt to find a homolog which produced an extensive foreign-body reaction? He also wanted to know if granuloma formation was used as the basis for the occlusion.

Dr. Woodward considered this a matter for experimental evaluation. He thought that a necrotizing cyanoacrylate (e.g. the methyl which is being used to occlude rabbit fallopian tubes) was capable of producing quite an inflammatory response and fibrosis; perhaps this could produce an acute inflammatory response and possibly rupture the tube. It is possible that a higher homolog that would produce a foreign-body response might also occlude the oviduct without an inflammatory response.

Dr. Richart said that he had studied methyl, ethyl, and isobutyl compounds without producing tubal rupture. Tissue responsiveness depends on the site and the surrounding tissue. Fibrous tissue produces one type of response, epithelium another. In epithelial tissue, methyl compounds were the only ones which caused a response, isobutyl compounds just remain against the epithelium. Species differences in responsiveness are striking; tubal epithelium of rabbit, rat, monkey, pig, and humans have been tested and demonstrate different levels of response. Preliminary indications imply that necrosis is necessary in order to produce fibrosis, for epithelium is protective unless it is eliminated. Fibroblast response seems to differ interspecifically.

Dr. Segal asked if the cyanoacrylates have an advantage over other necrotizing agents.

Dr. Richart explained that the occlusion of the oviducts required some type of chronic response. If acute chemical injury is produced and enormous amounts of tissue are destroyed, any small focus of epithelium that is left is capable of regeneration. In the rabbit, the methyl cyanoacrylate has been the most successful, presumably because it produces a chronic fibroblastic response which closes the fallopian tube. Attempts to produce fibrosis and tubal closure generally have been unsuccessful with single applications. In contrast, multiple applications in the human produce fibrosis. There appears to be some clinical evidence that indicates the need for repeated acute injuries, rather than a single acute episode.

The problem seems to be the innate capacity of the oviducts to regenerate, to recanalize, to maintain an open conduit. This is really what the structure is designed to do; it is most difficult to overcome this feature. The methyl compounds remain for a sufficient time so that they continue to produce necrosis and fibrosis; the epithelium is not able to recover the wound again before the appearance of fibroblasts.

Dr. Woodward said that one aspect of cyanoacrylates was that, unless specially treated, they remain *in situ* once they polymerize; if coconut oil were injected into the fallopian tube, there would be no possibility of predicting its migration. When cyanoacrylate is injected into the fallopian tube, it is almost impossible to get the monomer out beyond the tube; this is an advantage. This is more than stickiness; in a few seconds a liquid is converted into a high molecular weight compound.

Dr. Shubeck wanted to know what there was about the substance that made it adhesive. Once polymerization occurs, a higher homolog is produced and this results in the production of a nonreactive material. But what holds the tissues together?

Dr. Woodward replied that any roughness of the tissue surface is adhered to by the cyanoacrylate.

Dr. Shubeck still wanted to know why it stuck if the material is nonreactive.

Dr. Woodward explained that hydroxyl groups present in proteins probably contribute polymerization catalysts that are entrapped in the polymer. Many polymers are not adhesive in the process of polymerization; there probably is no satisfactory answer to the adhesive properties of the materials nor to the question of polymerization being an adhesion-producing process.

Dr. Shubeck said that the compound was self-adhesive during polymerization, but the question remained as to what was holding the cells against an essentially nonreactive material.

Dr. Roth thought that this was partially due to the hydroxy and amino groups. Obviously a relationship exists between surface and polymer formation, but what occurs at the very fine interface between polymer formation and substrate is not completely understood.

Dr. Segal asked why Scotch® tape sticks.

Dr. Woodward explained that adhesion was a function of surface wettability, in part. The contact angle between any surface and a potential adhesive is a function of wettability; as the contact angle decreases, the adhesion increases. For example, Teflon® is a nonwettable surface, and cyanoacrylates can be allowed to polymerize on Teflon. But the problem is really not that simple. Stainless steel wouldn't be considered to be an adhesive surface, yet blocks of the steel can be joined with methyl cyanoacrylate. The bond strength of this is such that several thousand pounds can be supported; this is a much higher bond strength than that in dermal-to-dermal adhesion. Although collagen contributes most of the tensile strength to skin and other organs, it is not a particularly good substrate for adhesion.

Dr. Neuwirth wanted to know what agents could be used to slow the polymerization rate of methyl cyanoacrylate to about thirty seconds.

Dr. Roth thought acetic compounds could be used; sulfur dioxide presently is used for inhibiting the formation of some polymers.

Dr. Prager asked how much time that gave.

Dr. Roth said it depended on the amount of material, but probably it would not be much more than thirty or forty seconds.

Dr. Neuwirth wanted to know if acetic acid was preferable.

Dr. Roth affirmed that it would be an aid, but he could give no information on the amount to add to achieve certain time limits.

Dr. Richart asked if polymer size were decreased when such agents were added.

Dr. Woodward stated that there was indirect evidence showing that if partial polymerization took place under controlled conditions with high sulfur dioxide concentrations, the mean molecular weight of the polymers would be lower than if the same polymerization had occurred with less sulfur dioxide.

Dr. Richart questioned if this changed the tissue reaction.

Dr. Woodward said the effect was not marked.

Dr. Zinsser cited Dr. Casells experiment with six dogs in which he used cyanoacrylates as a tissue glue on the exterior of a splinted vas as a method of producing a watertight closure. The results of the work appear promising, and the animals have been maintained for about a year and a half. This might prove to be a very good method of vasal repair, and the method involved no sutures.

Dr. Prager thought the experiment was interesting because he had been discussing the possibility of using polymers as an external seal in addition to sutures.

Dr. Zinsser expressed the personal opinion that there was too much tissue reaction to the cyanoacrylates employed.

Dr. Hulka stated that Dr. Clyman had been using very minute quantities of polymers for tubal reconstruction and was enthusiastic about the value of the method as opposed to sutures. Culdoscopic examination of some patients revealed the absence of surounding adhesions.

Dr. Prager asked if this was done without any sutures at all.

Dr. Hulka said he believed so.

Dr. Zinsser mentioned that he had been very encouraged with experiments employing highly polymerized gelatin to which other materials had been added. A firm gelatin block was obtained, and no tissue reaction was observed in the tissue implantation site. The material is not available commercially, but can be made in the laboratory; it is possible that it may be just as good as other compounds in the long run.

Dr. Thompson mentioned that he had had limited amount of experience with cyanoacrylates used in the corneal area of monkeys; so far he had obtained nothing more than a very superficial reaction. He wanted to know if inter-cross-linked gelatin had been used in this area.

Dr. Zinsser explained that cross-linked gelatin exhibited no tissue reaction after three or four weeks; it just melted away.

Dr. Prager questioned its use as a plug.

Dr. Zinsser said they had not used it as a plug, but merely for exterior application as a glue that was good for two weeks.

Dr. Schmidt demonstrated an electrode that was designed for producing occlusion of the vas; it has a metal tip and an insulating shaft and is similar to a #20 or #21 hypodermic needle. He has attempted sterilization by inserting the needle through the scrotum so as to impale the vas on its point, and then using electric current to heat the section of the vas and obliterate it. He has attempted the procedure on dogs, and it worked well. In humans, the vas was anesthetized, but the patients still complained of a heat sensation, and vasal occlusion was not obtained. Dr. Ko suggested a number of improvements.

If a hypodermic needle is inserted into a tube (with one wire emerging at the tip and another wire emerging about 2 mm behind, separated by an insulator) and the outside of the tube is coated with a resistance material, an electric current can be applied and heat generated. The heat generation can be controlled by the current, and the current can be applied in the form of a sharp pulse. In a short period of time, with relatively high temperatures (about 200-300° C), some burn could be produced at the inner surface of the lumen causing the lumen to collapse and fibrous tissue to form.

This is the basic concept. It is possible that the fibrous tissue could completely occlude the lumen and permit no fluid passage; this could be controlled by the extent of the burn. There is a possibility that regeneration could be such as to provide a bypass to the occluded tube. Another problem would be the location of the lumen, but trial and error should permit this localization.

It seemed possible to Dr. Ko that a device of this nature could be constructed simply and at low cost; operating techniques could be taught quickly.

Dr. Schmidt wanted to know if access to the lumen of the vas could be achieved from the outside.

Dr. Zinsser declared that the lumen of the vas could be hit from the outside fairly easily and that the position in the vas also could be determined. Unless the tissue were killed, epithelium could grow across the defect probably more quickly than fibroblasts could grow in circumference. This is a problem; also, it is not known how long a lesion must be induced. If a straight needle were used with this type of design, and about 3 cm of vas lining were necrosed, the time it took for the epithelium to grow 3 cm through the middle might be too long for the lesion to heal itself. Progressive, graded killing of the vasal epithelium has not been done. It is possible, on a theoretical basis, that there is some degree of destruction of the lining necessary to produce fibrosis.

Dr. Segal inquired for a consensus that the discussion revolved about changing or improving existing vasectomy techniques, with the two issues involved being simplification of the existing procedure and greater reversibility assurance. He felt that procedures utilizing advanced techniques would produce little in terms of simplification of vasectomy. It is difficult to simplify further the procedure that is employed in Indian vasectomy camps, where perhaps eighteen hundred sterilizations can be done in forty-eight hours.

Then the issue becomes one of increasing the likelihood of reversibility. He did not see how this could be accomplished when a clean surgical cut was replaced by tissue necrotization, either by cautery, chemical agents, or pressure. He asked for comments by urologists on his opinions.

Dr. Schmidt thought that one of the things to be gained was speed. The discussion involved the possibility of placing an electrode or similar device within the vas and completing the sterilization in two or three minutes without the need for an incision.

Dr. Segal inquired if this could be done without visualizing the vas.

Dr. Schmidt stated that the vas could be lifted under the skin and the skin could be stretched over it. The vas would then be between the operators fingers; he could then clamp, spear the duct, move the tip of the needle, and have the vas follow.

Dr. Segal wondered about mistaking the spermatic artery for the vas.

Dr. Schmidt said that the vas was so distinct a structure that you could be certain of making no error.

Dr. Zinsser took exception to Dr. Segal's contention. He thought that if it were possible to develop a procedure that took less than five minutes and could be used by operators of low technical skill, it would be a distinct advantage and a real breakthrough. He considered that the potential does exist for the development of such a technique.

Dr. Tietze returned to the question based on distinguishing between the vas and the spermatic artery. He wanted to know if such a simple differentiation were possible after the application of local anesthetics.

Dr. Schmidt said that the question only arose when there was a double blood supply; in this case the vas and the artery do interchange.

Dr. Brueschke pointed out that the relatively simple pulse doppler could be used to show if you have the vas or an artery under the skin.

Dr. Segal inquired if it would not be simpler to make the slit instead of employing all those additional procedures.

Dr. Brueschke said that he did not think so, for the incision could be construed as a time-consuming procedure. Arterial determination with the pulse doppler takes only a few seconds; it does require an additional instrument, but the equipment is small.

Dr. Southam asked Dr. Schmidt if any fluid was returned when a needle was inserted into the vas.

Dr. Schmidt stated that he did not obtain any; fluid could be detected but very little fluid was there.

Dr. Southam visualized this as the same as the difference between a simple vena puncture and a blood vessel cut-down.

Dr. Schmidt agreed that that was a good comparison.

Mr. McLeod felt that the psychological aspect was more important than the time saved, for it is simpler to get someone to have an injection than it is to persuade them to undergo surgery.

Dr. Zinsser returned to the concern about damaging the spermatic artery. He mentioned that, since blood would be returned if an artery were encountered, this would act as a safety factor. If a lumen exists, local anesthetics can be injected with the same needle used for the procedure. The vas usually is not manipulated without using local anesthesia, because patients do not like vasal manipulation, and it does cause a massive systemic reaction. Local anesthesia is definitely indicated in the proposed procedure.

Dr. Woodward suggested that cyanoacrylates, should be compared to cauterization in animal experiments to determine ease of performance.

Dr. Richart thought that there must have been experiments on dogs with direct visual cautery and chemical agents. The question was, did the procedure work or did the occlusion recanalize. In the oviduct, an acute injury can be produced and it can recanalize. Does this not occur in the vas because it is a much smaller structure?

Dr. Zinsser said that if the outer coating were well burned, there would be external granulation and no reanastomosis. The degree of injury would have to be graded carefully so that the muscularis and the mucosa were destroyed, but not the entire vas.

Dr. Richart inquired about literature on the use of chemicals for burning the lumen.

Dr. Zinsser told him that he did not know the papers.

Dr. Brueschke said that Dr. Lee had done work of this nature.

Dr. Lee reported that he had done experiments and printed material in 1964. His research was not successful because the burns were too extensive. With injections of diluted phenol, there were also extended burns and fibrosis. Epithelial regrowth occurred due to the incomplete injection of the chemicals. All in all, the results were unsatisfactory.

IV REVERSIBLE STERILIZATION

Ralph M. Richart, *Moderator*

Chapter 17

REVERSIBLE VAS OCCLUSION BY INTRAVASAL THREAD

HEE YONG LEE

Attempts to develop a new device for reversible vas occlusion in animal experiments have employed various techniques. These include injection of Biowax; insertion of a piece of plastic material; electrocoagulation; chemical cauterization; and the placement of nonreactive suture material in the vas. The nonreactive suture method has proved to be the most satisfactory technique.

A previous study has demonstrated that sperm passage can be blocked by placing either surgical nylon thread or surgical silk thread into the vas deferens as an intravasal thread (IVT); vasal patency can be restored by removing the IVT. In a small number of vasa, however, sperm passed through the dilated lumen with the IVT *in situ*; it is possible that this is a result of increased intravasal pressure caused by continued sperm deposition because of an imbalance between testicular spermatogenesis and spermatolysis.

ANIMAL EXPERIMENTS

Adult male dogs were employed: one group had surgical nylon thread placed in the vas; one had surgical silk thread placed in the vas; and the other dogs had a small piece of plastic material inserted intravasally.

The intravasal thread is nonreactive and nonabsorbable surgical thread, either nylon or silk. It is 1 cm long; and its diameter varies from that of chromic catgut Numbers 1 to 5, depending on the lumen of the vas. Two 8 cm strings of size 6-0 black filiform nylon are attached to one end (Fig. 17-1).

Intravenous sodium pentothal was used as the general anesthetic. A high, midscrotal incision was used to expose 2 cm of the vas. The filiform nylon threads attached to the intravasal thread were run through a straight-round needle; the intravasal thread was inserted into the vas from the distal to the proximal

194   *Human Sterilization*

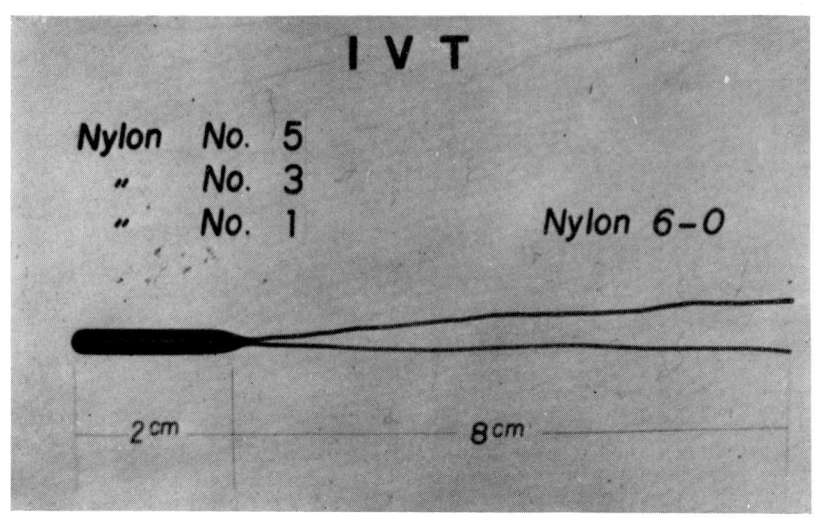

Figure 17-1. Photograph and dimensions of intravasal thread. Note that several gauges of nylon are used for the tip. Size is chosen depending on the lumen of the vas.

end by the straight needle. Then the filiform nylon threads were tied, not too tightly, just around the vas (Figs. 17-2 through 17-5).

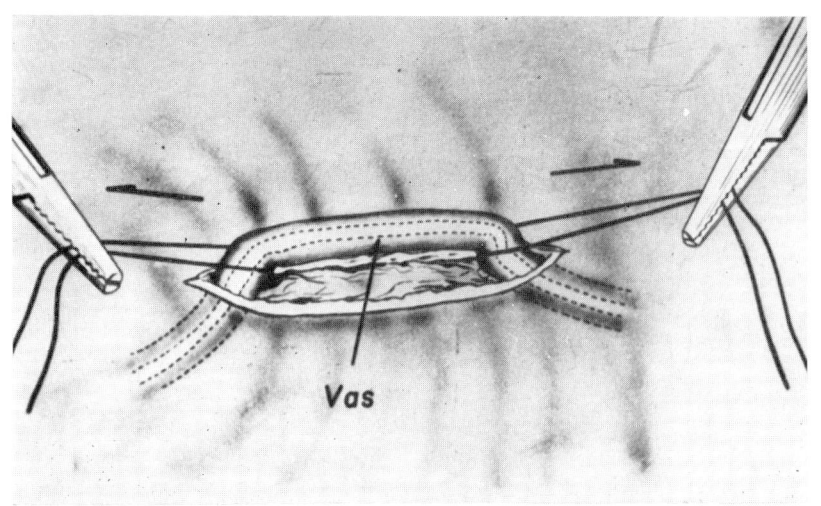

Figure 17-2, 3, 4, and 5. Sequential diagrams of technique of exposure of vas deferens, placement of intravasal thread and tying of attached nylon threads.

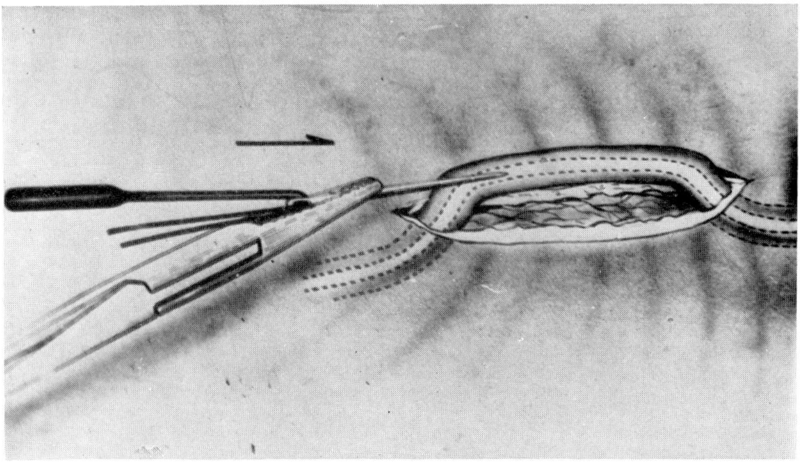

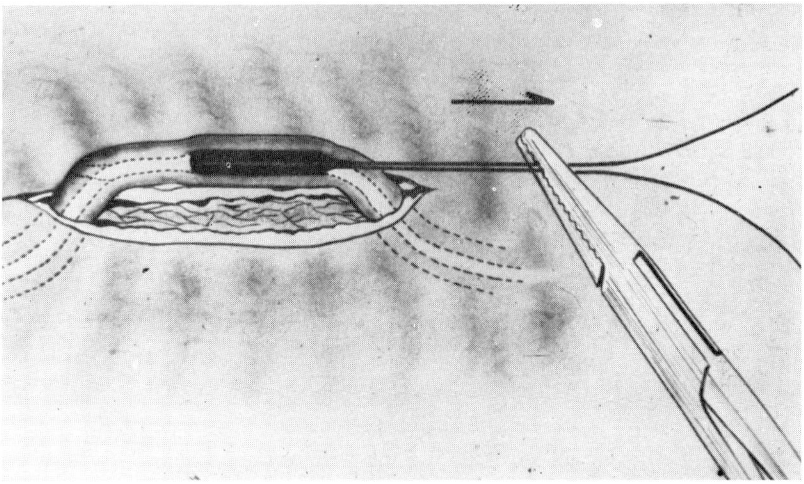

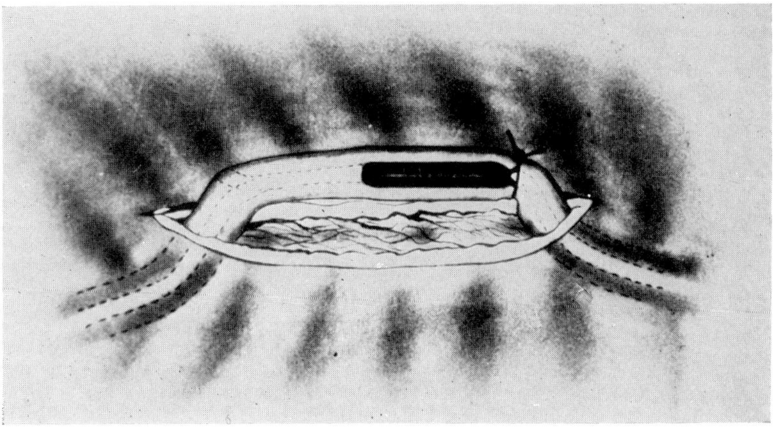

The filiform threads must be very fine in order to avoid permanent fistula formation due to long-term placement. They should be tied just tightly enough to hold the intravasal thread in place without choking the vas. These threads should be black or dark blue for easy identification in case removal of the intravasal thread is required. The filiform nylon threads which are attached to the proximal end of the intravasal thread function in the prevention of upward migration of the intravasal thread and in eliminating the necessity of using an incision for intravasal thread removal.

The same procedures were employed on the other side. Bleeders were clamped and tied as required. The scrotal incisions were closed by layers with silk sutures.

Three to six months after the insertion of the intravasal thread, semen analysis was performed. No sperm was present in the ejaculates except in a specimen from a dog in which there had been faulty intravasal thread insertion.

After these preliminary analyses certain animals were sacrificed, and the vasa were examined both radiographically and histologically. Vasography showed complete occlusion, except in the case of faulty intravasal thread insertion. Histologic examination revealed the following: of five vasa examined in the surgical nylon thread group, one revealed mild tissue reactions and the remaining four no significant changes; of the six vasa examined from the surgical silk intravasal thread group, one showed a moderate degree of tissue reaction, one showed a mild tissue reaction, and four showed no significant changes. In the animals in which a plastic material had been inserted, there was moderate tissue reaction in one, mild tissue reaction in two, and no significant change in one. The cells were well preserved and very few inflammatory cells were found. No significant changes had taken place in any of the materials that had been inserted.

Six months after the insertion of the intravasal thread, the remaining animals were studied for reversibility. The dogs were anesthetized by sodium pentothal; the vas was exposed as it was for the insertion; and the intravasal threads were removed by cutting and pulling the filiform thread with a pair of mosquito forceps. A 2–0 nylon thread was introduced into the previously occluded vasal lumen as an internal splint; the distal end of the splint was fixed to the scrotal skin. The nylon thread splint was used to prevent kinking of the vas due to extensive fibrotic contracture of surrounding tissues following the intravasal thread removal. The wound was closed in the usual manner. The splint was removed on the tenth postoperative day. (Figs. 17-6 and 17-7).

One to three months after the removal of the intravasal thread,

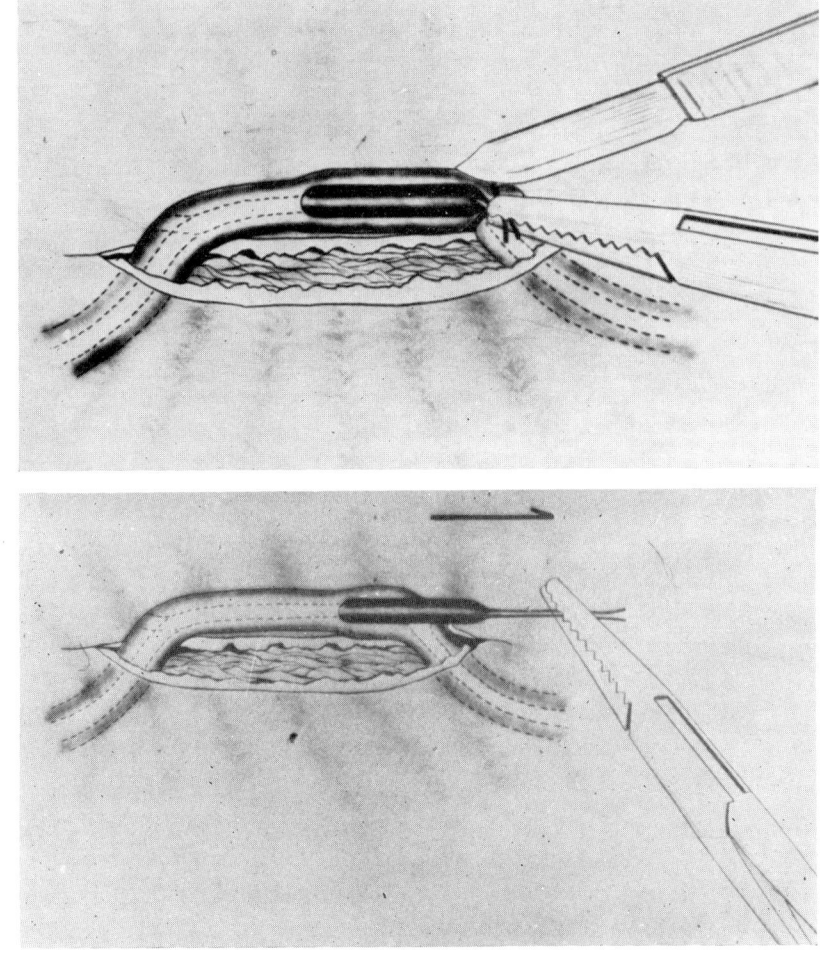

Figure 17-6 and 7. Diagramatic representation of removal of intravasal thread. The stay suture is cut and the intravasal thread is removed by pulling the attached nylon.

the remaining animals were sacrificed. Vasography revealed the following: where surgical nylon thread was employed (eleven cases), nine vasa recanalized, and two remained occluded; where surgical silk was used as the intravasal thread (eleven cases), nine vasa were restored to patency, while two remained occluded. In the eight animals in which plastic material had been inserted, four showed recanalization and four persistent occlusion. Tissue damage was produced where the intravasal thread had been too large; this resulted in vasal stricture following its removal. Excessive tension on the filiform threads produced severe vasal damage and eliminated the possibility of patency restoration.

Histologic examinations were performed in order to assess tissue reactions. Where surgical nylon was used as the intravasal thread (twelve animals), there was one case of moderate tissue reaction, one case of mild tissue reaction, and ten cases showed no significant changes. Where surgical silk thread was employed (twelve cases), one case showed moderate tissue reaction, two cases exhibited mild tissue reaction, and nine cases showed no significant changes. Of the ten animals in which plastic materials had been inserted, there were four cases with tissue reaction (two moderate and two mild) and six cases with no significant changes.

The scrotal portion of the vas is considered to be the best site for intravasal thread insertion because of the relative absence of the sheath. Occlusion of the vasal lumen with an intravasal thread large enough to cause vasal blockage, but not so large as to distend it, proved satisfactory. Surgical nylon thread appears to be the product of choice, for surgical nylon sutures left in the human long after abdominal surgery exert no harmful effects on living tissues.

Occlusion reversibility is accomplished easily by cutting and pulling the filiform nylon threads.

The intravasal thread insertion technique is technically as simple as that for an ordinary vasectomy. However, restoration of vasal patency following intravasal thread occlusion is simpler than the ordinary vasovasotomy.

The exact mechanism by which the intravasal thread stops sperm passage is unknown. It might act merely as a mechanical device to block the sperm transport route. It is possible that changes in local vasal peristalsis and intravasal environmental changes in the immediate area of the intravasal thread may interfere with sperm transport; however, they do not appear to play an important role in blocking sperm passage. Sperm may pass through the dilated vasal lumen with an intravasal thread *in situ*, and sperm passage can be restored upon removal of the thread. These findings reinforce the belief that the intravasal thread acts locally by mechanically occluding the route of sperm transport.

HUMAN STUDIES

Intravasal thread studies have been done on a total of 216 men. The device was placed in the vas under local anesthesia; a single (3–4 cm) scrotal incision was used.

Semen specimens in 195 cases contained no sperm (or fewer than 7 million per cubic centimeter) twenty-four days postoperatively or following three ejaculations. In 21 cases sperm reappeared in the ejaculate in the amount of 30.7 million per cubic centimeter approximately thirty-one days after the previous azoospermic state. Six cases whose ejaculates contained more than 60 million sperm per cubic centimeter were reoperated upon. In 4 of the 6 cases, sperm had passed through the dilated lumen of the vas with the intravasal thread *in situ*. It is possible that the vasal dilatation resulted from increased intravasal pressure caused by deposition or stasis of continued sperm production attributable to an imbalance between spermatogenesis and spermatolysis. In the two other cases, the distal end of the intravasal thread penetrated the vasal wall on one side and almost protruded through the lumen. Thus, the intravasal thread did not function as a plug. The normal course of the vas was found to be bent markedly at the site of penetration; this possibly might be attributable to extensive fibrotic contracture of surrounding tissues after the intravasal thread insertion. When the thread was placed close to the original aperature through which it had been inserted, the distal end of the intravasal thread might erode and penetrate the vasal wall.

To reverse the procedure, the vas was exposed in the same

manner as it was for the intravasal thread insertion. The thread was removed from the vas by cutting and pulling the filiform nylon thread with a pair of mosquito forceps.

Eight volunteers were studied as to reversibility about five months after the intravasal thread had been inserted; their semen had been azoospermic about one month postoperatively. After removal of the intravasal thread, semen specimens of 7 of the 8 cases contained an average count of 54 million viable sperm per cubic centimeter about one month postoperatively. This indicates that vasal patency can be restored properly and satisfactorily. In the remaining case, marked vasal fibrosis was noted and the vas was divided accidentally during the surgery for intravasal thread removal.

SUMMARY AND CONCLUSIONS

Intravasal thread was placed in the vas for the purpose of performing a reversible vasal occlusion.

In the majority of cases, sperm passage was inhibited as long as the intravasal thread remained in the vas. However, in a small number of cases, sperm passed through the dilated vasal lumen with the intravasal thread *in situ*. This failure was more evident in the human cases.

With the removal of the intravasal thread, patency of the vas could be restored. The filiform nylon thread holds the intravasal thread in place and permits its easy removal. Histologic studies demonstrated no marked vasal tissue reactions. Nylon thread remained inert after remaining in the vas for several months.

This preliminary study indicates that it is possible to produce reversible vasal occlusion with intravasal thread insertion. The relatively few cases in which sperm escaped through the dilated vasal lumen around the intravasal thread is a problem which must be overcome before the procedure can be presented as a fully proved technique. Further modifications of the procedure can lead to its widespread use as a practical method of producing reversible vasal occlusion.

Chapter 18

TUBAL STERILIZATION WITH CLIPS

MOTOYUKI HAYASHI

In order to evaluate the validity of tubal sterilization with clips under culdoscopy or culdotomy, a preliminary report on the silk ligature method by the vaginal route will be discussed. This will provide preliminary evaluatory data.

Silk ligature method: The data for this study were obtained from 6,887 questionnaires answered by 10,693 patients who had this surgical procedure performed between 1960 and 1967.

The majority of women ranged in age from 30 to 35 years; the second largest age group was in the 36 to 40 year old range. Specific ages of the patients were: under 25, 1.7 percent; 26 to 30, 21.7 percent; 31 to 35, 41.2 percent; 36 to 40, 26.4 percent; 41 to 45, 8.7 percent; and 0.2 percent were 46 or older.

The majority of women were multiparas with one to four children each. Number of children of women in the sample: zero, 0.62 percent; 1, 6.45 percent; 2, 47.10 percent; 3, 35.60 percent; 4, 8.28 percent; 5, 1.60 percent 6, 0.14 percent; 7, 0.21 percent; 8 or more, 0.06 percent.

Intravenous anesthesia with sodium pentothal was used in the majority of cases; dosages ranged from 0.5 gm to 1.5 gm (0.5 gm, 19.6%; 0.8 gm, 44.6%; 1.0 gm, 7.42%; 1.5 gm, 0.54%). Intratracheal intubation was not considered a necessity. Where spinal anesthesia was employed, xylocaine was the anesthetic of choice (24.1%). Also used were Percamine-S® (3.24%), Nupercaine® (0.23%), Tropacocaine (0.17%), and Percamine-L (0.09%). One death was attributed to anesthetic failure.

The peritoneum was opened anteriorly per vagina in the vast majority of cases (96%). Posterior section and anterior and posterior section combined were used also. The Madlener procedure was used in 73.1 percent of the cases; the Pomeroy technique was employed in 26.9 percent of the women.

The average operating time was 12 minutes; the entire time range of the procedure was from 5 to over 30 minutes.

There were postoperative pregnancies. These were attributed to tuboabdominal fistula (9), tubal rupture (6), ligature slippage (4), ligature relaxation (4), and tubal pregnancy (7).

Operative complications included hemorrhage, injuries to the bladder and/or rectum, and tubal rupture. This suggests the possibility that the vaginal route is a more difficult surgical procedure than the abdominal route. Postoperative complications included intra-abdominal hematomas and intraligamentous hematomas. There were two fatalities, one from hemorrhage and the other from anesthetic failure.

Postoperative somatic complaints included: lumbago, headache, shoulder stiffness, weight gain, heavy-headedness, dizziness, cold feet, abdominal pain, insomnia, and dyspareunia. Although the majority of patients experienced no libidinal changes (59.6%), 38.6 percent of the women reported increased libido, and 1.77 percent reported decreases in libido. It is possible that these reported changes are not significant but merely represent psychosomatic manifestations.

The silk ligature method is not recommended for it requires unusual technical skill; deep anesthesia, which can be dangerous; and can produce foreign-body reactions.

TUBAL STERILIZATION WITH TANTALUM, SILVER, OR PLASTIC CLIPS

Clinical work with this technique was done in the period between 1962 to 1968.

The principal animal experimental work was done by Drs. H.H. Neumann and H.C. Frick.[1] They employed tantalum and silver clips to occlude the oviducts of baboons and rhesus monkeys. There was no evidence of sloughing, irritation, or other inflammatory reactions. Of 18 clips applied, 2 slipped off the tissue; all the smooth-edged, machine-made clips remained *in situ*. Hydrosalpinx developed between the blocks when 2 clips were inserted. The results of patency restoration after the clips had been removed were not conclusive; some oviducts had patency restoration, some remained occluded, and there was evidence of mucosal damage and fibrotic changes.

Plastic clips also have been applied to rabbit oviducts for periods of from one to five weeks. This produced a slight inflammatory reaction and minimal side effects.

The clip method was tested in 82 human cases with culdoscopy and in 50 cases with culdotomy. The age distribution and the parity data of the patients was essentially the same as it was for the silk ligature cases.

For the cases performed under culdoscopy, local and inhalation anesthesia were preferred, but intravenous anesthesia was also used. The vast majority of culdotomy patients were spinally anesthetized, but intravenous anesthesia also was employed.

The stapling instrument consists of: a telescope; a light; and a freely movable grasping arc. This seizes and clutches the oviduct under direct vision and leads it between the jaws of the clamp. The instrument is inserted into the cul-de-sac through a cannula which is elliptical in cross-section and has a diameter of 9–12 mm.

Postoperative complications were the following: 2 ectopic pregnancies; 3 uterine pregnancies; 3 cases of hemorrhage; 1 peritonitis case; and 1 case of rectal fistula.

Sterility duration for the culdoscopy patients was the following: under 1 year, 5 cases; 1 to 2 years, 5 cases; 2 to 3 years, 8 cases; 3 to 4 years, 13 cases; 4 to five years, 21 cases; and 30 cases were sterile for more than 5 years. Culdotomy patients exhibited the following postoperative sterility: 1 to 2 years, 4 cases; 2 to 3 years, 9 cases; 3 to 4 years, 13 cases; 4 to 5 years, 11 cases; and over 5 years, 3 cases.

Where clips are used with culdoscopy, they remain *in situ*, but the procedure is difficult from a technical standpoint. In order for the clip method to have increased application, it is necessary that both the material and the design of the clips be improved. If modifications were made, it is possible that the clip technique could become the simplest, most reversible method of sterilization possible.

REFERENCE

1. Neumann, H.H., and Frick, H.C.: Occlusion of the fallopian tubes with tantalum clips. *Amer J Obstet Gynec*, 81:803, 1961.

Chapter 19

TEMPORARY OCCLUSION OF THE DUCTUS DEFERENS[*]

K.H. Moon and Ray G. Bunge

Bilateral vasectomy has been considered the only reliable procedure for permanent male sterilization, although surgical reversibility is possible. Low reversibility and pregnancy rates following surgical reanastomosis of the ductus deferens has caused vasectomy to lose popularity as a temporary sterilization technique. Therefore, in the last few years, a reversible procedure for fertility control in the male has been under study; and a number of promising procedures which can produce a transient sterility in experimental animals have been developed. These procedures generally are based on mechanical obstruction such as blockage of a portion of the vas with minimum damage; restoration of fertility occurs with the removal of the plugging material. Materials used were silicone-rubber, nylon wire, and silk sutures. In order to produce a reversible sterilization of the male, a nontoxic plastic device to block the lumen of the vas has been developed. Fertility is restored by its removal. The results of the insertion of the device and its subsequent removal from the ductus deferens in dogs is reported here. The surgical procedure for insertion and removal also are discussed.

MATERIALS AND METHODS

Thirteen adult male dogs varying from 15 to 25 kg in weight were used for this study. All of the animals were able to ejaculate when masturbated. Semen samples were examined simply for the presence of sperm. All of the animals had been proved to be normospermic on two or three occasions before surgical experimentation. A plastic device was made of inter-

[*] Gratitude and appreciation are expressed to A.W. Bauger, who prepared the device used in the study.

medic polyethylene tubing, P.E. 50 (I.D. 0.023″, O.D.O.038″). It was 7 cm long, with both ends tapered by heat treatment (Fig. 19-1). The midportion, which occluded the lumen of the ductus deferens was about 3 cm long. One end of this device was threaded into a straight sewing needle (Sharps 7, Arms needle, Redditch, England) and then placed in a Steri-Vas Gas sterilizer.

PROCEDURE FOR THE INSERTION OF THE DEVICE INTO THE VAS

Under general anesthesia, the scrotal skin was prepared. The ductus deferens was palpated through the right scrotal sac and was made to lie just under the skin surface by digital pressure. Two towel forceps then were applied around the vas (Fig. 19-2).

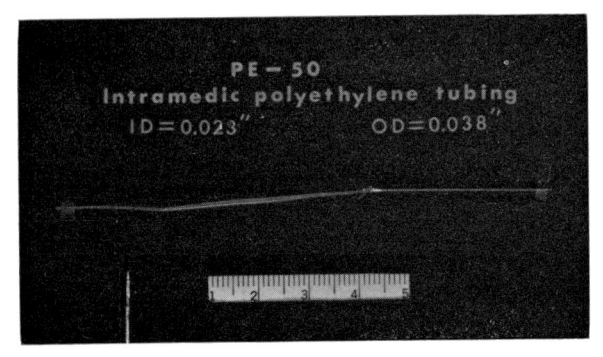

Figure 19-1. Configuration of plastic device for human ductus deferens.

A small incision was made over the ductus deferens between the two clips, and the tissue over the ductus was separated by blunt dissection. The ductus was isolated with minimal interference to its vascular supply (Fig. 19-3). When the distal portion of the exposed ductus was stretched digitally, a transluscent whitish streak appeared; this represented the lumen (Fig. 19-4). A straight needle carrying the device was inserted into the lumen. Both ends of the device, which were out of the ductus, were clamped with silver clips (Fig. 19-5). The clips prevented mobilization of the device in the vasal lumen and also acted as a mark for identification at the time of removal. The same procedure was done in the left ductus deferens, and the wound then was closed.

206   *Human Sterilization*

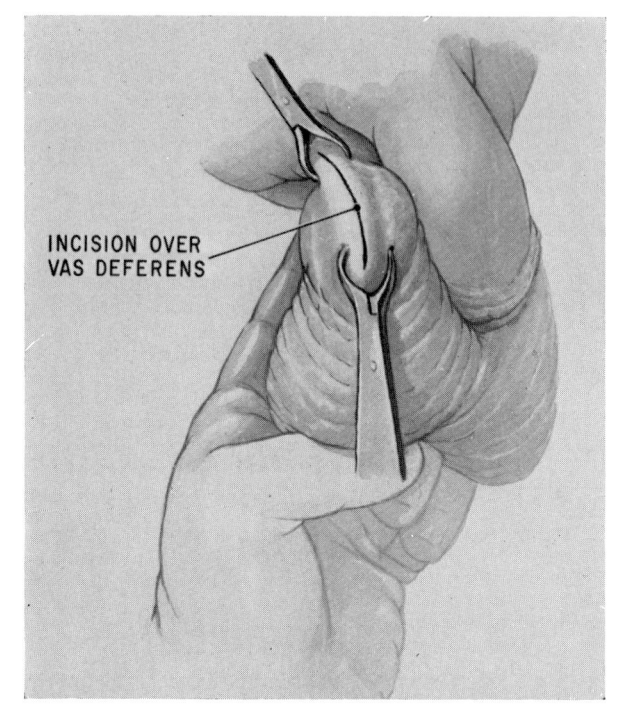

Figure 19-2. Ductus deferens fixed with towel forceps and in position for incision.

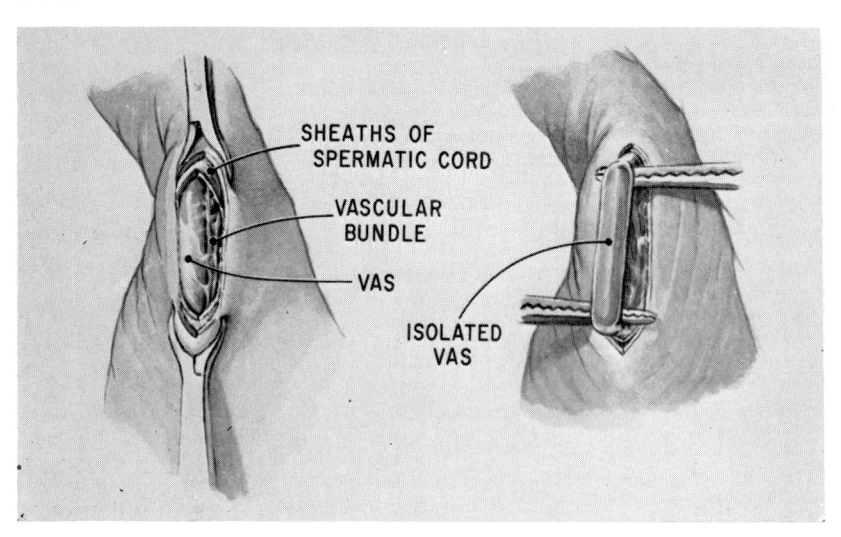

Figure 19-3. Isolation of the ductus deferens.

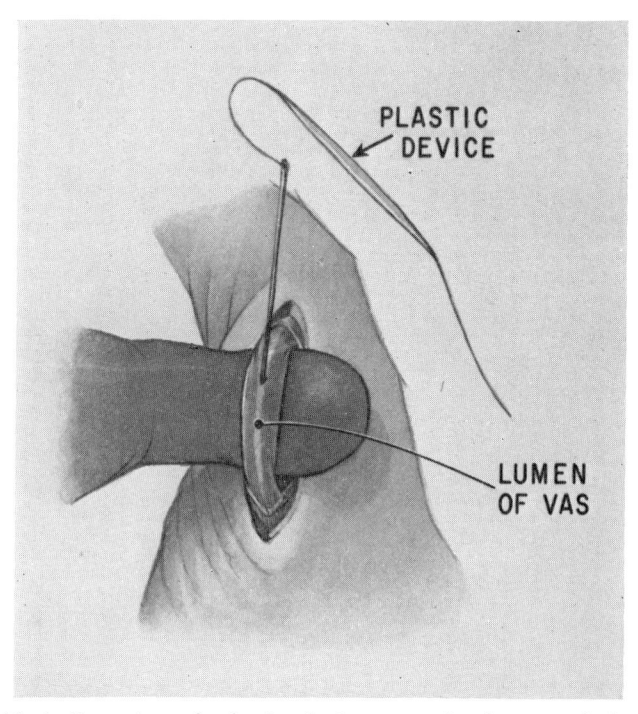

Figure 19-4. Insertion of plastic device into the lumen of the ductus deferens.

In general, semen was collected two weeks following the insertion of the device; thereafter, two more ejaculated specimens were examined at one-week intervals. Success of this procedure is indicated when there is a constant azoospermic condition in the period of observation. The reversibility of this procedure was tested by the presence of sperm after the removal of the device from the ductus.

PROCEDURE FOR REMOVAL OF THE DEVICE FROM THE VAS

After the customary scrotal preparation, both clips were identified by digital palpation of the scrotal skin. A surgical incision exposed the vas; the device was located by the identification of the two clips. The ductus was isolated from the surrounding

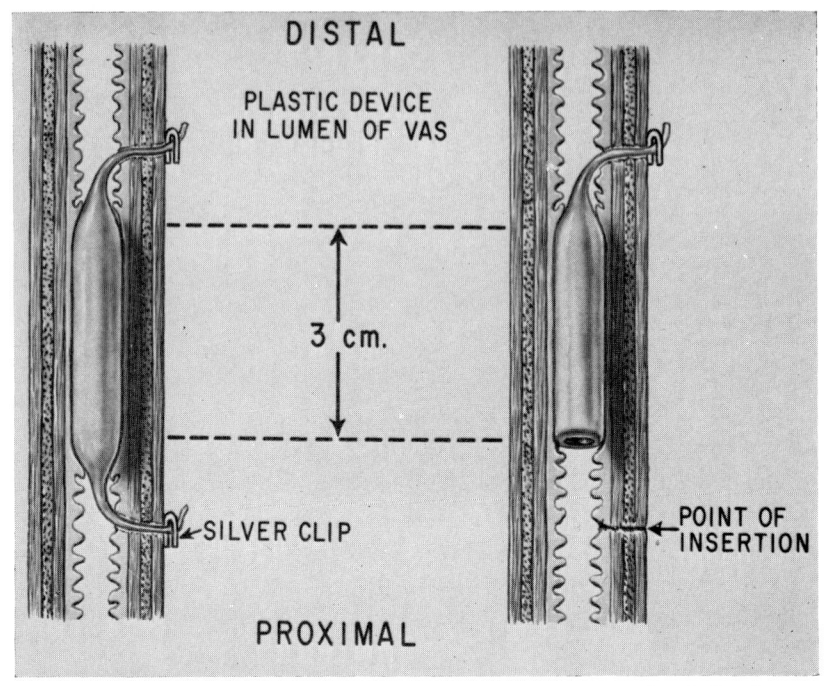

Figure 19-5. Left. Two silver clips are applied at both ends of the device. Right: Modified plastic device; only one end is fixed with a silver clip.

tissue. One end of the device with its silver clip was pulled out after the release of the other clip. The scrotal skin was closed in the usual manner. Semen examinations were performed at two, three, and four week intervals after the removal of the devices to confirm the presence of sperm.

HISTOLOGIC STUDY

In order to observe the local tissue reaction, occluded areas of the ductus were examined histologically four weeks after the insertion of the device.

RESULTS

As is shown in the table consistent azoospermic conditions were obtained in 12 out of 13 dogs—two, three, and four weeks after the insertion of the devices. One case which failed to

TABLE 19-I
SEMEN EXAMINATIONS AFTER INSERTION AND REMOVAL OF THE DEVICE

Dog Number	After Inserting Device 2 Weeks	3 Weeks	4 Weeks	After Removing Device 2 Weeks	3 Weeks	4 Weeks
1	−	−	−	+	++	++
2	−	−	−	+	++	++
3	−	−	−	++	++	++
4	−	−	−	+	++	++
5	−	−	−	+	++	++
6	−	−	−	+	++	++
7	−	−	−	+	++	++
8	−	−	−	++	++	++
9	−	−	−	++	++	++
10	++	++	++			
11	−	−	−	++	++	++
12	−	−	−	++	++	++
13	−	−	−	++	++	++

Code: + Means less than 10 sperm in high-power field; ++ means more than 10 sperm in high-power field; − means no sperm in high-power field.

produce an azoospermic condition was shown to have had an incomplete occlusion in the right ductus, with motile sperm beyond the occluded area. Also, the occluded area was only 1 cm long. Complete occlusion in the left ductus was proved by both the absence of sperm beyond the occluded area and injection of indigo dye. The length of this occluded area was 3 cm. Therefore, it is apparent that nonocclusion of the right ductus was the cause of failure.

SEMEN CHARACTERISTICS AFTER THE REMOVAL OF THE DEVICE

All 12 dogs which had successful occlusion with the plastic device showed recovery of sperm two weeks after its removal. At this time there was low viability, poor activity, and a reduced number of sperm; however, sperm viability, activity, and number improved significantly by three weeks, and a normal picture was obtained at four weeks postremoval.

HISTOLOGIC STUDY

The tissue of occluded areas of the ductus was examined histologically (Fig. 19–6). The lumen of the occluded area

3. Kothari, M.L., and Pardenani, D.S.: Temporary sterility of the male by intra-vasal contraception device (IUCD): A preliminary communication. *Ind J Surg*, 29:357, 1967.
4. Segal, S.J.: *Annual Reports*. The Population Council, New York, 1965, p. 26.

Chapter 20

THE SCOPE OF LIQUID PLASTICS AND OTHER CHEMICALS FOR BLOCKING THE FALLOPIAN TUBE

B. RAKSHIT[*]

Chemical blockage of the fallopian tubes with the idea of replacing laparotomy for female sterilization was attempted as early as 1964, and was reported in 1965.[*] The procedure was used initially in elderly patients who required hysterectomy but who had healthy and patent fallopian tubes. Blockage was demonstrated with quinine and urethane solutions. Recently, the use of liquid plastics which solidify upon the addition of a catalyst has been promising. The scope of the methods used and the possibility of reversibility need further investigation.

METHODS

The liquid silicone plastics (manufactured by Dow Corning) used in this study become solid upon the addition of a catalyst. Solidification time depends upon the amount of catalyst used; a dilution proportion for the catalysts which allows a working time of ten to fifteen minutes has been determined. Barium sulfate (15%) is added to make the plastic radio-opaque. Ten ml of the mixture are put into a syringe fitted to a wide-bore uterine cannula of a size suitable to the size of the cervical os. (Fig.

---

[*] The author wishes to express appreciation to Drs. H.L. Saha, S.R. Mukherjee, and S.C. Laha of R.G. Kar Medical College for their assistance with the college facilities; Dr. H.L. Saha also granted permission for the experiments and assisted with funds. R.K. Lahiri and Dr. D.K. Roy are thanked for their assistance in the fertility trial conducted at the Calcutta Zoo. Appreciation is given to Professors S. Sarker and R.K. Pal for their assistance in animal experiments; and to the house staff of R.G. Kar Medical College for their aid, especially Drs. T. Dasmahapatra, G. Mansukhani, and Ajoy Moitra. Dr. E. Mullison and Dow Corning Center for Aid to Medical Research are thanked for supplying liquid plastics free of cost and distributing information.

20–1). The plastic and the catalyst for each injection are stirred briskly within the syringe. The piston is inserted, the air gap is disbursed, and the liquid level is adjusted to reach the tip of the cannula. (Fig. 20–2).

The cannula is inserted into the uterine cavity through the cervix; care should be taken to maintain a tight fit at the cervical

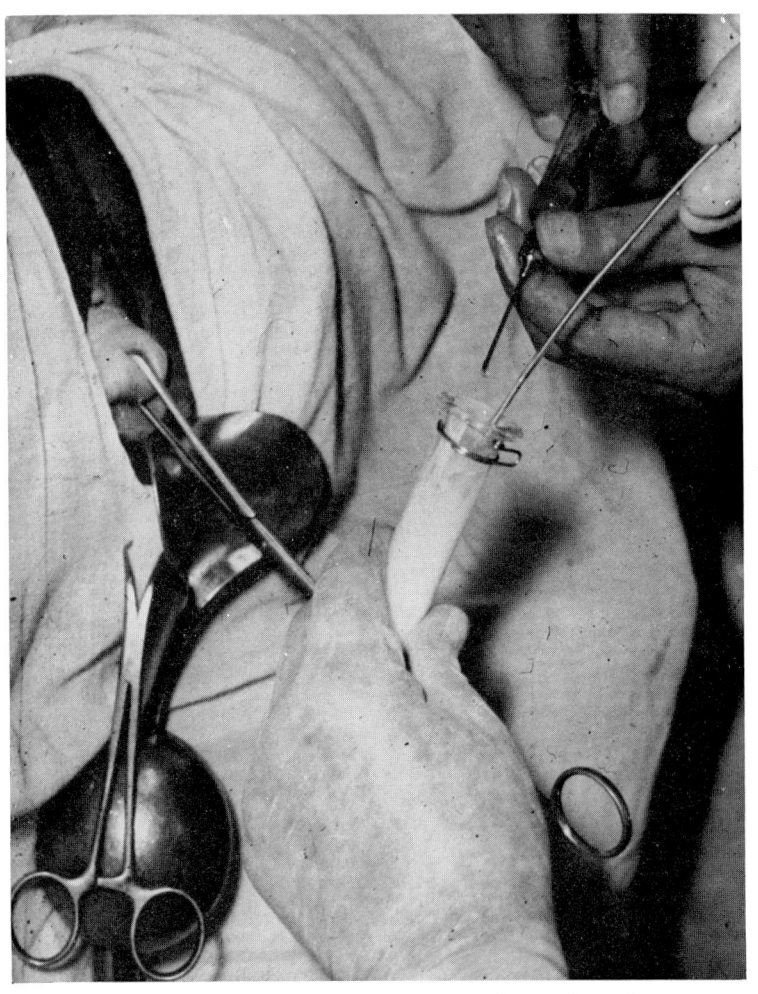

Figure 20–1. Plastic and catalyst being inserted into hypodermic syringe which has been fitted with wide bore cannula.

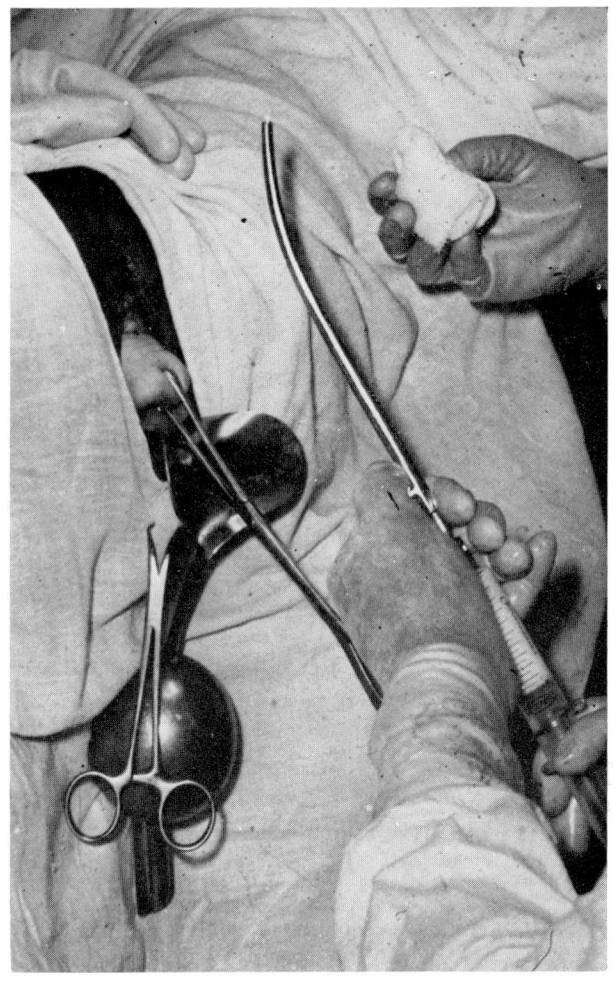

Figure 20-2. Plastic level is adjusted to reach tip of cannula.

os (Fig. 20-3). About 5 to 6 ml of the solution are injected. The cannula is withdrawn and both the syringe and cannula are washed immediately in xylol before the liquid can set. The plastic pours out of the uterine cavity after the cannula is withdrawn. (Fig. 20-4). To facilitate cleaning the uterine cavity, the cervix is dilated and sponged with gauze on a uterine dressing forceps. Before the plastic is injected, the same cannula is utilized for an

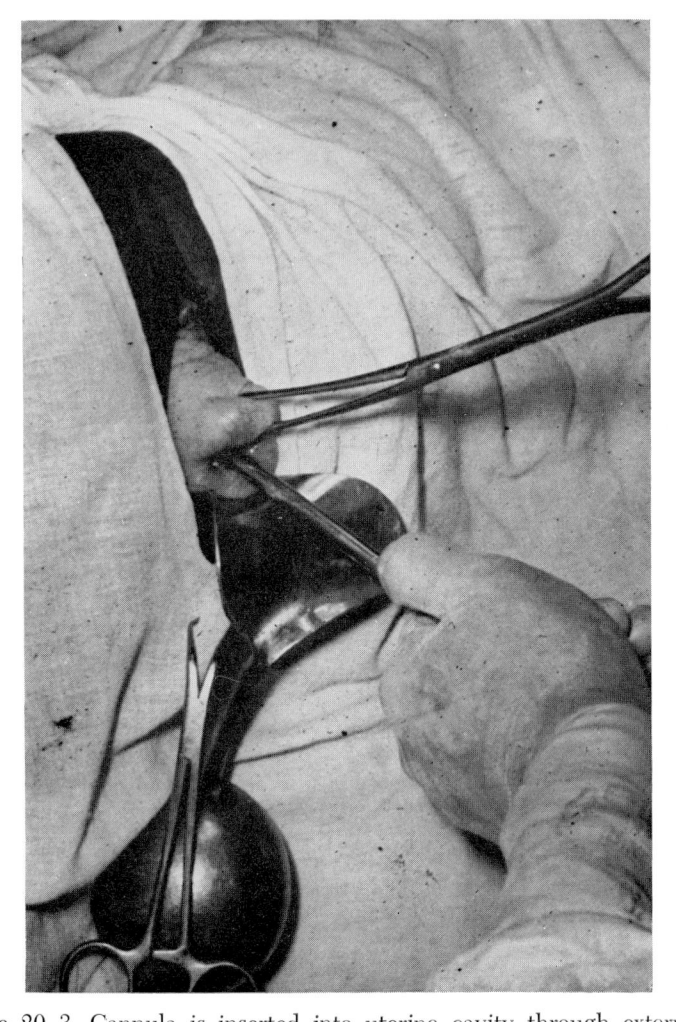

Figure 20-3. Cannula is inserted into uterine cavity through external os.

insufflation. Plastic injection is undertaken only when there is positive insufflation.

In a series of previously published cases[2,3] all attempts were made through the cervix. The few failures were due to: loosely fitting cannulas; doubtfully positive insufflation tests at high pressure; the use of too much barium sulfate, making the solution too thick; and blockage of the cannula. In later trials, attention to these points prevented failures.

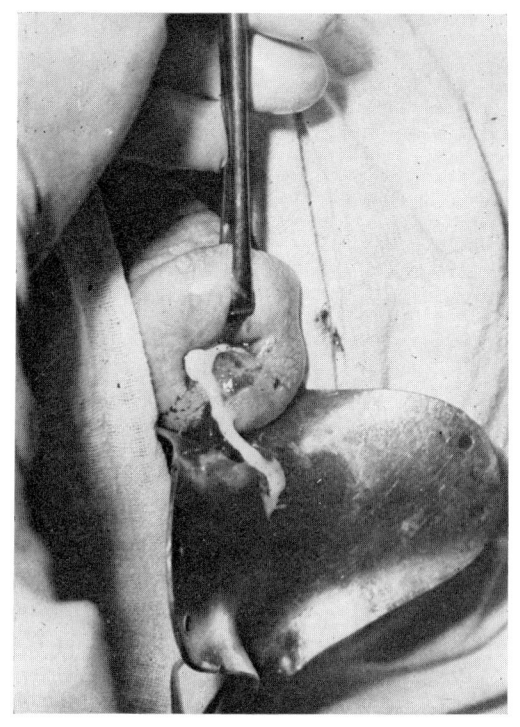

Figure 20-4. Plastic runs from uterine cavity following withdrawal of cannula.

In some cases during tubal ligation by the abdominal route, plastic has been instilled through the abdominal ostium of the tube; ligation is done only near the uterine end, with or without resection of a small portion of the tube. The object of this was to study possible tubal rejection of the plastic; to study the possibility of patency restoration by removal of the plastic; and to use plastic by the abdominal route in place of tubal ligation in order to prevent the adverse sequelae of ligation and resection.

ANIMAL EXPERIMENTS

Surgery was performed on 15 rabbits; 3 died during anesthesia, and 2 died within two to three postoperative days. Two animals were injected with sodium morrhuate, and liquid plastic was used with 8 rabbits (S-521 in 5 cases and 68–110 fluid in 3 cases).

The 2 animals injected with sodium morrhuate showed complete fallopian tube blockage and no uterine damage. x-ray studies of the rabbits injected with plastics showed that the plastics had been rejected in 6 of the 8 animals after 2 weeks. Fertility trials of plastic-injected rabbits at the Calcutta Zoo demonstrated that 4 cases with x-ray negative shadows conceived within six weeks; 2 cases with x-ray positive shadows conceived after eighteen weeks, apparently with subsequent rejection of the plastic.

Reversibility studies with rhesus monkeys failed; this may be attributable to the very narrow and small oviducts of these monkeys. Studies of reversibility are being conducted on langur monkeys at present.

HUMAN EXPERIMENTS

Vaginal instillation studies with S-521 were done on 14 women; 6 of these had salpingectomy, hysterectomy, or ligation and 8 had intact oviducts. There were 9 satisfactory blockages, 3 doubtful cases, and 2 failures. Follow-up showed no rejection up to nine postoperative months; there was 1 pregnancy in a case with a doubtful shadow in the x-ray.

Vaginal instillation studies with S-5392 in 6 cases with salpingectomy, hysterectomy, or tubal ligation gave no satisfactory blockage results; 4 cases were doubtful and 2 were negative.

Abdominal instillation of S-521 was attempted in 7 women; 3 of these cases had intact oviducts, 2 had simple ligation, and 2 had ligation with loop removal. There was no rejection up to eleven months postoperatively. Pregnancy occurred in 1 of the cases with previous simple ligation. Reversibility studies have not been attempted to date.

The animal experiments demonstrate that the material is harmless to the tissues. Even when the chemical is spilled, subsequent laparotomy demonstrated no adhesions.

Liquid plastics have been used in 27 women; 20 cases have had vaginal instillation through the cervix, and 7 cases have had the plastic inserted through the abdominal ostium of the fallopian tube at laparotomy.

Cervical instillation with Silastic-521 demonstrated 9 satisfactory blockages, 3 doubtful cases, and 2 unsatisfactory cases. Spilling into the peritoneal cavity occurred in only 1 case.

The results with the 6 cases in which Silastic-5392 was used were unsatisfactory. The material is very sticky, and it solidifies very quickly. A small quantity of the plastic was found to have entered the oviduct in 4 of the 6 cases studied.

Follow-up studies by x-ray on all cases who did not have salpingectomy shows that the material has not been rejected; one patient has retained the plastic for eleven months (Fig. 20-5).

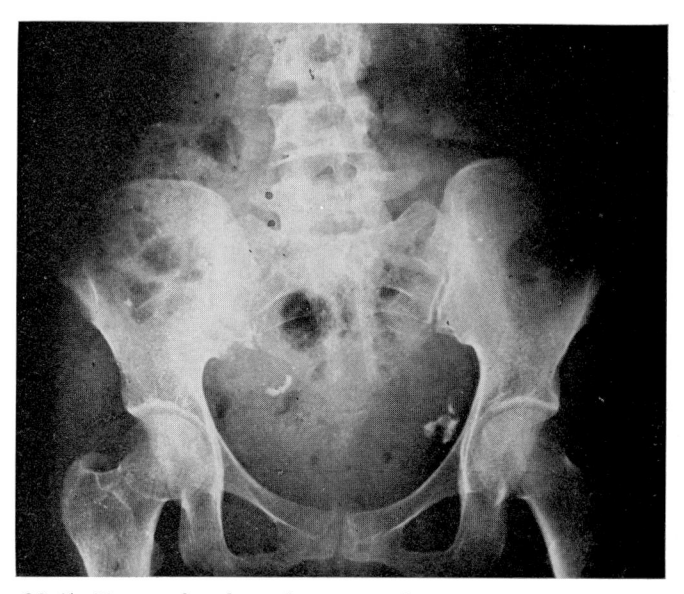

Figure 20-5. X-ray of pelvis showing radio-opaque impregnated plastic material in fallopian tubes.

None of the cases who have been instilled with plastic without tubal ligation or excision has conceived in a period of up to two years.

Since the Indian government is paying an incentive fee for sterilization, it is difficult to get volunteers to subject themselves to plastic-instillation experiments. It is anticipated that future studies will be made with these materials.

DISCUSSION

Liquid plastics appear to be harmless to both human an animal tissues. Many of these materials are being used in plastic and blood vessel surgery.

The plastics can be inserted blindly through a tight-fitting uterine cannula to reach the fallopian tubes and solidify there. When the chemical solidifies, it assumes a segmented appearance because of tubal peristalsis. It is simple to empty the uterine cavity; x-rays have demonstrated no plastic within the uterus and there is no danger in case of spillage.

The material spilled into the peritoneal cavity in only one case in these studies. High viscosity and rapid solidification tend to prevent such complications. Spillage into the peritoneal cavity in this series was attributed to solidification failure due to a stale catalyst. In animal experiments, deliberate spillage into the peritoneal cavity was permitted, but no adverse tissue reaction or adhesions were found. Spilling will not occur if the proper amount of both plastic and catalyst are employed.

The lumen of the oviduct is completely filled with plastic; blockage is complete, and no danger of ectopic pregnancies is anticipated. Since the material is soft and pliable, it does not cause pain, damage the tubal wall, or restrict tubal movement.

Future experimentation with the method is necessary. It is important to demonstrate that the plastic can be removed from the tube abdominally, and that tubal patency and fertility can be restored. Even if patency restoration is not possible, plastic instillation is superior to tubal ligation for sterilization purposes.

It is possible that plastic instillation can be accomplished without the use of anesthesia. Some trial cases with chemical irritants have been conducted without anesthesia. If the need for anesthesia is eliminated, it might be possible to establish blockage with plastics as a mass, large-scale contraception method.

If the plastic is not removed from the uterus by dilatation and sponging, the major portion of the liquid flows out spontaneously. It is anticipated that the remaining liquid, even the solidified portion, will be extruded spontaneously.[4]

It is necessary to demonstrate that effective contraception can be achieved by plastic instillation rather than tubal ligation by any route. Animal and human experiments are necessary to establish this point. Tubal ligation involves more postoperative care and involves such known complications as menstrual disorders, pelvic pain, and hydrosalpinx formation. Even if anesthesia were required for plastic instillation, it would still be preferable to tubal ligation. No anatomical alteration is made, for the plastic is pliable and soft and adapts to tubal movements; tubal perforation appears to be very unlikely.

The method is not intended to replace intra-uterine contraceptive devices, but it should replace tubal ligation. It is possible that abdominal instillation will have to be used, but the vaginal route should be the aim in procedure improvement.

Attempts at sterilization by the plastic instillation method have not been made before Shubeck[4] tried intra-uterine mold formation. Pitkin[1] instilled sodium morrhuate after abdominal ligation in order to produce fibrosis of the remaining portion of the tube without hydrosalpinx formation. Much additional work is needed in the method; experiments with monkeys are already being undertaken.

REFERENCES

1. Pitkin, Roy M.: Sodium Morrhuate for tubal sterilization. *Obstet Gynec*, 28:680, 1966.
2. Rakshit, B.: Intratubal blocking device for sterilization without laparotomy. *Calcutta Med J*, 65:90, 1968.
3. Rakshit, B.: Experiments on tubal blocking for sterilization without laparotomy. *J Obstet Gynec India*, XVIII, No. 2, April, 1968.
4. Shubeck, Frank: Use of polymerizing plastics in pregnancy prevention. Preliminary report. *Obstet Gynec*, 25:724, 1965.

Chapter 21

OCCLUSION OF THE VAS DEFERENS WITH SILASTIC

Kenneth A. Laurence

The recent development and availability of medical grade elastomers prompted the investigation of the possibility of utilizing such substances as a means of creating a temporary occlusion in the vas deferens as a means of fertility regulation. It was considered that such an occlusion could be made a reversible method, and as such, would be a more acceptable method for males than the permanent method which now exists.

ELASTOMER

Medical grade liquid Silastic S-5392 (Dow Corning) was mixed with a catalyst immediately prior to its introduction into the lumen of the vas. The Silastic was introduced, in 0.05 to 0.08 ml amounts, via a 1.0 cc disposable tuberculin syringe with a 23 gauge needle. Immediately after the introduction of the material was initiated and the flow of spermatozoa could be observed, an artery forceps was used to prevent further movement of the elastomer. This created a ballooning of the vas deferens in that area. A second artery forceps then was placed on the vas to prevent a backwash until the liquid Silastic had vulcanized. This solidification process generally occurred within three to four minutes, after which time the forceps were removed.

ANIMALS

For the injection of the animals, general anesthesia (Diabutol) was used. Through a longitudinal abdominal incision, the testes and the vas deferens were exposed and made ready for a bilateral introduction of the Silastic. Later, the reproductive organs were returned to their proper position.

Three species of animals were employed for this study. Twenty young adult male rats (Holtzman) weighing between 220 and 250 gm and 10 males weighing more than 600 gm were used for testing the ability of the Silastic plug to prevent pregnancy during cohabitation with a female.

Twelve male guinea pigs, of the Rockefeller University strain, weighing between 600 and 750 gm were electroejaculated[1] after the introduction of the vas plug. This permitted an evaluation of the semen sample in respect to seminal fluid volume, cellular condition, and number of spermatozoa in the ejaculate.

Twelve adult male white New Zealand rabbits, weighing 4 to 5 kgm were used similarly to test the quality of the ejaculate as was done with the guinea pigs. These rabbits had been trained previously to service an artificial vagina.

The male rats were placed with a female partner in the state of proestrus. The following morning, the vaginal lavage was examined for the presence of spermatozoa and/or vaginal plug. This was considered day one of pregnancy. Each mated animal was thereafter followed daily to determine if the mating was fertile.

Each experimental male rat was mated three times weekly for a period of two months, and then once a week until the termination of the experiment, usually four to seven months later. The guinea pigs were electroejaculated twice weekly for periods up to four months, while the rabbits were ejaculated thrice weekly for seven to nine months. For sperm counting, the electronic method, employing a model B Coulter Counter, was used. For the guinea pig sperm counts, the settings for the instrument were Amplification 2, Aperature Current 1. For the rabbit sperm counts, the settings were Amplification 2, Aperature Current 2.

HISTOLOGY

At the termination of the experiments, the animals were sacrificed; the testes, seminal vesicles, prostate, and the vas were weighed and then fixed in Bouins solution. Later, histological sections were prepared at 7μ and stained with hematoxylin and eosin.

RESULTS

Rats

After the introduction of the Silastic into the 220–250 gm animals, fertile matings were observed for at least three contacts. After the three fertile matings, for a period of almost three months all matings resulted only in pseudopregnancy. Soon after, however, a number of pregnancies began to occur. At this time, surgical intervention into the vas revealed that the plug either had been dislodged from the original site or had been expelled completely. From further observations, it became apparent that as the animal grew in body size, the vas increased slightly in size as well, and therefore it was no longer able to retain the vulcanized Silastic in position. For this reason, the larger 600 gm male rats were used for the continuing studies. Again, after three to four fertile matings, all ensuing matings resulted in pseudopregnancies until the matings were discontinued some seven months later. In all cases, at autopsy, the testes appeared functional and unimpaired. All organs remained within the normal and expected weight range at the time of sacrifice.

Guinea Pigs

After the occlusion of the vas of the young adult guinea pigs, an average of six ejaculates were required before the samples were free of spermatozoa. The sperm counts did not drop abruptly to azoospermic levels, but instead gradually were reduced to sperm-free levels by the sixth ejaculate.

Similar to the results with the young adult male rats, the vas plug eventually was displaced from its original site and permitted the passage of viable spermatozoa into the ejaculate. As time passed, the number of sperm present in the ejaculate increased to normal preocclusion quantities. The azoospermia lasted for only a few months before the return to normal counts. The ejaculate volume remained within the normal range during the entire experimental period.

Rabbits

With the occlusion of the rabbit vas, from five to seven ejaculates were required before azoospermic levels were reached. During a period of nine months of observation, the plug was displaced in two of the rabbits. The plugs, however, never were completely expelled. In these two cases, the plug moved to a different area and permitted the passage of viable sperm in low quantities. The counts were reduced from a total count of 90 to 100 million to less than 1 million. Nevertheless, in a few mating experiences, successful pregnancies ensued even with the low total sperm count.

Although the testes (Fig. 21-1) appeared normal after a period of nine months, the epididymis was always abnormally

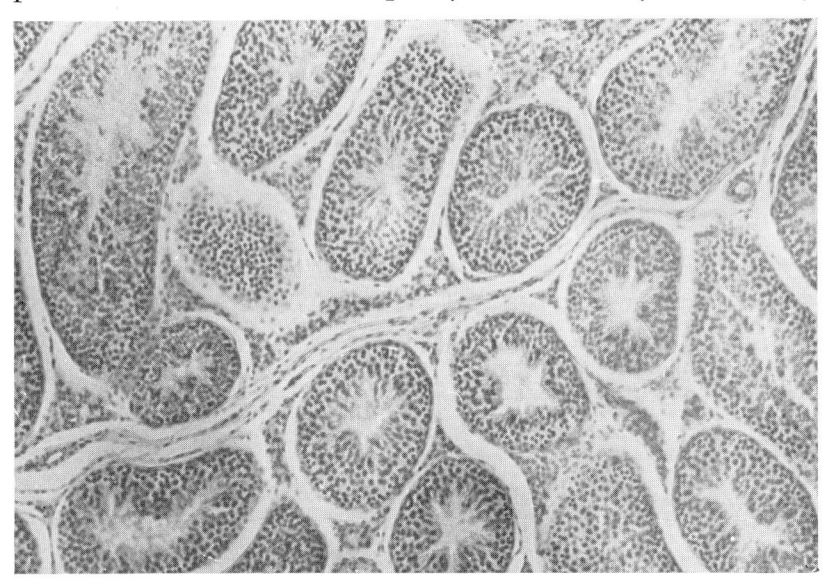

Figure 21-1. Rabbit testes removed nine months after vas occlusion. Notice that spermatogenesis has not been interrupted ($\times$ 33).

large and filled completely with spermatozoa. The section of the vas between the epididymis and the plug was filled with spermatozoa, and the lining of the vas was slightly compressed (Fig. 21-2). At the site of injection, where the Silastic first begins to occupy the area, some of the spermatozoa were compressed and trapped against the wall of the vas (Fig. 21-3). In the area where the Silastic had enlarged the lumen, no sperm could be found; the lining of the vas was severely compressed (Fig. 21-4). In the areas immediately after the plug, no sperm could be found; the lining of the vas remained normal with no apparent compression of the cellular lining (Fig. 21-5).

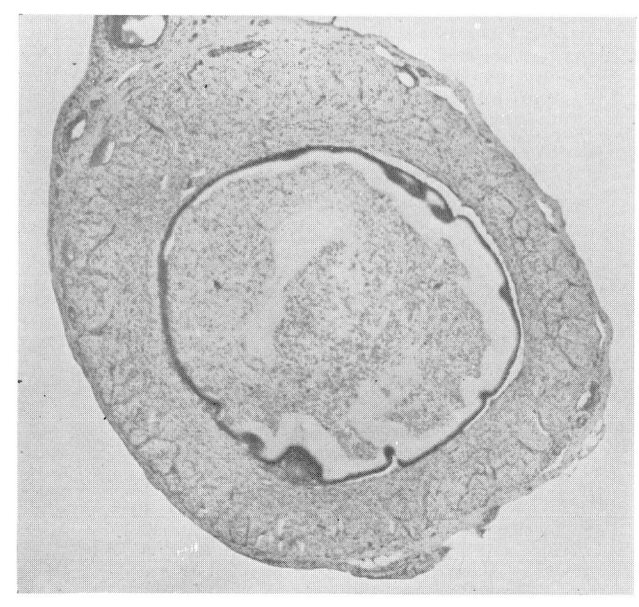

Figure 21-2. Rabbit vas removed from an area between the epididymis and the vas plug ($\times$ 30).

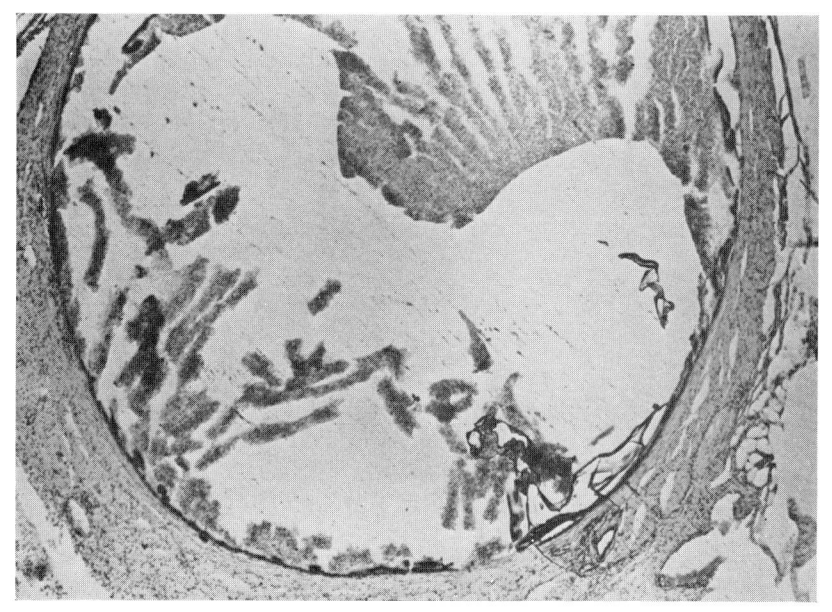

Figure 21-3. Area of the vas into which the silastic was first injected. Fragments of the silastic are apparent in the section ($\times$ 40).

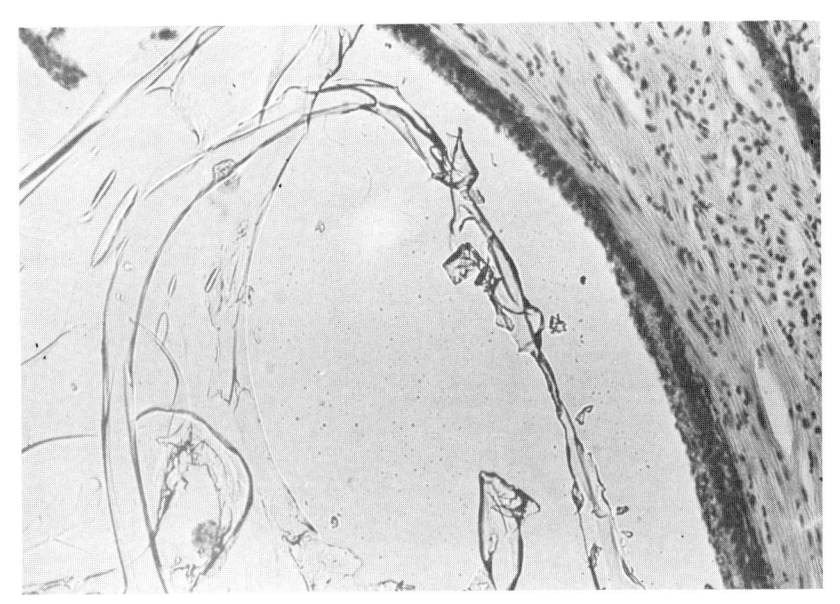

Figure 21-4. Area of the vas deferens directly in contact with the silastic plug.

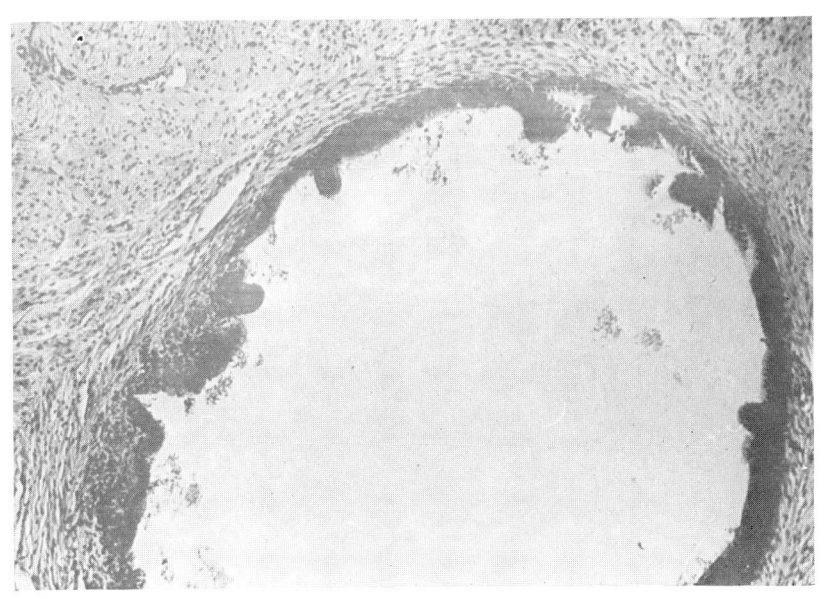

Figure 21-5. Area of the vas beyond the plug. Notice the lack of spermatozoa and the normal condition of the cellular lining. Some cellular debris is present in the lumen.

On occasion, inflammatory cells were found in the muscle layers of the vas. No other pathology associated with the plug could be observed, other than the enlargement of the epididymis.

DISCUSSION

It is obvious from these few studies that the elastomers only can be effective in occluding the vas if they are introduced into fully developed animals of any species. It is also obvious that the plug, in order to remain effective, must be fixed in place with no movement within the lumen. Since the Silastic forms with the contour of the tissue, any forced movement of the plug, therefore, will not match exactly to the contour of its new position. This will permit the passage of the dammed-up sperm through minute faults and grooves in the vulcanized plug. Pregnancies can occur even when the sperm counts are reduced to what might be considered subfertile levels.

Nevertheless, these studies suggest, as have the studies of Hrdlicka[2] and Hefnawi,[3] that it is possible to safely occlude the fallopian tube or the vas deferens without impairing these structures permanently. It is now a matter of finding a method of preventing the slightest movement of the introtubal device. If this can be accomplished, a place for vas occlusion in the armamentarium of temporary, reversible male sterilization methods can be anticipated.

REFERENCES

1. Laurence, K.A., and Carpuk, O.: The counting and sizing of guinea pig spermatozoa. *Fertil Steril, 14:*451, 1963.
2. Hrdlicka, J.G., Schwartzman, W.A., Hasel, K., and Zinsser, H.H.: New approaches to reversible seminal diversion. *Fertil Steril, 18:*289, 1967.
3. Hefnawi, F., Fuchs, A.R., and Laurence, K.A.: Control of fertility by temporary occlusion of the oviduct. *Amer J Obstet Gynec,* 99:421, 1967.

DISCUSSION: REVERSIBLE STERILIZATION

Ralph M. Richart, *Moderator*

Dr. Pai mentioned that Drs. Kothari and Pardanani were colleagues of his and he considered himself responsible for encouraging their experimentation with temporary vas occlusion. There were only a few animal experiments and some human ones, about thirteen cases to date. Results demonstrated consistently that sperm started reappearing after a certain period and that the sperm count was not totally suppressible. He wanted to know if Dr. Moon or Dr. Lee had had similar experiences. It was his opinion that the vas dilated once the lumen was occluded. The size of the material should relate to the size of the lumen. It was his considered opinion that no matter what device was inserted, the lumen of the vas would dilate with the passage of time and permit the escape of sperm.

Dr. Lee admitted that he was confronted with this problem. About ten percent of the intravasal thread patients had dilatation, and sperm counts reverted to almost preinsertion status; this represented a ten percent failure. He was now considering such factors as intravasal thread size, shape, and length in terms of correlating them with the dilatation.

Dr. Tietze wondered if he had considered using a cone-shaped device which was not tethered by a thread; as the proximal end dilated, the cone would slip further down the vas. He wanted to know if the idea was feasible and made sense.

Dr. Ko brought up Dr. Moon's mention of the fact that one of the criteria was minimum tissue reaction. The basic simplified picture was that of an elastic tube to be blocked. There is a pressure differential between the two sides; no matter what is used for blockage, the lumen seems to expand. Initially the leak would be small, but it would tend to increase. One method of counteracting this reaction would be to force the blocking material to adhere to the wall of the tube. If the blocking material were coated and then inserted, it might be possible to make the surfaces rough or porous and force tissue growth. This would make the inserted matter an integral part of the tube. However, it would present problems in removal. He suggested a Dacron coated sleeve incorporating a device such as a screw which could produce a tight plastic-to-plastic or metal-to-metal seal. If this were inserted, the Dacron would integrate with the tissue wall. If removal were desired, force could be used to break a portion of the locking device; it could be unscrewed and the Dacron sleeve could be permitted to remain.

Dr. Hulka mentioned that there had been a number of recent devices for occlusion of the vas. One interesting instrument was a dumbbell-shaped plastic appliance; it can be inserted into the lumen of the vas as easily as the intravasal thread. A suture is placed around the stricture of the dumbbell to prevent motion. He did not know if the method worked. He agreed with Dr. Ko about the use of Dacron. It has well-established biological usefulness in establishing contact between plastic and tissue; it is used in heart surgery and in ophthalmology. It may be applicable to the vas also. Mr. Rabelski suggested etched Teflon as a usable material. He supplied Teflon samples which were normally quite inert insofar as their adhesiveness to plastics. Preliminary studies inserting the Teflon into the skin of rats to test for tissue reaction indicated that the Teflon was about as adherent as Dacron, cotton fibers, or Avona. He thought it was quite feasible to insert an obstructive device into the vas; if the healing powers of the body were taken advantage of, occlusion would occur and subsequent leakage could be avoided. The problem of reestablishing patency involves occlusion reversal with a valve or a turning device that could open or close the lumen without surgery. He thought these concepts were feasible and worthy of study, but he did not know if they would work.

Dr. Zinsser stated that he had used Dr. Segal's injected silicone and was not satisfied with the results. Seven hogs and nine dogs were injected with silicone; blockage persisted for about two and a half years in the hogs and two years in the dogs without any leakage. However, after eight or nine months, the silicone, although it had not produced any tissue reaction, showed signs of degeneration. Some of the plugs were severely discolored and would fragment when pulled. In spite of this, no leakage of sperm appeared.

Electroejaculation was possible on the hogs, and masturbation on the dogs. Leakage was prevented because the silicone was deteriorating and swelling; the dilatation was tremendous. If a 3 cm plug had been inserted, a 2½ to 3 cm plug could be removed; it showed longitudinal shrinkage. Why shrinkage went in one direction or another is not known.

Dr. Zinsser continued by saying that he had four human cases who were blocked prevasectomy with 1½ mm silicone thread prevulcanized at high temperature. He wanted to stress the dimensions of the thread, for some investigators wish to use 1 mm thread, which he considers too small. An important problem is swedging a 1½ mm thread onto a straight needle; this has not been accomplished as yet. The threads that were used were inserted through the eye of a round needle; it is very difficult to get that through the vas lumen without tearing a fairly large hole and cutting the silicone. It is possible that the ultimate result will be gluing the silicone into the hole in the swedge needle; just crimping it tends to cut a great many of the nylon threads. The insertion can be made without a skin incision, and if insertion into the lumen is 3 cm, the plastic will militate against dilation for quite a long time. At present 2 groups in India are studying the procedure; it is hoped that there will be 6 groups by the end of the year. Silicone thread is being shipped to India and also is being used in preprostatectomy cases to obtain short-term information. The long-term follow-up has been discouraging.

Testicular histology returned to normal very rapidly in the dogs and hogs from whom the silicone plugs had been removed. Patency was proved in all animals by radiographic techniques. All of the animals were mated at least three times. Not a single pregnancy resulted, quantitative tests of the semen looked good, although sperm counts in the dogs are highly questionable. The testes appeared normal histologically, although thymidine uptake of both dog and hog testes was still less than thirty percent of normal for as long as four months after the occlusion was removed. The question of what vasal occlusion for two or more years does to testicular function is still open.

Dr. Schmidt expressed the opinion that the research was at-

Dr. Laurence said he had not.

Dr. Zinsser stated that there probably were tremendous interspecific differences in testicular changes resulting from vasal blockage and that it was most important to study humans now. The hog sections looked rather severely damaged, but the dog and rat sections did not. There is not sufficient good testicular biopsy material taken very early after complete vas occlusion.

Dr. Bunge stated that he had seen 11 cases of congenital absence of the ductus deferens and he did not recall any severe histologic changes. He was going to review these cases, for these represented a circumstance in which there was no duct and definite obstruction over a long period of time.

Dr. Zinsser said that he had 2 cases that showed no changes. The biopsies were so good that he wanted to examine the epididymis but was unable to do so.

Dr. Cohen mentioned Dr. Tietze's speculation on the possibility of sperm storage for sterilization patients who might want to change their minds. Since Dr. Bunge had had a sperm bank for many years, it might be feasible for that segment of the population that wanted to father a child for X number of years to do so.

With regard to Dr. Hayashi's paper, Dr. Shubeck explained that a new clip made the procedure a little easier. The silver clips do not occlude the tube and sperm can pass both ways. He said that in the 4 cases in which he and Dr. Decard had used clips, they had obtained 3 pregnancies in spite of the fact that the clips were intact.

Dr. Tietze questioned Dr. Hayashi's first series of women with ligational operations. He noted that the great majority of pregnancies that occurred followed tubal ligation in connection with the interruption of early pregnancy. He thought it would be interesting to know whether failure was more common after hysterectomy and ligation than it was after puerperal ligation. He also wanted to know if the times mentioned included the time for the abortion also, or if it was the specific time it took to perform the sterilization surgery.

Dr. Hayashi explained that the times mentioned referred only to the sterilization procedure.

Dr. Tietze stated that the first question related to the number of operations that were postpartum, postabortum, and interval.

Dr. Hayashi said that he thought that two-thirds of the patients were not pregnant, and one-third were pregnant.

Dr. Tietze recalled that there were 2 failures after puerperal sterilization, 2 failures in nonpregnant patients, and that all the other failures were in connection with abortions. He wanted to know the same distribution for the other cases.

Dr. Hayashi said it was still one-third pregnant and two-thirds nonpregnant. He thought that the procedure could be performed during abortion surgery or pregnancy; it is possible that the pregnancy rate following the abortion is higher.

Dr. Tietze agreed but said that still left the question of the puerperal cases unanswered.

Dr. Taylor asked why the anterior approach was used instead of the posterior cul-de-sac approach. He thought that most Americans would consider the anterior approach infinitely more difficult.

Dr. Hayashi stated that a special surgical team of 43 gynecologists had been used; they were very skillful and had consulted with a sterilization specialist. They preferred the anterior approach and constructed a special appliance for the procedure. It took about twelve minutes to operate.

Dr. Taylor wanted to know if there were many bladder injuries.

Dr. Hayashi said that there were 41 bladder injuries out of 6,887 cases and one death because of hemorrhage.

Dr. Richart then opened discussion on oviduct occlusion with plastic materials.

Dr. Shubeck said that he had done work with plastics in 84 cases, but not to block the tubes; in 2 cases the material was expelled or did move. It is easy to have the plastic flow out of the tubes, but it is technically difficult to get the proper proportion of Silastic to go into the tube and cure before part of it runs out into the peritoneal cavity. He thought the idea was good but it did produce a little anxiety concerning technique; it is most important to get the proper mix with catalyst so that the plastic will flow properly within the needed working-time interval.

Dr. Clyman expressed concern about using high pressures in the uterine cavity. It is possible for it to get into the vascular tree, and there is the possibility of embolic phenomena as well as venous obstruction. He mentioned that Dr. Rakshit's roentgenograms demonstrated obstructions in the uterine cavity and wanted to know if postoperative laparotomies had been performed.

Dr. Rakshit explained that some oviducts removed during hysterectomy showed the material in the tubes.

Dr. Clyman asked if there was one case of projection out of the tube.

Dr. Rakshit said there was.

Dr. Richart commented on the disparity between the number of sterilizations and the number of reanastomosis procedures performed. He questioned the need for developing reversible sterilization procedures and wanted to know if it was worth spending a great deal of effort on reversal.

Dr. Pai thought that reversibility was a must from the standpoint of patient confidence. Some of the patient resistance encountered is due to this problem. It is necessary to explain to the patient that it is possible, but not always certain, that the sterilization can be reversed.

Dr. Prager wondered if reversibility studies were worthwhile if the few patients who would not accept sterilization if it were not reversible were the only ones under consideration. He thought that this might apply to the United States, but wondered if it was realistic when the large number of sterilizations in India were being considered.

Dr. Pai noted that few sterilizations were done in the United States because the need was not felt. But the fact that population control is a global problem means that America's need will count. At the moment it does not exist, either for the middle or the poor classes, but the need will come. Every other contraceptive method has a reversibility factor; this is an important component.

Dr. Neuwirth stated that there was no occlusion procedure that was a hundred percent effective; the patient cannot be given a guarantee that he is going to be sterilized. There is reversibility; it is just a question of degree. He thought that Dr.

Richart's question had to be approached from that point of view. There has been an underlying assumption that reversibility means a hundred percent reversibility; a hundred percent assurance of sterility cannot even be given.

Dr. Darbari replied from the viewpoint of a worker in a country with a mass sterilization program. Improved techniques have improved the percentage of successful sterilizations. Reversibility is necessary for patient morale. If a sterilized patient lost all his children by death or if he remarried, he would be most anxious for reversal. If the government had a reversal program, it would be excellent for the patients.

Dr. Tietze agreed that the real concern was with the degree the belief in the possibility of reversal increases the initial acceptance of sterilization surgery. He suspected that, in practice, the number of reanastomoses would always be minimal in terms of the number of sterilizations performed. The question was will more men and women accept the operation and accept it at an earlier stage in their reproductive careers if it is reversible. A population control problem in India and other countries has been that sterilization has been done on individuals with large families who are fairly well advanced in age; the demographic effect of this is relatively small. Apparently this is no longer true in Dr. Pai's program in Greater Bombay.

Dr. Phatak thought that the problem of reversibility had to be considered in relation to the psychological security of a segment of the population. In India, large numbers of individuals accept sterilization after they have had two children. The average age of sterilized women ranges between twenty-four and twenty-eight years. Under these circumstances, women with two children who are sterilized because it is more convenient than accepting an intra-uterine contraceptive device or taking pills have problems if they remarry, if children die, or if the family finances improve. Under such conditions, they might want to have additional children. It is important that there be some possibility of reversal; in fact, it seems absolutely necessary to work on the possible production of a hundred percent reversibility.

Dr. Segal declared that the various aspects of the problem should be considered as a unit. It should be borne in mind that sterilization is not considered the only method of family planning; methods that are known to be reversible are available for individuals who desire that characteristic. He thought that there were four major objectives: simplification of the operative procedure; reversibility; saving hospital bed space, in the case of female sterilization; and the implementation of programs that would permit the use of paramedical personnel in place of physicians, who are very scarce in some areas. Insofar as female sterilization is concerned, it does not seem possible that a method will be developed which would eliminate the need for a physician, perhaps even a highly specialized physician. He agreed with Dr. Pai that there was a need for reversibility where family changes produced a desire for another child or for such individuals who would be reluctant to undergo a procedure that could not be reversed. If the over six million male sterilizations in India were considered, he thought that it was not worthwhile to be concerned about the possible twenty thousand men who might want sterilization reversal. If the lack of reversibility was a problem, then these individuals should be encouraged to get good medical advice and employ a contraceptive procedure that allows for reversibility. He said that he was somewhat discouraged in regard to what was being done to simplify sterilization surgery, especially vasectomy. Some of the films that are presented distort the complexities of routine male sterilization surgery, but the new procedures did not seem to be a great improvement or more simple than the customary methods of female sterilization.

Dr. Tietze thought that the entire field of birth prevention should be considered; this, of course, would include a discussion of abortion. It was his opinion that a great deal of emphasis had been given to maximum effectiveness and minimum acceptance because of a desire to avoid interventive abortion. If physicians were not concerned with abortion, the logical procedure would be to promote contraception methods that are reasonably effective and reasonably or highly acceptable. Pregnancy incidence would be reduced and unwanted pregnancies could be aborted. Permanent sterilization would be undertaken when the individuals felt that they were reasonably certain that they did not want any additional children. He considered that part of the search for a reversible surgical sterilization could be attributed to dissatisfaction with methods of contraception that had not provided the requisite effectiveness to eliminate the need for induced abortion. Legal and administrative changes necessary to include abortion in accepted population control programs should be considered.

Dr. Segal questioned the moral considerations of abortion, especially for those of the Moslem or Catholic faiths. He agreed that it was a logical approach to the problem, but that acceptability of abortion would have to be increased; he felt that it was fundamentally unacceptable at present.

Dr. Tietze commented that abortion was acceptable to the elite classes in certain countries and was available everywhere to women who sought it. He said he knew of no place in which more induced abortions are performed than Latin America.

Dr. Thompson stated that abortion was more complex procedurally than most sterilizations and probably had a higher mortality rate. This also might have to be repeated two or three times in the same individual.

Dr. Pai said that, along with the idea of effectiveness and acceptance, he personally felt that reversibility should be included as an important criterion of any family planning program. He agreed that the implementation of large-scale abortion programs would involve much difficulty and money. This is very true in India, where mistakes have led to nonacceptance of family-planning programs. He commented on the fact that the problem of antepartum tubal ligation had not been discussed. He thought everyone was speaking of postpartum tubal ligation and postabortion tubal ligation. He could well imagine women who were highly motivated for family planning, especially when they became pregnant; then they would seek abortion. He wanted to know if a simplified tubal ligation technique could be used on pregnant women who were seeking abortion.

Dr. Tietze wanted to know if he meant aborting the women and then sterilizing them.

Dr. Pai said that abortion could not be done legally in India, but tubal ligation could be done. This has been attempted in one hospital where a physician has done hundreds of ligations. When women appear for abortion, they are highly motivated to use family planning; when they return to their rural homes, where tubal ligation services are not available, the motivation is lost and family limitation suffers. If tubal ligation could be done on these pregnant women, they could well return to their homes for delivery, but future pregnancies could be prevented. He wanted to have opinions on undertaking tubal ligation during pregnancy.

Dr. Thompson commented that the situation was a supreme indication for vasectomy.

Dr. Pai asked what would happen if the husband were not ready. He thought that the women who begged for abortions had husbands who resisted the idea of sterilization.

Dr. Phatak stated that a colleague of hers did a series of tubectomies during pregnancy. She said that if tubectomy were undertaken before the uterus was too high, the procedure was quite simple. As pregnancy advances, tubal ligation was associated with more hemorrhage and tissue destruction.

Dr. Hulka commented on the current and realistic association between sexuality and fertility; this implied that, in order to produce an effect on fertility, such procedures as contraception or sterilization must be used. Reversible sterilization, either chemical or surgical, would disassociate sexuality from fertility; fertility would be associated with a positive action, rather than vice versa. He was interested in the concept of infertility as a norm, with the production of fertility by a voluntary act; this is directly germane to the population problem.

Dr. Zinsser then inquired if foaming Silastic had been used in an attempt to produce blockage.

Dr. Richart noted that this apparently had not been attempted.

Dr. Tietze asked if there was any systemic substance which would be excreted by the oviduct whose action on the tube could be implemented by systemic injection.

Dr. Richart commented that there had been a suggestion of employing iron particles, which might be picked up by the tube and then placing the patient in a strong electromagnetic field, and attempting to produce blockage by heat but this has not been attempted. It was also noted that work was being done in trying to characterize, immunologically and chemically, some of the tubal fluid components in an attempt to determine if there are components which are peculiar or unique to the oviduct. Then the specific induction of permanent or reversible sterilization could be attempted immunologically. Also, a microencapsulation technique had been suggested for toxic chemicals but no experiments have been performed.

Dr. Southam asked Dr. Tietze about women who failed to conceive after having used every known contraceptive method. Inflammatory disease developed in some users of intra-uterine devices; complications develop among users of birth control pills; injected patients have problems. She wondered if the number of involuntarily fertile individuals following sterilization exceeded the number of involuntarily infertile individuals after the discontinuance of the so-called reversible contraceptive devices.

Dr. Tietze said that he could not think of any contraceptive method which was followed by even fifteen percent infertility after discontinuance. He did not include those patients who had had blockage injections, for this he considered sterilization rather than contraception.

Dr. Southam stated that that was not her point. In India 138 requests for reversal were made after six million sterilizations. She knew 138 women who had discontinued birth control pills and wanted to conceive but could not. So she thought that the absolute number should be considered.

Dr. Tietze said he thought that the real problem of fertility after a sterilizing operation was absolutely negligible. What is important is the problem; if people believe that sterilization is non-reversible, they are constrained from accepting it early enough.

Dr. Rakshit said that although reversibility was sought in about one in a million of the sterilization cases, one out of a thousand individuals would like to know that the method was reversible.

V BIOENGINEERING TECHNOLOGY (B)

Denis J. Prager, *Moderator*

Chapter 22

FIBER OPTICS FOR VISUALIZATION AND ILLUMINATION

ROBERT E. INNIS

Fiber optics usually refers to the techniques of conveying light from one location to another through a particular configuration of glass or plastic fibers. In this paper we are concerned with bundles of long fibers, both flexible and rigid, which are used to transport visible light. Some properties of fiber optics will be discussed, and some applications to medical problems of visualization and illumination will be described.

The technology of modern fiber optics goes back about fifteen years to papers which described fiber bundles as image-carrying devices. A recent bibliography showed that in the intervening period more than three hundred papers and articles have been published, some sixty of which are concerned with medical applications of fiber optics.

PRINCIPLES

The mechanism of light conduction by optical fibers is based upon the phenomenon of total internal reflection which occurs at the interface between two transparent optical media of different refractive indices when the incident light is coming from the higher index side. If the media are free of optical absorption and the interface is smooth and clean, the reflection is indeed perfect. Thus, when light enters a fiber at one end, it will be contained within the fiber by multiple internal reflections, propagated down the fiber length, and emitted at the other end.

In optical fibers, the core of the fiber is made of a material with a higher refractive index than the coating, so that total internal reflection takes place at the core-coating interface for light rays internally incident at oblique angles (Fig. 22-1). The coating serves two purposes: it preserves the integrity of the

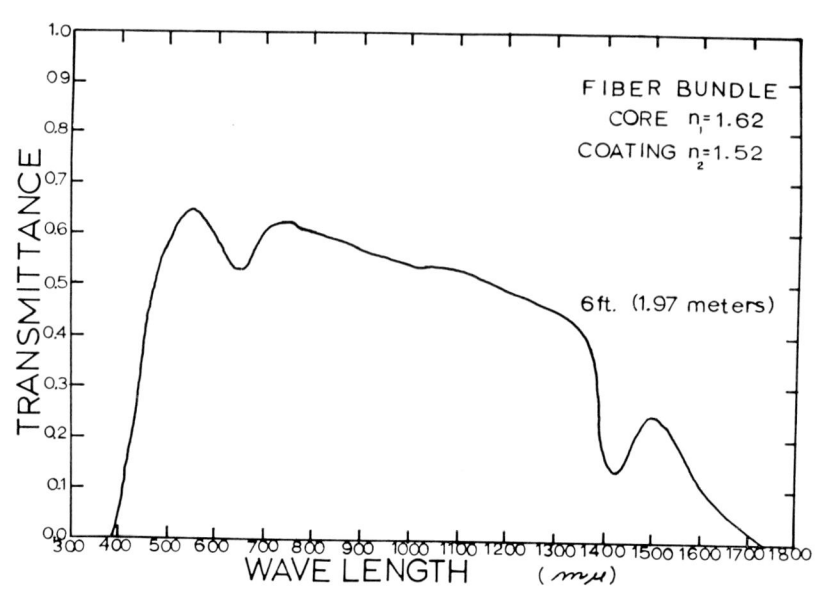

Figure 22-3. Transmittance of a 6 foot long fiber bundle (end losses not included).

will be transmitted by optical fibers of this glass combination. As a rule of thumb, 50 percent of the incident light is lost for each 7 feet of length. In general, the higher index glasses absorb the blue-violet light and tend to be yellow in appearance. Another factor which affects the transmittance of fiber bundles is the loss of usable cross-section in a bundle due to space between fibers and space occupied by coating material.

FLEXIBLE FIBER BUNDLES

Coated fibers may be bundled together to form highly efficient flexible light or image conductors. If only light is to be conducted, there is no need to coordinate precisely the fiber ends; such bundles often are called *light guides*.

For further transfer, the fiber ends must be coordinated precisely to prevent distortion and/or resolution loss. Since the fiber size limits the resolution, it is desirable to utilize the smallest fiber size possible; however, the smaller the fiber size, the more difficult it becomes to achieve precise coordination.

Fiber Optics for Visualization and Illumination

Fibers can be made so that one filament comprises a number of optical elements. Such fibers, called multifibers, permit fabrication of small diameter optical elements in a size that can be handled. Figure 22-4 is a photomicrograph of the ends of a row of flexible multifibers where the individual element size is 10 microns. Image resolution of over fifty line pairs per millimeter have been observed with these multifiber bundles. Other con-

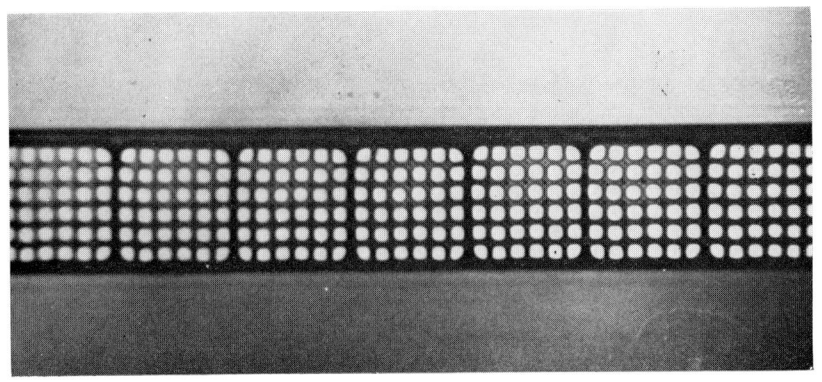

Figure 22-4. Photomicrograph of a row of flexible multifibers (individual fiber elements size is 10μ).

figurations have been employed including a square cross-section multifiber with 100 elements, each about 5 microns in diameter. Such multifibers permit fabrication of high-resolution visualizing systems.

FUSED FORM OF FIBER OPTICS

The technique of multifiber construction can be extended to produce bundles with many elements. By fusing and drawing together several hundred elements, a multifiber rod having a large number of perfectly aligned optical channels can be formed. Such a bundle is commonly called an *image conduit*. By combining a number of such conduits, and repeating the fusing-drawing process, a fiber rod with many thousands of optical channels can be fabricated. Although such structures are rigid, they can be bent easily with heat from a torch or oven (Fig. 22-5).

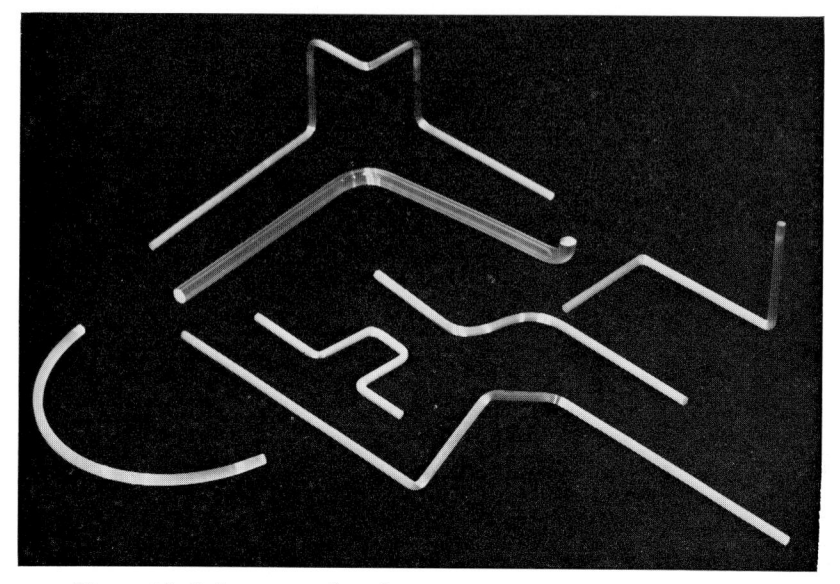

Figure 22-5. Image conduits bent into a variety of configurations.

FIBER OPTICS AS MEDICAL ILLUMINATORS

Fiber optic light guides have been used in medical applications for illuminating areas that are inaccessible to conventional light sources, and have supplanted the electric light bulbs used is some conventional endoscopes. Fiber optic illuminators permit the source of illumination to be located at a distance from the site of examination so that problems of inadequate lighting and local heat production are eliminated. In addition, typical optical fibers filter out the infrared and ultraviolet radiation that may be present. Thus, a medical fiber optic illuminator provides an intense *cold light* at the site of interest.

Among the early fiber optic illuminators was an instrument for intracardiac illumination. It consisted of a curved stainless steel probe, 3 mm in diameter and 15 cm long, which contained one large clad rod. The probe coupled optically to a flexible fiber bundle, which, in turn, coupled to a source of illumination. The illuminator was a 20 watt, 6 volt tungsten lamp and an optical system which focused the light on the end of the fiber bundle so as to fill the N.A. of the fibers. The unit was designed to transilluminate the ventricular septum during open heart surgery for septal defects. It has been used clinically.

Another instrument which provides a novel means for transillumination is called a ureteral transilluminating catheter. In this device, basically a transparent ureteral catheter with the end hermetically sealed, the distal 27 cm of transparent catheter emit visible light which comes from the ends of optical fibers terminating all along this length. The catheters have been made in sizes 4 or 5 French (⅓ or ⅝ mm in diameter) and about 1 meter long. They couple to an illuminator which provides an intense beam of light that is focused on the fiber bundle so as to fill the N.A. of the fibers. This instrument has been used clinically in surgery involving the ureters.

FIBER OPTICS IN CARDIAC ENDOSCOPY

A small diameter fiber optic endoscope was developed to visualize the aortic valve *in vivo* without the need for thoracotomy. Heart catheterization techniques are employed to advance the endoscope into the aorta, over the aortic valve. A specially constructed balloon, fastened to the tip of the instrument, clears the blood and permits visualization of the structure in contact with the transparent balloon.

The initial approach to visualizing heart structures *in vivo* in the presence of blood was to develop a rigid fiber optic endoscope. A rigid instrument was chosen because of the simplicity of construction and the relatively low cost. Figure 22–6 shows the first model of the experimental cardioscope. It was essentially a straight piece of stainless steel tubing 3.8 mm diameter with a right-angle bend near the proximal end. The insertable portion was 52 cm long. Within the steel sheathing were the imagery, illumination, and insufflation systems. The image relay bundle (image conduit) contained 76,000 fibers, each 175 microns in diameter. The instrument had a fixed objective lens of 2.6 mm focal length. The field of view was 18 mm diameter at a working distance of 22 mm; resolution at this working distance was 5 line pairs per millimeter.

A flexible instrument was later developed to fulfill the require-

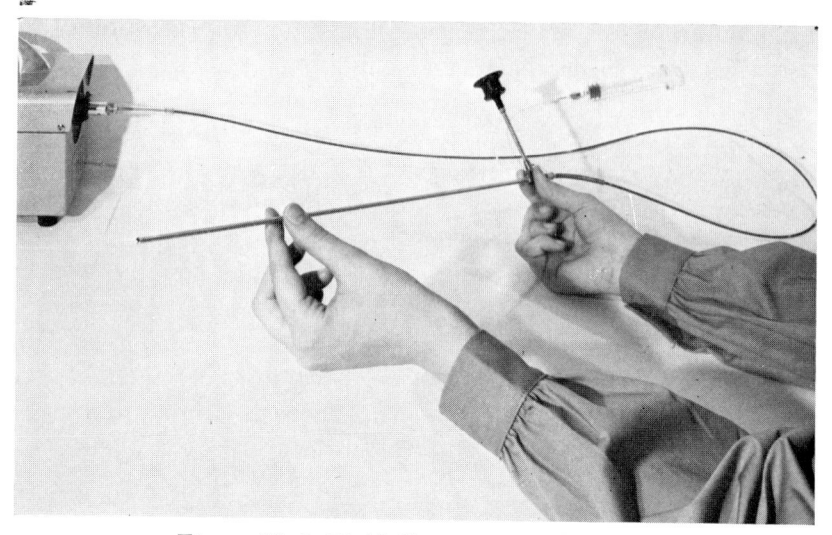

Figure 22-6. Rigid fiber optic cardioscope.

ments of heart catheterization techniques. Figure 22-7 shows an early flexible cardioscope. It was 4 mm in diameter and flexible for about 80 cm of length. The imagery system consisted of an objective lens of 2.8 mm focal length and a flexible fiber relay

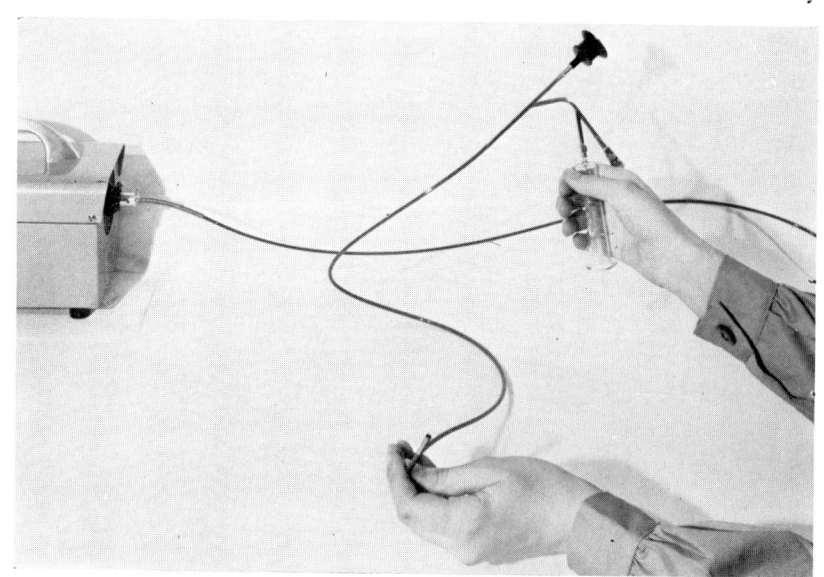

Figure 22-7. Flexible fiber optic cardioscope.

bundle composed of multifibers with elements 5 microns in diameter. There were approximately 70,000 image points. The field of view was 12 mm at a working distance of 22 mm. Resolution was 8 line pairs per millimeter. The illumination system employed about 100 monofibers, each 50 microns in diameter.

REFERENCES

1. Siegmund, W.P., Innis, R.E., Koester, C.J., and Gamble, W.J.: Fiber optics principles and applications in medicine. *Ann NY Acad Sci, 157*:47, 1969.
2. Potter, R.J.: History and evolution of fiber optics. Society of Photo-Optical Instrumentation Engineers, Seminar Proceedings, Vol. 14, pp. 9–28, 1968.
3. *The Science of Color.* Committee on Colorimetry, Optical Society of America, New York, 1953, p. 41.
4. Bernhard, W.F., Innis, R., and Gross, R.E.: Transillumination of the ventricular septum. *New Eng J Med, 257*:909, 1962.
5. Innis, R.E., and Jaffee, S.R.: U.S. Patent #3,131,690, 1964.
6. Gamble, W.J., and Innis, R.E. 1967: Experimental intracardiac visualization. *New Eng J Med, 276*:1397, 1967.

Chapter 23

PRODUCTION OF CLINICALLY USEFUL INTERACTIONS OF LASER RADIATION WITH TISSUE

C.H. Swope

The word *laser* is an acronym standing for *light amplification by stimulated emission of radiation*. It consists of a host material to which an impurity has been added, and is normally contained in a cylinder (a solid rod for solid materials and a glass tube for gases or liquids) placed between two mirrors which are in parallel alignment; one mirror totally reflects the light, the other reflects it partially.

When energy is introduced into a laser, some of the energy is absorbed by impurity atoms which become excited. The excited atoms are then capable of releasing energy (*spontaneous emission*) as they return to the unexcited state. As a result, "packets" of light (photons) are emitted. Some of these photons will approach other excited atoms, causing them to emit energy (*stimulated emission*). This interaction occurs again and again so that a large number of photons are produced in a short time. Some photons will be emitted in the direction of the mirrors where some light will escape, but some will return to course through the material and interact with more atoms.

This is an amplification process. Originally there was one photon, now there are many. As many of them escape from the cavity, they provide a useful output of energy. The energy is monochromatic, with the wavelength unique to the laser material, and the energy is unidirectional being contained in a narrow beam.

The energy required to excite the impurity atoms varies from laser to laser. For example, it may be light from a flash tube for solid lasers or an electric discharge through a laser gas.

The most common commercial lasers are ruby, neodymium,

argon, krypton, carbon dioxide, helium–neon or diode lasers. The diode lasers are solid lasers which are very tiny. Ruby and neodymium lasers can produce a large amount of energy in short periods of time. The argon ion laser is a gas laser; it operates continuously and can produce about one watt of power. The krypton laser is very similar to the argon laser. In fact, the two gases can be mixed in a common laser to produce many wavelengths covering most of the visible spectrum. The carbon dioxide laser is particularly interesting for medical purposes; its wavelength is in the infrared where most biological materials absorb very strongly. The helium–neon laser is a gas laser with an output primarily at 633 nanometers; because it produces little power, it is unlikely that it would interact with a biological system on any clinical scale.

Methods of laser operation vary: Q-switched, long-pulsed, and continuous are the most common. The Q-switched laser yields very short pulses on the order of 10^{-8} seconds. Long-pulsed lasers have pulses of light energy of about one millisecond in duration; continuous lasers operate constantly. Another operation method is mode-locking, which makes possible pulses down to 10^{-12} or 10^{-13} seconds. This has potential utility for biological systems but is not in clinical use at present.

While the development of the medical use of lasers is active, it is still in a primitive stage.[1] A notable exception to this, however, is the development of the laser photocoagulator, a commercially available instrument.[2] The experience and data generated in connection with laser photocoagulation can serve as a guide in developing laser instrumentation for other areas of medical interest.

For the purposes of this discussion, the laser can be considered a source of monochromatic light (ultraviolet, infrared, or visible) which is capable of being concentrated to very high power density levels. Lasers have several other properties that are very interesting, but not important, in discussing the interaction of laser energy and biologic tissue.

There are two types of interaction of optical energy with tissue that are most likely to occur—photochemical and thermal. Photochemical interaction has been observed particularly with enzymes and proteins.[3,4] However, no clinical application of laser-induced photochemical processes has been developed yet.

Thermal interaction is characterized by the absorption of optical energy by the tissue and its conversion to thermal energy, with a corresponding temperature rise. This interaction can have a range of effects on the tissue depending on many parameters. The efficiency with which the tissue absorbs the laser energy, the rate at which the energy is delivered, and the thermal parameters of the tissue (e.g. thermal conductivity and specific heat) will determine the maximum temperature rise and the time required to achieve it. With pulsed lasers the energy can be varied so as to produce the disruption of a few cells, the production of a typical thermally-induced lesion, or an explosive destruction of tissue. Excessive overexposure can result in extensive damage to healthy tissue. For example, if the site of the pathology is highly absorbing to the laser light, but is located above or below relatively transparent healthy tissue, explosive reactions in the pigmented tissue will cause mechanical damage to the surrounding tissue even though the laser energy did not directly interact with it. This has made the laser treatment of pigmented tumors very difficult, because viable tumor tissue often is found dispersed throughout neighboring healthy tissue after laser irradiation. This illustrates the need to produce a carefully controlled interaction between the laser and the pathological tissue.

In applying the laser to sterilization, the desired tissue reaction probably will be that of lesion production without excessive hemorrhaging, explosive effects, or widespread heating. In most potential applications for the laser, a very localized site of specific tissue damage is desired. The characteristics of the lesion depend considerably on the absorption characteristics of the tissue and on the laser used. Noyori et al.[5] described the nature of lesions produced in the retina by a long-pulsed ruby laser. A series of papers by Campbell and co-workers[6] describe lesions in the retina produced by a Q-switched ruby laser, long pulsed neodymium laser[7] and a continuous wave (cw) argon ion laser.[8] The second paper of the series described corneal lesions produced by a cw carbon dioxide laser (see Table 23-I).[9] When a long-pulsed (approximately 0.7 msec) ruby laser[5] produced a clinical

TABLE 23-I
MOST COMMON LASERS

Laser	Material Solid	Material Gas	Operation Q-Switched	Operation Long Pulsed	Operation Continuous (cw)	Wavelengths	Typical Output
Ruby	X		X	X		694.3 nm	0.1-500 Joules
						347. nm*	
Neodymium	X (Glass or Yag)		X	X	X	1060 nm	0.1-1000 J (pulsed)
						530 nm*	1 Watt (cw)
Argon Ion		X		X	X	458,477,†488,†	10^{-3}-1 Watt (cw)
						497,5017,515†	(Total)
Krypton		X		X	X	350,476,520†	10^{-2}-1 Watt (cw)
						568,647†	(Total)
CO_2		X			X	10600 nm	10-1000 Watt (cw)
He-Ne		X			X	633 nm	10^{-4}-5 × 10^{-2} Watt
Diode	X		X	long pulsed	at rapid rep. rate	800-1000	10^{-3} Watt (average)

* Frequency doubled wavelength—usually obtained only with Q-Switched mode.
† Wavelengths at which most of the power occurs.

exposure in the retina, it radically changed the retinal architecture. The pigmented epithelium was redistributed among retinal layers. Within days, exudate which had appeared soon after irradiation, disappeared and a fibrous plaque formed; this was responsible for the desired chorioretinal adhesion. With more laser energy, more exudate and disruption of the pigmented epithelium and cells of the nuclear layers were observed; the retina often was elevated by the presence of a subretinal gas bubble. With higher energy, retinal layers fractured and the bubble escaped into the vitreous. With still more energy, a retinal hemorrhage developed.

With the Q-switched ruby laser,[6] the energy necessary to produce retinal lesions was lower, but it was delivered in a much shorter pulse (0.4×10^{-4} times that of the long pulse or $25 \times 10^{-9} - 30 \times 10^{-9}$ sec). The lesions were somewhat similar to those produced by the long-pulsed ruby, except that the relative range of energies from a minimal lesion to a retinal hemorrhage was much smaller.

Campbell *et al.* also described lesions with long-pulsed neodymium lasers.[7,10] Roughly speaking, the retinal lesions were very similar to those produced by the long-pulsed ruby laser, but more energy was required to produce them. This increase in energy can be understood primarily on the basis of the absorption characteristics of the ocular media, retinal layers, and pigmented epithelium, and the difference in wavelength between the ruby laser (0.694 μm) and the neodymium laser (1.06 μm).

The argon ion laser was used to produce small retinal lesions.[8] Pulse durations were 50 or 100 msec ($\sim$100 times that of the long-pulsed laser). The lesions were similar to those produced by the long-pulsed lasers; however, there was a relatively-less violent disruption of the chorioretinal architecture, although subretinal hemorrhaging could be produced. The span in energy from mild lesions to severe lesions was larger than it was for pulsed lasers.

These observations qualitatively demonstrate that, even with 50 to 100 msec pulse durations, the temperature rise in the pigmented epithelium occurred rapidly, and the thermal stress was great. The appearance of the gas bubble even implies some vaporization of the material. The nature of the lesions demonstrates the importance of the many parameters. In the retina, most of the absorption of the energy takes place in the thin, highly absorbent layer of pigmented epithelium where extraordinarily high temperatures easily can be developed rapidly. With this in mind, it is not surprising that the initial result is that resembling a small explosion. On the other hand, because the pigmented epithelium is so thin, long time-exposures would require considerably more energy due to the conduction of heat away from the lesion site. Several thermal models have been suggested and, at least qualitatively, account for many of the observations.[11]

Thus, for the retina at least, the wavelength of the laser and the absorption characteristics of the tissue, the structure of the tissue, the rate at which the energy is delivered, the size of the irradiated area, and the total energy delivered are all important parameters in the production of a lesion and the nature of its post-irradiation development. However, complex as the situation seems to be, most of the observed effects appear to be primarily thermal; it is thought that a sufficiently sophisticated thermal model could explain many of the observations quantitatively.

Because so many tissue and laser parameters are involved, the nature of a lesion is difficult to predict; on the other hand, proper variation of the parameters can assist in producing the desired type of lesion. For example, absorption can be varied by the use of specific dyes. Lasers are available today at various wavelengths, and to some extent, the laser can be chosen to be compatible with the absorption of the tissue.

The parameters of power, energy, wavelength, and mode of operation cannot be selected independently; the range of variation in these parameters generally is fixed for a particular laser. Table 23-I describes some of the common types of lasers. Many more exist, but they are not yet generally available.

As the table shows, lasers vary greatly in the values of the parameters with which researchers are concerned. There are more subtle differences not shown in the table which govern the degree to which a particular laser can be modified to enhance one or more characteristics. For example, the thermal conduction of the host material will play an important role in a laser's pulse repetition rate, and the degree of simplicity in the design of the laser system depends on whether or not the laser material is transparent to its own radiation.

For many applications, the problem of delivering the laser energy to the work site will arise. In these cases, the use of a fiber optic delivery system is intriguing. A previous paper by Innis[12] describes the manner in which light propagates along an optical fiber and the ways in which it might be used to conduct light to and from remote locations in the body. Fiber optic systems can conduct laser light also. Problems do exist with fiber durability when the fiber is subjected to the intense laser radiation and high thermal gradients produced at the work site. But these problems generally are not insurmountable and some interesting partial solutions have been found.

For example, one serious problem is getting the light into the optical fiber without high loss or damage to the end of the fiber. With pulsed lasers, this is the limiting constraint in conducting a high-powered pulse. The problem is still serious with cw lasers, but because the power level is lower, damage to the fibers is less likely to occur. One way to avoid this difficulty is to use fibers made of laser glass and to make the fiber act as the laser. Several fibers can be grouped together to form a composite, flexible laser.

Devices utilizing this concept have been constructed and used in applications associated with the eye, the ear, and the skin.[10,13] For the eye,[10] 54 laser fibers were used in a probe whose flexible length was about 60 cm. This probe was used to produce lesions in the eyes of rabbits by transcleral irradiation. The laser emission was at 1.06 μ with a pulse duration of about 0.8 msec. Energies up to 1.8 joules into 0.78 sq mm were delivered at the probe tip. Auxiliary fibers were included in the probe to carry visible light so that by means of an opthalmoscope the probe tip could be located properly with respect to the retinal pathology.

For the ear studies[13], a probe utilizing a single 300 μ laser fiber was used. Lesions were produced in the cochlea of squirrel monkeys for the purpose of destroying the audio response at certain frequencies. Each monkey's hearing was tested functionally, and the production of lesions inferred by the detection of a hearing loss in the animal. The results indicate that, while a hearing loss throughout the audio range was produced, the maximum loss occurred in the desired range between 5000 and 8000 Hertz.

The results of the experiments with the skin[1] have been negative to date. The problem is to destroy the root of a hair with a fiber laser probe. While lesions have not been produced, a probe has been constructed and operated successfully. The device used a 50 μ fiber in a 125 μ sheathing of stainless steel. The tip was easily inserted into the hair follicle, and delivered up to 3 mjoules. Figure 23-1 schematically shows the construction of the probe. The probe did deliver over 100 joules/cm^2 at the tip *in situ* on a reasonably reliable basis.

A specific proposal on the use of a laser in the area of sterilization is outside the scope of this paper. However, production of lesions by lasers in small tubes such as the vas deferens in the male and oviducts in the female, for the purpose of occlusion is feasible. Another approach might include the production of

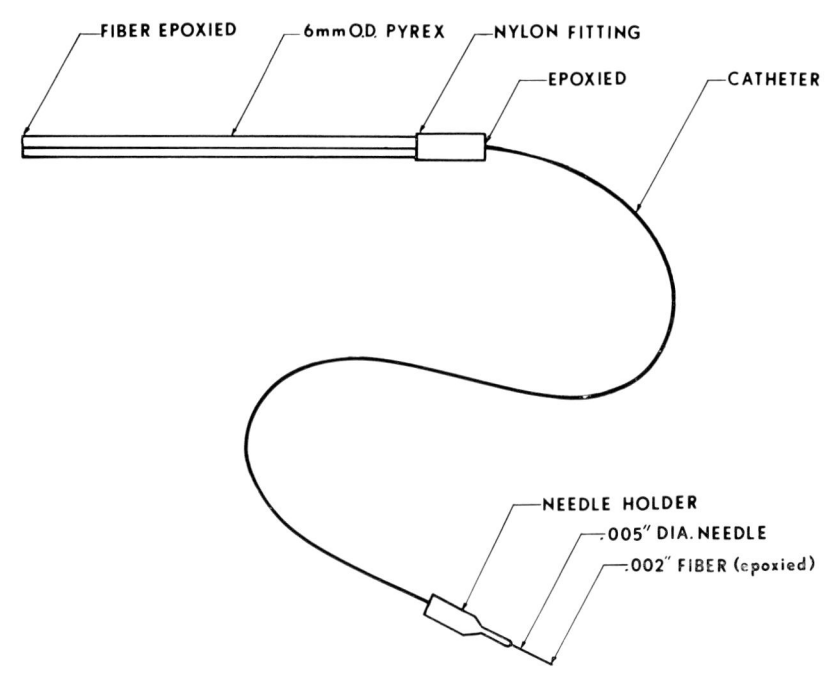

Figure 23-1. Schematic construction of fiber laser probe.

lesions in certain areas so as to create an inhospitable environment for sperm or egg cells. The possibility of inducing permanent or long-term changes in a part of the reproductive system by laser-induced photochemical reaction does not seem likely at first glance, but it should not be ruled out without careful study.

The further development of laser fiber optic technology for use in solving problems in connection with a particular biomedical problem, including sterilization, will be expensive and difficult. It will require the closest cooperation of the optical scientist and the life scientist and their respective support groups. However, the rewards to be gained from such an effort certainly justify the investment.

REFERENCES

1. Fine, S., and Klein, E.: Lasers in biology and medicine. *Laser Focus Mag*, 5:28–36, 1969.
2. Campbell, C., Koester, C., Curtice, V., Noyori, K., and Rittler, C.: Clinical studies in laser photocoagulation. *Arch Ophthal* (Chicago), 74:57–65, 1965.
3. Gerraets, W., Burkhart, J., and Guerry, D.: Enzyme activity in the coagulated retina: A means of studying thermal conduction as a function of exposure time. *Acta Ophthal Supp*, 76:79–93, 1963.
4. Chan, G., Berry, E., and Gerraets, W.: Alterations of soluble retinal proteins due to thermal injury. *Acta Ophthal Supp*, 76:101–108, 1963.
5. Noyori, K., Campbell, C., Rittler, C., and Koester, C.: The characteristics of experimental laser coagulations of the retina. *Arch Ophthal*, 72:254–263, 1964.
6. Campbell, C., Rittler, C., Swope, H., and Koester, C.: Ocular effects produced by experimental lasers: I. Q-switched ruby laser. *Amer J Ophthal*, 66:459–470, 1968.
7. Campbell, C., Rittler, C., Innis, R., and Shiner, W.: Ocular effects produced by experimental lasers: III. Neodymium laser. *Amer J Ophthal*, 66:614–632, 1968.
8. Campbell, C., Rittler, C., Swope, H., and Wallace, R.: The ocular effects produced by experimental lasers: IV. The argon laser. *Amer J Ophthal*, 67:671–681, 1969.
9. Campbell, C., Rittler, C., Bredemeir, H., and Wallace, R.: Ocular effects produced by experimental lasers: II. Carbon dioxide laser. *Amer J Ophthal*, 66:604–614, 1968.
10. Campbell, C., Noyori, K., Rittler, M., Innis, R., and Koester, C.J.: The

application of fiber laser techniques to retinal surgery. *Arch Ophthal,* 72:850–857, 1964.
11. Ham, W., Williams, R., Mueller, H., Guerry, D., Clarke, A., and Gerraets, W.: Effects of laser radiation on the mammalian eye. *Trans NY Acad Sci, 28*:517–526, 1966.
12. Innis, R., Chapter 22 in this volume.
13. Wilpizeski, C., Sataloff, J., Innis, R., and Shiner, W.: Audiometric effects of pulsed laser irradiation of the squirrel monkey inner ear. Presented at the 76th Annual Meeting of the Acoustical Society of America, Cleveland, Ohio, November, 1968.

Chapter 24

TISSUE RESPONSES TO POLYMERIC IMPLANTS: THE CYCLOACRYLATES[*]

STEPHEN C. WOODWARD

Nonreactive polymeric materials have been used as non-absorbable sutures, as replacements for defective parts such as heart valves, and as contraceptives such as intra-uterine devices. Generally, such polymers as nylon or polyethylene behave as "inert" foreign bodies. Their usefulness depends upon bland local responses without development of neoplasms, and fabrication which permits effective long-term function. Nonreactive polymers enjoy widespread and increasing uses in medicine.

By contrast, except for catgut sutures and topical hemostatic agents such as fibrin, few biodegradable polymers have been available for surgical applications, despite their usefulness in hemostasis and wound closure. Cyanoacrylate tissue adhesives include highly reactive and necrotizing polymers as well as inert, well-tolerated ones. Their study has stimulated the development of new test systems to quantify local toxicity of reactive implants.[1,2] This presentation will describe host responses to cyanoacrylates. Their unique physiochemical characteristics perhaps will result in the selection of a cyanoacrylate to occlude portions of the human reproductive system; methyl α-cyanoacrylate already has been employed in rabbits to occlude the oviduct.[3]

CYANOACRYLATES AS REPLACEMENTS FOR SUTURES

Alpha cyanoacrylates are particularly suited as tissue adhesives, partly because of their accidentally-discovered[4] polymerization

---

[*] American Cyanamid Company, Ethicon, Incorporated, Minnesota Mining and Manufacturing Company, and the United States Army Biochemical Research Laboratories contributed the α-cyanoacrylates. Studies were supported in part by United States Army Research Contract DA-49-193-MD 2646. John B. Herrmann and A.R. Katz collaborated closely in these studies.

characteristics (Fig. 24–1). Polymerization, which often occurs within seconds, is catalyzed by weak bases such as hydroxyl groups present within moist living tissues. Rapid polymerization, which is associated with considerable local evolution of heat,[5] can be retarded, and rapid accumulation of heat diminished, by incorporating acidic moieties such as sulfur dioxide into the monomer.[5] Since cyanoacrylates require no catalyst other than hydroxyl groups (which are abundant within tissues), the possibility of toxic local reactions to catalysts is eliminated.

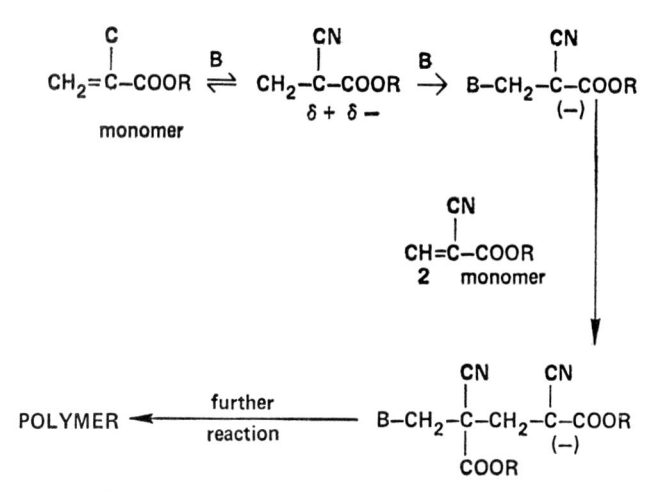

$$CH_2=\overset{\overset{C}{|}}{C}-COOR \;\rightleftharpoons\; \underset{\delta+\;\delta-}{CH_2-\overset{\overset{CN}{|}}{C}-COOR} \;\xrightarrow{B}\; B-CH_2-\overset{\overset{CN}{|}}{\underset{(-)}{C}}-COOR$$

$$\underset{2\;\;\text{monomer}}{CH=\overset{\overset{CN}{|}}{C}-COOR}$$

$$POLYMER \;\xleftarrow{\text{further reaction}}\; B-CH_2-\overset{\overset{CN}{|}}{\underset{COOR}{C}}-CH_2-\overset{\overset{CN}{|}}{\underset{(-)}{C}}-COOR$$

Figure 24–1. Polymerization of Alkyl-2-cyanoacrylates. B represents the initiating base. Sequential addition of monomer units forms polymer chain.

Bonding to biological substrates such as dermal collagen provides bonds requiring 1,000 to 2,000 gm/cm^2 for disruption; disruption of such bonds usually takes place by fragmentation of the collagen substrate. These adhesive properties make skin graft fixation or even arterial anastomosis with cyanoacrylates relatively easy once one has learned carefully to control where the monomer is applied.

Initially, only methyl α-cyanoacrylate was available, and its efficacy as a tissue adhesive was greeted with enthusiasm by surgical investigators. Since 1960 about three hundred publications related to surgical applications of cyanoacrylates have appeared.[6] Most of these are reports of experiments in which cyanoacrylates have been employed as replacements for sutures in a variety of applications. Enthusiasm has wained somewhat recently.

This may be due largely to the intense local necrosis which develops at sites of application of methyl α-cyanoacrylate, the first cyanoacrylate available, and the most widely studied material. Inflammation represented an interesting and, at first, unexpected local effect. Since polymerized cyanoacrylates are soluble only in a few organic solvents, such as nitro-methane,[4] they might have been expected to behave inertly.

CYANOACRYLATES AS HEMOSTATIC AGENTS

In a recent experiment performed by Herrmann, Osterhaut, Woodward, and Leonard,[7] cyanoacrylate monomers were sprayed upon the cut surfaces of the liver in ten adult beagle dogs to control hemorrhage, following resection of the tips of various liver lobes (Table 24-I). Temporary occlusion of vessels supplying the hepatic pedicle was applied; following this, methyl, n-butyl, and neo-pentyl α-cyanoacrylates were applied in succession to sections of liver lobes. Polymerization was rapid, especially with n-butyl, and blood loss was only moderate. Hemostasis and blood loss were scored 0 to 4 plus. Employing n-butyl and neo-pentyl monomers, a single spraying produced good hemostasis. Methyl, its pH intentionally lowered to increase its spreading properties, polymerized slowly and was the least effective hemostatic agent. Adhesions were graded 0 to 4 plus, and were not conspicuous at sacrifice, seven or fourteen

TABLE 24-I
RESULTS OF SPRAYING CYANOACRYLATES UPON CUT SURFACE OF LIVERS IN DOGS

	Methyl	n-Butyl	neo-Pentyl
Surface Areas (cm^2)*	3.60	3.53	3.30
Polymerization Times (sec.)*	28.2	3.64	6.11
Blood Loss (a)†	33.5	20.00	16.00
Hemostasis (a)†	16.0	29.5	34.5
Adhesions at Sacrifice (b)†	23.0	29.5	22.0

* Mean values, 10 determinations.
† Sums of scores, 10 resection sites; higher values indicate greater blood loss or more effective hemostasis, (a) $p \leq .001$, by χr^2, ref. 11, (b) $p \leq .10$, by χr^2, ref. 11.

days later. At both seven and fourteen days, surfaces sprayed with methyl were inflamed and vascular (Fig. 24–2A and B). Little of the polymer was identified even at seven days, but its pyogenic effects, including continuing accumulation of neutrophils and development of a wide zone of granulation tissue were obvious. By contrast, n-butyl and neo-pentyl polymers elicited a

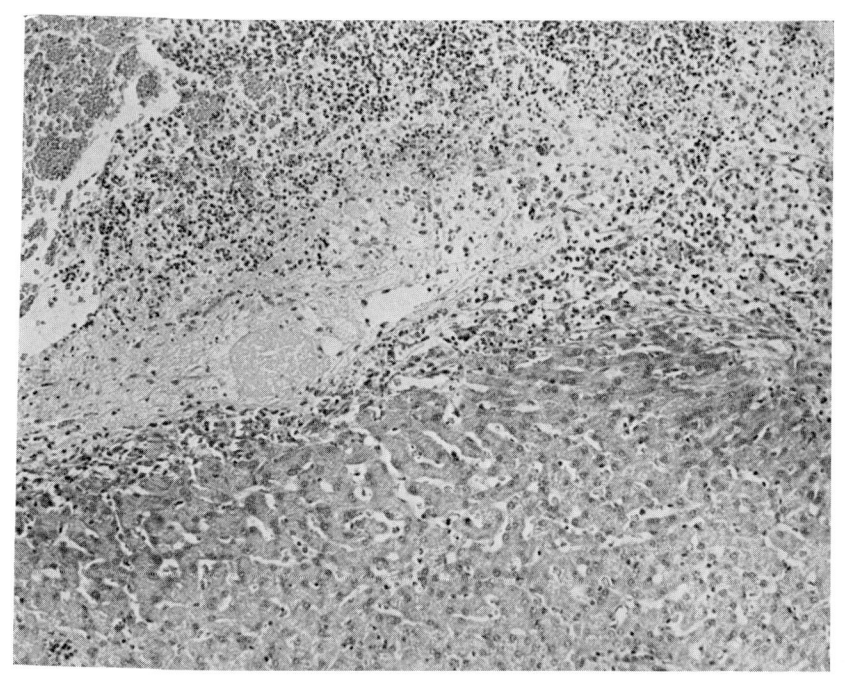

Figure 24–2A. Methyl, seven days. Intense pyogenic response including mass of fibrin over liver surface, Bottom center (H & E, × 100).

foreign-body response, with little attendant inflammation (Fig. 2C and D). These polymers were in close proximity to hepatic cells. Unlike methyl, n-butyl and neo-pentyl deposits did not appear to undergo appreciable resorption within two weeks.

EFFECTS OF CYANOACRYLATES UPON FIBROPLASIA

Favorable results generally cannot be achieved when a toxic necrotizing cyanoacrylate is substituted for sutures in surgery.[8]

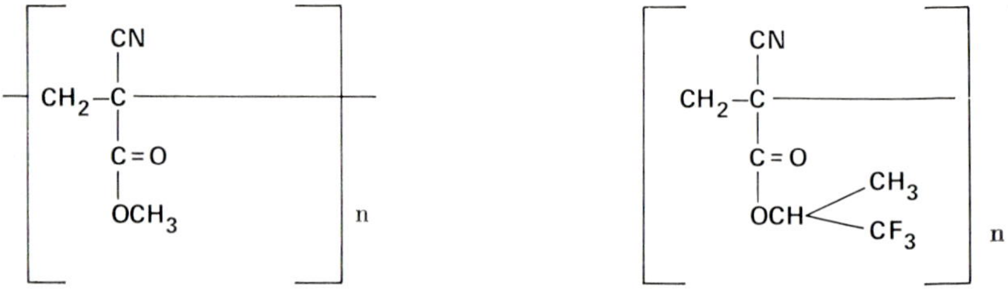

$$\left[\begin{array}{c} \text{CN} \\ | \\ \text{CH}_2-\text{C} \\ | \\ \text{C}=\text{O} \\ | \\ \text{OCH}_3 \end{array} \right]_n \qquad \left[\begin{array}{c} \text{CN} \\ | \\ \text{CH}_2-\text{C} \\ | \\ \text{C}=\text{O} \\ | \\ \text{OCH}\!\!<\!\!\begin{array}{c}\text{CH}_3\\ \text{CF}_3\end{array} \end{array} \right]_n$$

Polymerized methyl α-cyanoacrylate

Polymerized Trifluorisopropyl α-cyanoacrylate

Figure 24-3.

is an inert porous disc which can be used to harvest newly developing granulation tissue. The disc can be evaluated gravimetrically and biochemically in terms of its collagen content. Collagen content is determined from the content of hydroxyproline, an identifying amino acid for collagen. The sponge also can be examined histologically in terms of local inflammatory responses to local polymer deposits. In this experiment 50 mg doses of cyanoacrylate monomers were incorporated into test sponges. Six sponges were implanted in each animal: two untreated control sponges and two test sponges containing each cyanoacrylate. Hydroxyproline content measurements at seven days showed reduced values for cyanoacrylate-containing sponges as compared with the controls.

Dry tissue weights represent the constant dry weight of the sponge developed under vacuum minus the sum of initial weights of the sponge and polymer. The negative dry tissue weight noted

TABLE 24-II

TOXICITY AND RESORPTION OF METHYL-α-CYANOACRYLATES (METHYL-) AND β,β,β TRIFLUOROISOPROPYL-α-CYANOACRYLATES (BETA) WITH A SPONGE GRANULOMA TECHNIQUE*

	Methyl-	Beta	Control
Hydroxyproline Content (mcg)	23.8 ± 5.7	23.0 ± 1.9	32.2 ± 8.2
Dry Tissue Weight (mg)	−34.9 ± 1.7	10.9 ± 2.9	14.9 ± 2.0
Hydroxyproline Concentration (mcg/mg dry tissue)	—	—	2.2 ± 0.4
Cyanoacrylate Lost From Implant (weight in mg)	45.0 ± 2.8 (84%)	9.1 ± 4.2 (18.7%)	—

* Seven day study with 10 rats and 50 mg doses. Means ± standard error.

for methyl at seven days provides direct evidence of cyanoacrylate resorption, since such implants had lost weight during their period of implantation. Small amounts of fibroconnective tissue were visible within these sponges. In the case of beta, while dry tissue weights were less than those observed for the controls, no direct evidence of resorption was found. Using the hydroxyproline concentration of dry tissue in control sponges, the actual weight of dry tissue required to provide the hydroxyproline content values observed for cyanoacrylate containing sponges can be estimated. The hydroxyproline concentration is assumed to be the same in control and test sponges. Employing this reasoning, it is possible to estimate the weight of cyanoacrylate which has been lost from the implant. It appears that eighty-four percent of methyl and eighteen percent of beta had disappeared from the implant site by seven days.

Table 24-III provides fourteen day data from this experiment. Methyl test sponges continued to have low collagen content values. As at seven days, fourteen day methyl sponges had lost weight after implantation. About seventy-six percent of the methyl polymer had been resorbed; results were not dissimilar from seven-day results. By contrast, beta and control sponges showed a six-fold increase in collagen content values from seven-day levels. About fifteen percent of beta polymer had been resorbed.

Control sponges were infiltrated by vascular granulation tissue and were firmly bound to adjacent structures at fourteen days. Methyl sponges were edematous, swollen, and surrounded by a pyogenic membrane at seven and fourteen days. Beta sponges

TABLE 24-III
TOXICITY AND RESORPTION OF METHYL-α-CYANOACRYLATES (METHYL-) AND β,β,β TRIFLUOROISOPROPYL-α-CYANOACRYLATES (BETA) WITH A SPONGE GRANULOMA TECHNIQUE*

	Methyl-	Beta	Control
Hydroxyproline Content (mcg)	28.8 ± 4.4	179.6 ± 57.9	161.0 ± 57.5
Dry Tissue Weight (mg)	-37.6 ± 0.9	16.0 ± 3.1	18.8 ± 0.7
Hydroxyproline concentration (mcg/mg dry tissue)	—	—	7.9 ± 2.5
Cyanoacrylate Lost From Implant (weight in mg)	41.3 ± 1.2 (76%)	8.1 ± 2.7 (14.5%)	—

* Fourteen day study with 10 rats and 50 mg doses. Mean ± standard error.

showed a response intermediate between the control and the methyl sponges. Beta sponges were slightly swollen, but partly infiltrated by developing granulation tissue. Microscopically, methyl sponges were edematous, almost devoid of granulation tissue, and inflamed at seven and fourteen days; the polymer was present as refractile plates. Beta sponges contained fibroblasts and collagen; however, moderate numbers of acute inflammatory cells were seen at sites of polymer deposition. Beta polymer resembled the irregular, amorphous polymers which result from polymerization of the higher alkyl homologues of methyl.[2,5]

Table 24-IV summarizes the results from a number of sponge

TABLE 24-IV
RESORPTION AND TOXICITY OF 50–60 MG DOSES OF CYANOACRYLATES IN FOURTEEN-DAY SPONGE IMPLANTS IN RATS

Cyanoacrylate	Percent Control Hydroxyproline Content	Percent Cyanoacrylate Loss
Methoxyl-ethyl†	32	81
Methyl†	13	80
Ethyl†	22	65
βββ Trifluoroisopropyl†	100	15
n-Heptyl	94	9
n-Pentyl	100	3
neo-Pentyl	88	0
Cyclopentyl*	86	0
n-Propyl*	100	0
n-Hexyl and higher homologues	100	0

* Acute inflammation, marked.
† Acute inflammation, marked.

implant experiments with various cyanoacrylates over the last six years. Some of these experiments are supported by direct measurements employing isotopically-tagged cyanoacrylates.[2] A dichotomy is shown. Those α-cyanoacrylates such as methoxyethyl, methyl, ethyl, and beta, which are rapidly resorbed from sponge implants, generally also are associated with continuing acute inflammatory responses within the implants. These inflammatory responses usually are accompanied by inhibition of collagen elaboration. Thus, these cyanoacrylates appear to be unsuited for application to sites where elaboration of collagen is necessary, that is, sites of wound repair. In marked contrast, their inflammatory and necrotizing effects, coupled with their physiochemical properties, may make one or more of these

The Cyanoacrylates

highly reactive adhesives uniquely suited for occlusion of the oviduct, or possibly the vas deferens.

The reverse is represented by other materials listed in Table 24-IV. Long-chain alkyl cyanoacrylates such as n-hexyl, do not inhibit collagen elaboration and also are not appreciably absorbed. These materials generally evoke a foreign body reaction, mild chronic inflammation, and minimal or no local necrosis (Fig. 24–4). It was assumed that a simple structure-activity relationship could be described, in which the degree of foreign-body reaction, lack of inflammation, and retention in tissues were functions of increasing alkyl-site chain length. The relationship is not this simple. Table 24-IV groups cyanoacrylates in order of decreasing local resorption. A third member of the alkyl series, n-propyl, is low on this list.

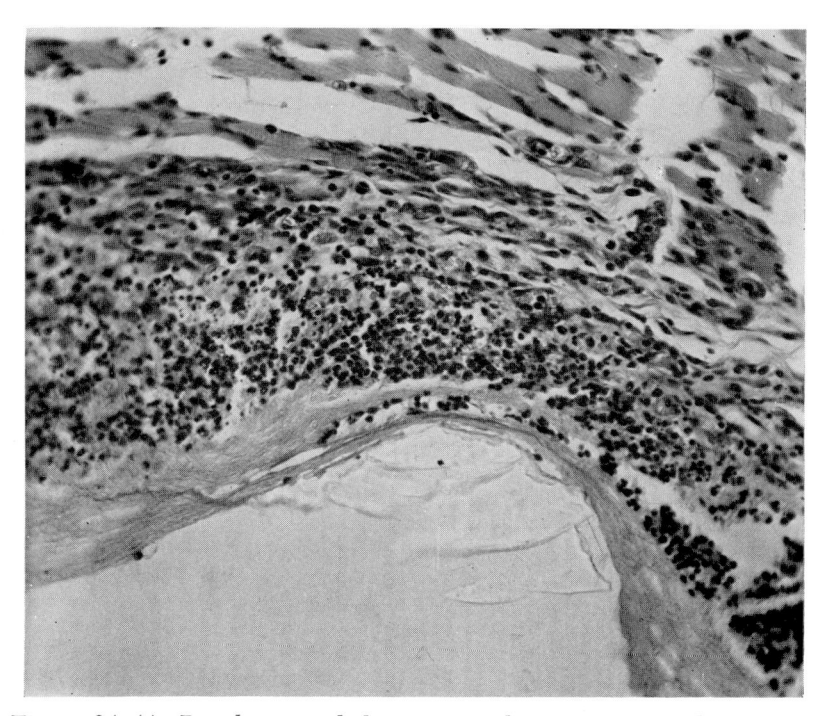

Figure 24–4A. Periphery, methyl sponge implant, twenty-one days. Plate-like polymer fragments at edge of implant are surrounded by fibrin, necrotic debris, and inflammatory cells (H & E, × 250). Photographed at Walter Reed Army Institute of Research, Washington, D.C.

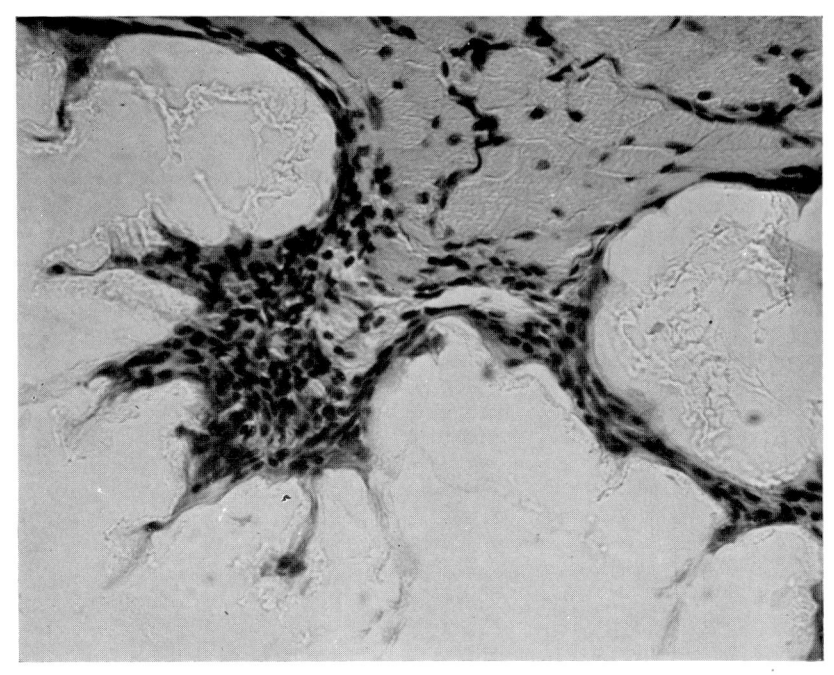

Figure 24–4B. Periphery, n-pentyl sponge implant, twenty-one days. Irregular, fibrillar polymer deposits are surrounded by giant cells. Almost no inflammation is present (H & E, × 400).

CONCLUSION

α-cyanoacrylate tissue adhesives are effective hemostatic and wound-closure agents possessing novel adhesive properties. Some α-cyanoacrylates are necrotizing and pyogenic, making their possible use in occlusion of the oviduct or vas deferens an interesting possibility worthy of experimental study.

REFERENCES

1. Herrmann, J.B., and Woodward, S.C.: The effect of cyanoacrylate tissue adhesives upon granulation tissue formation in Ivalon sponge implants in the rat. *Surgery*, 59:559, 1966.
2. Woodward, S.C.: Physiological and biochemical evaluation of implanted polymers. *Ann NY Acad Sci*, 146:225, 1968.
3. Corfman, P.A., Richart, R.M., and Taylor, H.C., Jr.: Response of the rabbit oviduct to a tissue adhesive. *Science*, 148:1348, 1965.

4. Coover, H.W., Jr., Joyner, F.P., Shearer, N.H., Jr., and Wicker, T.H., Jr.: Chemistry and performance of cyanoacrylate tissue adhesives. *Soc Plastics Engineers J, 15*:413, 1959.
5. Woodward, S.C., Herrmann, J.B., Cameron, J.L., Leonard, F., Brandes, G., and Pulaski, E.J.: Histotoxicity of cyanoacrylate tissue adhesives. *Ann Surg, 162*:113, 1965.
6. Methyl 2-cyanoacrylate monomer. *A Biodegradable Plastic Tissue Adhesive.* Medical Research Department, Somerville, N.J., Ethicon, Inc., 1966.
7. Herrmann, J.B., Woodward, S.C., Osterhaut, D., and Leonard, F.: Unpublished observations.
8. Herrmann, J.B., Katz, A.R., and Woodward, S.C.: Experimental anastomosis of small arteries employing alkly-cyanoacrylates. *J Biomed Mat Res, 1*:395, 1967.
9. Herrmann, J.B.: Granulation tissue development and collagen elaboration within polyvinyl alcohol sponge implants of various sizes and shapes in rats. *Fed Proc, 26*:516, 1967.
10. Herrman, J.B., and Woodward, S.C.: The effects of a fluoroalkl cyanoacrylate tissue adhesive upon granulation tissue development, fibroplasia and hemostasis. *Ann Surg,* In press.
11. Siegel, S.: *Nonparametric Statistics for the Behavioral Sciences.* New York, McGraw Hill, 1956, p. 166.

Chapter 25

MICROELECTRONICS AND IMPLANT INSTRUMENTS

WEN H. KO

The phenomenal growth of microelectronics in recent years is due to the strong demands of the space program, the military, and industry. However, the impact of this technology is certainly not limited to these areas. The interaction of microelectronics with biomedical sciences will not only accelerate the growth of biomedical research, but also will provide many interesting problems and challenging stimulations for electronics engineers. This article discusses the application of microelectronics to biomedical instrumentation. Examples of implantable microelectronic circuits for telemetry and stimulation are given to illustrate the potentialities of microelectronic instrumentation in medical research.

BRIEF REVIEW OF MICROELECTRONICS

As the name implies, microelectronics refers to extremely small electronic circuits or systems. At the present time, the technology has been developed to such an extent that circuits containing a few thousand component parts may approach the density of cells in the human brain. Similarly, the corresponding theory has developed to a point where it can predict and explain accurately the electronic and atomic behavior of solid-state devices used in microelectronics. The packaging density, the number of electronic components (resistors, transistors, diodes, capacitors, etc.) per unit volume, is approaching a million per cubic centimeter. Typical packaging densities of currently available electronic circuits are shown in Figure 25-1. The implication of this development in solid-state circuits and theory to the life sciences is not fully recognized and cannot be overemphasized.

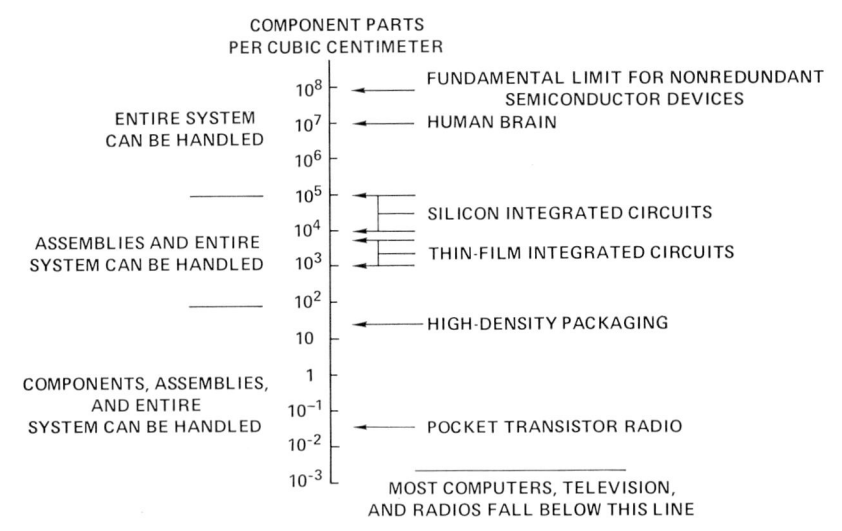

Figure 25-1. Packing densities of various microelectronic systems.

Fifteen years ago almost all electronic circuits were constructed from vacuum tubes and other conventional components. In a typical circuit (Fig. 25-2a), the vacuum tube itself occupies a large portion of the total volume. This type of circuit, with an average component density of 10^{-2} components per cc, still is used in many conventional electronic instruments.

The development of the transistor in 1948 and its subsequent improvement, have allowed it to replace the vacuum tube in most conventional circuits. A typical transistorized electronic circuit is illustrated in Figure 25-2b. Further reduction in size and mass can be obtained by miniaturization of each of the individual components such that they can be packed closely together. This *high density packaging* is illustrated in Figure 25-2c. Pocket radios and hearing aids currently are being made by this technique. It is possible to manufacture circuits with component densities as high as a hundred per cubic centimeter in this way.

These methods of building electronic circuits consist of taking individual components and assembling them. This process puts a lower limit on the size of each component, since very small parts are difficult to make and to handle. Furthermore, the need for interconnections and individual handling greatly increases

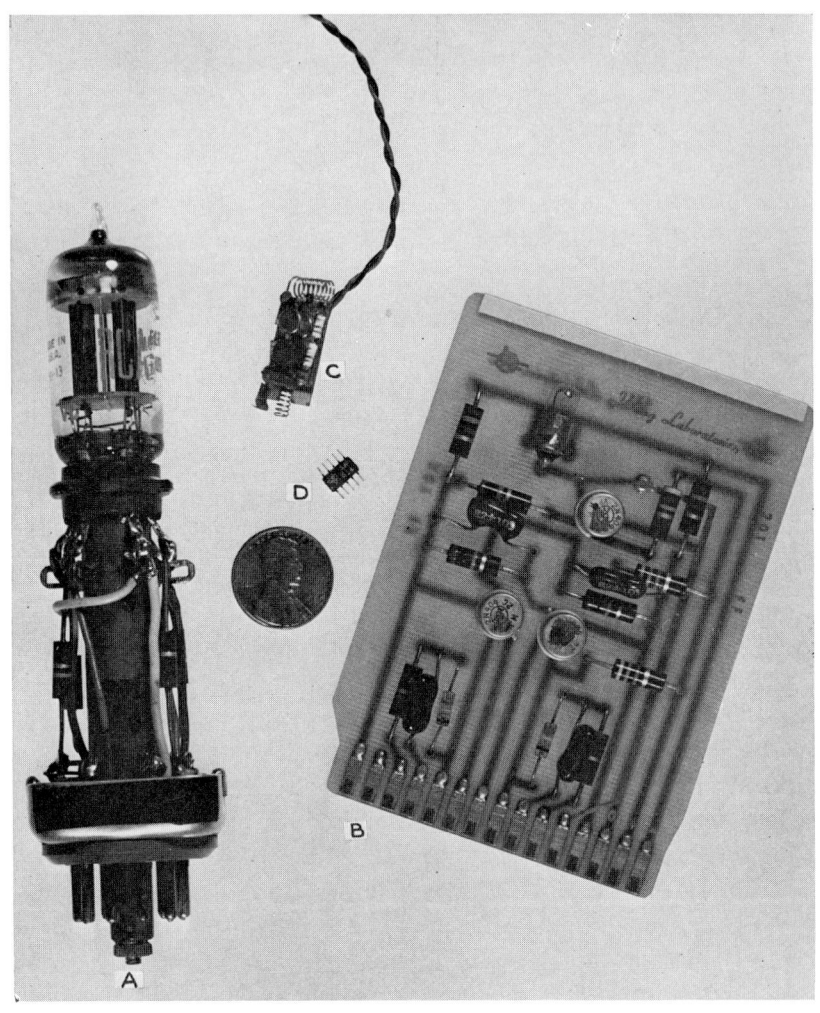

Figure 25–2. Examples of conventional and microelectronic circuits: a) conventional tube circuit; b) conventional transistor circuit; c) high-density packaged circuit; d) monolithic silicon integrated circuit.

the probability of failure. Thus, it has become necessary for electronics engineers to reshape their thinking completely to achieve further miniaturization. The result of this is the *integrated circuit* shown in Figure 25–2d. This circuit, which can perform the same functions as the others in Figure 25–2, is smaller than a conventional transistor package. Through the use of integrated circuit techniques, component densities of 10^4 to 10^5 components per cubic centimeter are being achieved.

Integrated circuits are constructed so that the components and their interconnections are integral parts of the substrate upon which the circuit is situated. There are two types of integrated circuits. In *thin-film integrated circuits* the components and connections are in the form of thin films of metals, insulators, and semiconductors with thicknesses of about one micron. These components are deposited on an insulating substrate in specific geometric patterns that give them the requisite electrical properties to form electronic circuits. In the *monolithic semiconductor integrated circuits* the substrate is a chip of single-crystal semiconductor such as silicon. Again, by depositing layers of specific patterns of impurities within the semi-conductor and thin films on its surface, it is possible to fabricate the entire circuit into a small silicon chip. A combination of thin-film and monolithic integrated circuits usually is called a *hybrid integrated circuit*.

The typical dimensions of the silicon chip are 0.5–2 mm square by 0.25 mm thick. Each chip contains from ten to hundreds of components. Several hundred circuits can be made simultaneously on a slice of silicon an inch in diameter and then separated into individual pieces and packaged. A typical wafer of integrated circuits is shown in Figure 25-3.

Published literature gives a more detailed discussion of fabrication techniques and their characteristics.

ADVANTAGES AND PROBLEMS OF INTEGRATED CIRCUITS

Besides the great size and weight reduction per electronic function, integrated circuits have the following important advantages over conventional circuits:

Better Reliability

For integrated circuits, extremely accurate internal connections are made at the same time that the components are manufactured. The mechanical strength-to-mass ratio of the entire circuit is increased greatly, so that integrated circuits can withstand

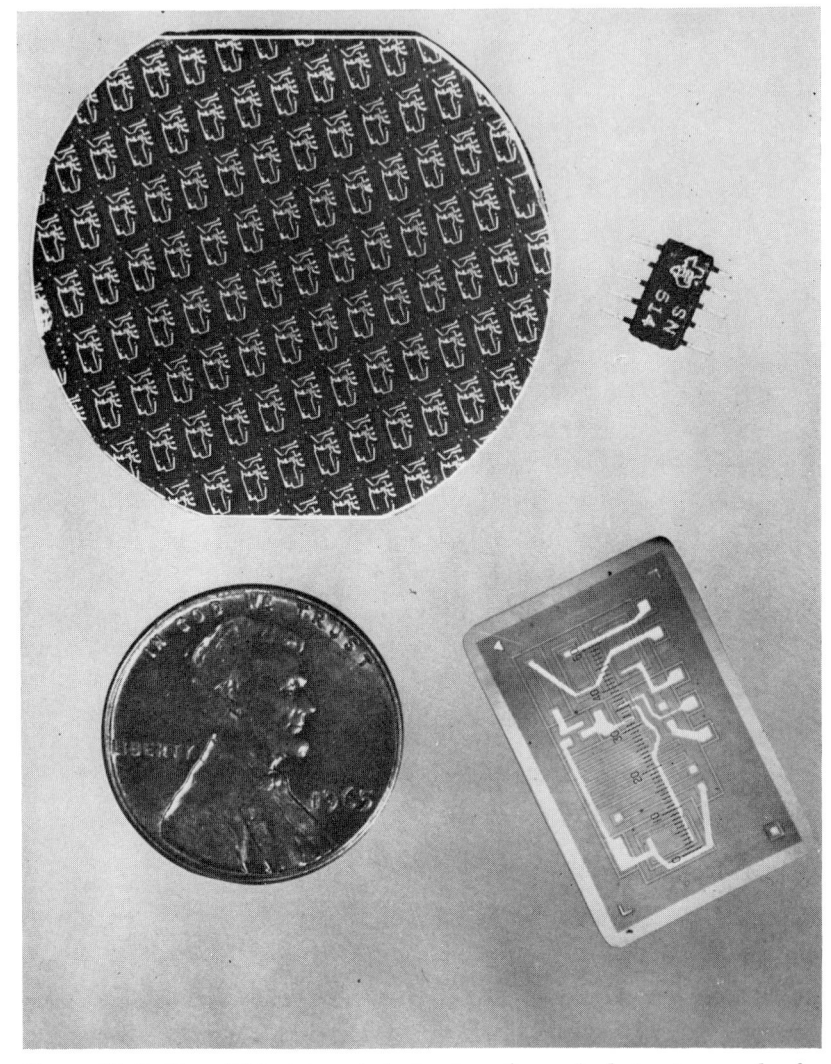

Figure 25-3. Monolithic integrated-circuit wafer and photomicrograph of a single chip.

twenty thousand times the gravitational pull of the earth. The failure rate of monolithic integrated circuits has been shown to be below ten parts per billion element hours. Such increased reliability makes more complex systems possible.

Better Performance

When the speed of electronic circuits is increased from one operation per millisecond (10^{-3} sec), to one per microsecond (10^{-6} sec), or one per nanosecond (10^{-9} sec), the time that the signal takes to travel through the circuit no longer can be considered infinitesimal. There will be a time delay due to the propagation of the signal in the circuit itself. This propagation time is reduced greatly when circuits are close together and very small.

Lower Cost

Although integrated circuits are made with costly, elaborate, and precise processes, many circuits can be made at one time; once a circuit is developed, it can be mass produced. At present, many integrated circuits are available at fractions of the cost of equivalent conventional circuits.

From the user's standpoint, integrated circuits have the following disadvantages: a) they cannot be repaired; b) the user is constrained to design his system using available integrated circuits, to avoid the high costs of custom design and the production of small quantities of integrated circuits.

MICROELECTRONICS AND BIOINSTRUMENTATION

The most apparent application of microelectronics is in the area of implant instrumentation. Because instruments made by microelectronic techniques are small and have a long life, they can be implanted or attached to the surface of a subject to measure or stimulate the response of the subject under study. This is the concept of implant electronics.

It is now possible to make extremely small telemetry systems which can be surface mounted, ingested, or implanted. They can relay information from the signal source to some remote data handling and recording equipment, eliminating the use of restraining wires. In the field of biotelemetry, many significant results are reported in the literature. For example, with implant telemetry, deep body temperature can be measured accurately to 0.05°C; and the heart rate of a mouse or a larger animal can be monitored twenty-four hours a day for weeks or years, while the subject resumes its normal activity.

The counterpart of telemetry is stimulation. It is well known that the brain, nerve, and muscle systems can be stimulated by electrical impulses. With microelectronic circuits these stimulators can be implanted in the body and made to respond to external commands. The cardiac pacemaker is a well-publicized example.

If a stimulator, and a telemetry unit are combined as shown in Figure 25-4, a closed-loop control system can be used in experi-

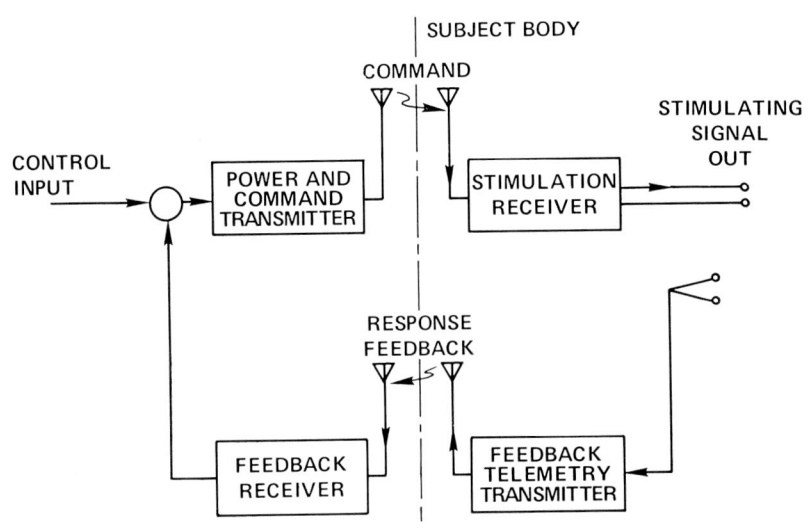

Figure 25-4. Schematic diagram of a closed-loop control system for implant bio-instrumentation.

ments to produce a particular response to a stimulation. An external electronic circuit can compare the telemetered response to the desired value and then adjust the stimulation level electronically until the response reaches the set amount. This type of system can be mounted on the surface or implanted in the body of the experimental animal.

For many existing instruments, the reduction of size and weight produced by integrated circuits might be desirable, but not essential. However, other improved performance characteristics of microelectronic circuits are also significant. In recording body signals, many experiments have to be made in a shielded room to avoid noise and interference of wire systems. If a microelectronic amplifier is used at the sensor or transducer location, the signal can be amplified before noise or interference gets into the system. A few models of such amplifiers have been constructed in our laboratories for electromyographic (EMG) measurement, and the results indicate that they are practical and very desirable.

With the continuing development of microelectronic technology, previously unavailable complex instrumentation systems for biomedical research are now becoming technologically feasible. Owing to improved reliability and small size, redundancy may be incorporated. These complex systems not only can serve useful instrumentation functions, but will permit a better understanding of life systems. Many interesting systems can be proposed. A few examples follow.

Current studies on the use of ear or shoulder muscles, not employed in normal activity, to control paralyzed limb muscles indicate that partial recovery of the limb function is possible. The ear muscle sends a coded command to the electronic circuit, which applies a stimulating signal to the paralyzed limb muscles. The desired response of the limb is achieved by closed-loop control systems through visual feedback. Such an electronic system can be made portable.

A new type of pacemaker capable of measuring the heart condition and making a simple diagnosis is being considered. It will be a monitor when the heart is functioning properly, but will start to pace as soon as the heart is not behaving normally. When the condition is severe, it will send an alarm to the person, asking him to call his doctor.

Surgical monitoring procedures for long operations can be automated. The condition of a patient can be monitored by a pattern-recognition system. Prior to surgery the system will be trained to recognize *normal* patterns (ECG, EEG, blood pressure, respiration, oxygen content of blood etc.) characteristic of the patient. During surgery, the equipment will scan these measurable parameters at a fast rate making constant comparisons with the normal patterns so as to determine the patient's condition. Whenever a danger sign appears the doctor will be informed and proper attention may be directed to the correction of the symptoms. The same system can be used in intensive-care units.

A man-machine direct communication system can be designed to bypass a defective sensory device or defective body limb. It seems possible to communicate with the central nervous system through the use of implanted electronic devices. Commands or notions of the subject can be transmitted through the implanted electronic device to an external computer unit which will interpret the signal or command and operate a machine. At the same time, the response of the machine can be fed back to the brain through the implant device. A part of such a system can be used as a sensory aid for the blind or deaf. It can also be a means of man-machine communication for a mute or paralyzed person.

Microelectronic technology is a result of a basic understanding of solid-state physics and its application to electronic devices and circuits. Similar methods can be used to develop new transducers for biomedical systems. Microelectronic amplifiers and signal processors could become an integral part of the transducer itself. In addition, the low power requirements of some special microcircuitry make it possible to consider biological sources of power to operate the sensor and associated electronic devices.

The microelectronic applications suggested above can be developed, but will demand considerable electronic engineering and life science efforts.

IMPLANT BIOTELEMETRY

To illustrate the potentiality of microelectronic bioinstrumentation, some of the implant telemetry research initiated at Case Western Reserve University will be discussed. These devices are designed by simple microelectronic techniques. Much improvement is expected when advanced facilities and skills are available for this research.

In implant-telemetry systems, the receiving units generally are standard and commercially available. Therefore, nearly all the research and design efforts are concentrated on the transmitting units which must be designed to meet the special requirements of each experiment. The generalized criteria for an implant transmitter can be summarized as follows:

1. Small size and weight (less than a few percent of the subject's size and weight).
2. Minimum body reaction (packaged with nontoxic materials and with proper shape to reduce tissue reaction).
3. High sensitivity (microvolts) and wide dynamic range to handle signals ranging from microvolts to millivolts
4. Good fidelity (signal frequency response from DC to several kHz or higher).
5. Low power consumption and long lifetime.
6. Reliable, rigid, and easily handled.
7. Suitable transmission range to permit the free movement of the subject.
8. Comply with regulations for radio transmission set up by the Federal Communications Commission.

SINGLE CHANNEL TELEMETRY SYSTEMS

It is desirable to explore the possibility of using new solid state electronic devices and technology in biotelemetry to meet the above general criteria and to obtain better performance, such as wider frequency range (from DC to 20 kHz); better sensitivity (microvolts) without amplifier stages and lower power consumption (microwatts) than thus far achieved. Six models of single-channel telemetry transmitters using tunnel diodes and transistors have been developed at Case Western Reserve University. They are identified as the K-1 to K-6 transmitters. Models K-1, K-2, and K-5 are high-density packaged units using discrete circuit components. Model K-3 is a thin-film circuit, and model K-5 is a multiple-chip silicon integrated circuit. Model K-6 has a hybrid integrated circuit unit assembled in a conventional flat pack and a monolithic integrated circuit unit. The performance specifications of K-1, K-5, and K-6 transmitters are listed in Table 1.

TABLE 25-I
PERFORMANCE OF K-1, K-5, AND K-6 TRANSMITTERS

	K-1	K-5	K-6
Size without battery	1.3 × 1.3 × 0.4 cm	0.8 dia. × 0.2 cm	1 × 0.6 × 0.3 cm
Weight without battery	1.7 gm	0.44 gm	0.5 gm
With battery	2.8 gm RM-400	1.44 gm RM-320	1.5 gm RM-320
Power consumption	1.3V, 1.2mA	1.2V, 1.2mA	1.2V, 0.4mA
Rf frequency (may be extended from 50 to 500MHz)	80–100 MHz	100–250 MHz	100–250 MHz
System noise (in shielded room, 1-kHz bandwidth)	1.5uV	3.5uV (at 100k input)	5uV, r.m.s.
Input sensitivity (6 db S/N)	1.uV	7.uV (10k input)	10uV
Dynamic range (limited by receiver)	2×10^3	10^3	10^3
Frequency response	0.1Hz-20kHz	0.1Hz-20kHz	0.1Hz-20kHz
Input impedance	5 to 8k	300 k to megohms	300 k to megohms
Transmission	5uV at 12 ft (with 4-in lead)	5uV at 4–8 ft. (without leads)	5uV at 4–8 ft. (without leads)
Carrier-frequency temperature stability	Poor	Better than 0.05%/°C	Better than 0.05%/°C

A study of powering the K-series transmitters by radio induction at 1 and 3.5 MHz is being made. A cage (30 × 24 × 14 inches) with coils wound around its outside and powered by a 150-W power oscillator, has been constructed. The detector unit, with three mutually perpendicular coils and rectifiers, has an over-all package size of a 1 cm diameter sphere, all the filtering components are placed within the sphere (Fig. 25–5). A smaller cage (18 × 14 × 14 inches) powered by a 30-W oscillator also has been tested and found to be satisfactory. The absorbed power density within the cage is about the 10mW/cm^2 safe limit set by government and industrial agencies. The power received by the detector is about 2mW.

A rechargeable battery can be used to power these implant transmitters, and a simplified radio frequency power detector (3/18 × 1/4 × 1/16 inches) can be used to convert external radio frequency power to charge the battery.

It also has been demonstrated that the transmitter can be powered by a silicon photocell with an area of 1 cm^2, a few feet from a 100 W lamp. It can be powered by a single thermocouple at a temperature difference of several hundred degrees centigrade or a thermopile operating at a 10° C temperature difference. From the literature, it appears that this amount of power can be generated in the body by chemical and mechanical reactions. Studies aimed at operating the transducer by body power are being undertaken.

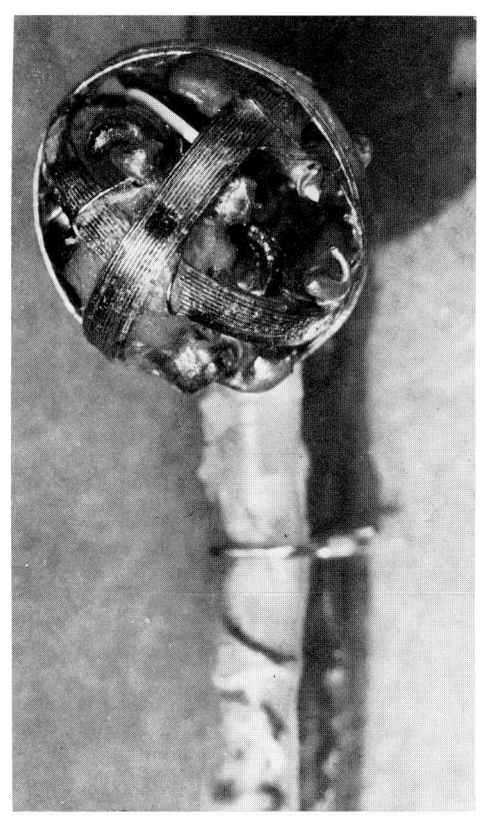

Figure 25–5. Structor of the implantable radio-frequency induction power detector.

K-5 and K-6 transmitters were implanted in animals to measure EMG, ECG, pressure, temperature, and stress. For the electrical signals, the input sensors can be platinum or stainless steel electrodes, either mounted one on each side of the transmitter package or extended through flexible cables to a remote location for ECG. The assembled transmitter is covered with an epoxy coating for sealing and then encapsulated in Dow-Corning medical grade Silastic 382. After encapsulation, the transmitter weighs about 1.5 to 2.5 gm.

The power supply can be packaged either with the transmitter or separately. When mercury cells are used, a miniature, bistable, magnetically actuated switch is included to spread the useful battery life over longer periods of time. The switch may be turned on or off by means of a DC magnetic field produced by a permanent magnet held up to six inches from the switch, or by a magnetizing coil.

A series of sixty K-5 and K-6 transmitters have been surgically implanted in rabbits, rats, and mice. Twenty-four of the transmitters were implanted directly in the right rear quadriceps muscle of adult albino male rabbits weighing between 3 and 6 kg. Standard surgical techniques were used to secure the transmitter and sensor electrodes within the longitudinal incision in the muscle. The power supply was located subcutaneously near the transmitter.

Using such systems, electromyographic signals were observed following the animal's recovery from the anesthesia (Fig. 25-6).

ECG signals from rats, rabbits, and mice were telemetered by implanting the transmitter and power supply subcutaneously on the backs of the animals below their necks. Wires connecting the transmitters to electrodes in the chest area were passed beneath the skin, and small incisions were made on the chest wall to suture the electrodes to the skeletal muscle to prevent their migration.

For some electrode placements, respirations rate as well as ECG was observed as periodic variations in the baseline. The signal quality of the radio-powered unit is comparable to that from the battery-powered unit. Figure 25-7 shows the photograph of a rat with a K-5 transmitter implanted on its back.

The lifetime of the electronic circuits should be indefinite for radio frequency-powered transmitters. A typical unit implanted in a rat has operated for 200 days. The major existing problems seem to be the packaging material and techniques.

M-SERIES TELEMETRY UNITS

For monitoring temperatures or other slow varying parameters, the M-1 to M-3 series of telemetry units was engineered. The

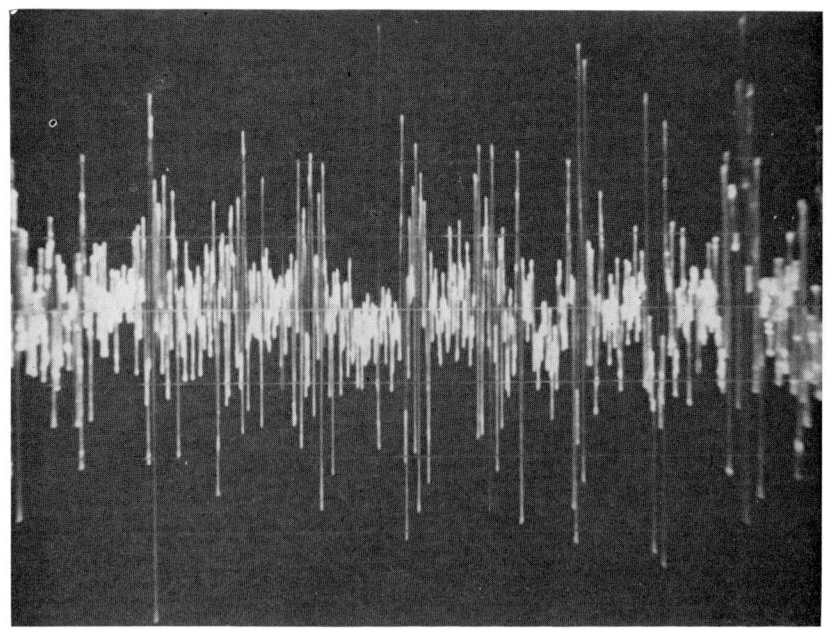

Microelectronics and Implant Instruments 289

Figure 25–6. EMG signals telemetered from the right rear quadriceps of a rabbit.

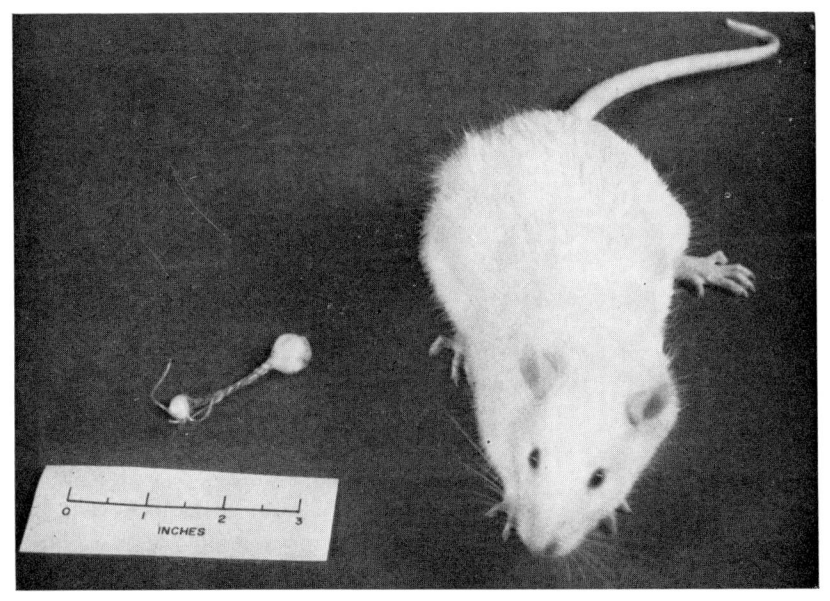

Figure 25–7. Rat with a K-5 transmitter implanted on its back. Another transmitter is shown for comparison.

emphasis is on the micropower consumption and simplicity in circuits. The M-1 unit occupies 0.4 cm volume and weighs 1.6 gm, including a 100 day battery supply. The improved M-3 unit is designed to operate at 1–5 μw power at a range of ten to thirty feet and with better battery voltage stability. This unit is packaged in two flat packs by the hybrid integrated circuit technique and radiated at frequencies of 100 to 200 MHz. The continuous operating lifetime of a battery for the M-3 can be one to two years.

MULTIPLEX SYSTEMS

A two channel, temperature and heart rate, micro-power telemetry system was constructed and demonstrated in our laboratory. The complete transmitter consumes 20 to 30 μw of power at 2.6 volts and can have a range from five to twenty feet.

A six-channel FM/FM multiplex system for metabolic studies was designed and built to monitor temperatures, respiration, ECG, and muscle spasms on the surface of a patient. It weighs 15 gm and has dimensions of 6.2 × 6.2 × 1.5 cm without battery. The time and temperature stability is better than 0.5 percent for 24 hours and for ± 10°C variation. Data were recorded twenty-four hours a day on a human patient for a two-week period and have yielded useful information on body rhythms.

A four-channel time-sharing multiplex system has been designed and evaluated in animals. Improved six-to-ten-channel systems are being developed. Without batteries, the four-channel transmitter occupies 0.4 cubic inch and weighs less than an ounce. These systems are designed for general purpose telemetry. For example, the four-channel transmitter may be used to transmit respiration and vector cardiograms or to transmit respiration, one-channel ECG, temperature, and heart sound.

IMPLANT STIMULATION

The stimulation of the brain, nervous system, and muscular system with surface or implanted electrodes is well known. Studies indicate that implant stimulation is a feasible method with which to control muscles that otherwise are useless.

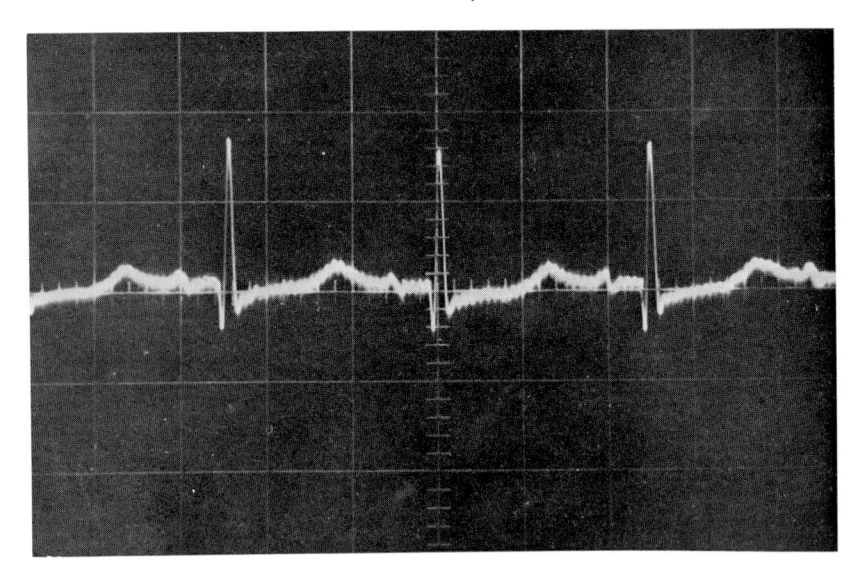

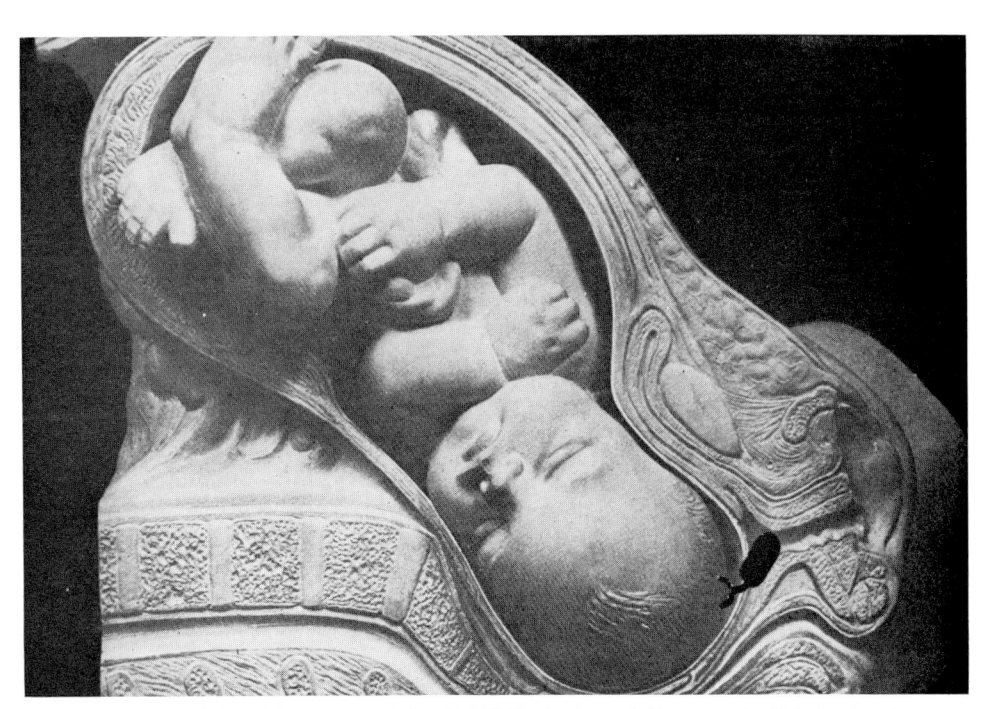

Figure 25-8. Telemetry of fetal ECG during delivery: a) ECG signal telemetered at the receiver output, b) placement of K-6 transmitter.

A radio-powered passive implant stimulator ($\frac{3}{8} \times \frac{1}{4} \times \frac{1}{8}$ inches) was designed and successfully evaluated in an animal. The unit converts the radio power from the external commanding transmitter into stimulating pulses for the muscle or nerve stimulation.

An implantable active stimulator to be controlled by external radio waves currently is being designed.

The pulse rate and duration of the stimulating signal will be controlled by the incoming radio wave, which also will supply the DC power for the electronic circuit. This is the first step towards the control system previously described.

APPLICATIONS

The telemetry and stimulation units are being used for monitoring and control experiments in medical research. A few examples are the following: monitoring fetal ECG during delivery, as shown in Figure 25–8; monitoring stress in a hip-joint orthotic nail head in a human patient; monitoring animal heart rate or temperature for air and water pollution studies and hibernation of animals; and stimulation of sections of the central nervous system for hibernation study and blood hypertension studies.

The application of these concepts and techniques to medical research and clinical cases is limited only by the creative speculation of each researcher.

REFERENCES

1. Koenjian, E.: *Microelectronics.* New York, McGraw-Hill, 1963.
2. Engineering Staff, Motorola Inc.: *Integrated Circuits.* New York, McGraw-Hill, 1965.
3. Bierman, H.: *Microelectronic Design.* New York, 1966.
4. Herwald, S.W., and Angello, S.J.: Integration of circuit function into solids. *Science, 132:*1127–1133, 1960.
5. Perugini, M.M., and Lindgren, N.: Microminiaturization. *Electron, 33:*78–107, 1960.
6. Wallmark, J.T., and Marcus, S.M.: Minimum size and maximum packing density of non-redundant semiconductor devices, *Proc IRE, 50:*286–298, 1962.

7. Hittinger, W.C., and Sparks, M.: Microelectronics. *Sci Amer, 213*:56, 1965.
8. Haggerty, P.E., et al.: Integrated Electronics. *Proc IEEE, 52*:1400–1669, 1964.
9. Ko, W.H., and Neuman, M.R.: Implant biotelemetry and microelectronics. *Sciences, 156*:351, 1967.
10. Cacares, C.A., Cooper, J.K., and Mackay, R.S.: In Cacares, C.A. (Ed.): *Biomedical Telemetry.* New York, Academic Press, 1965.
11. Slater, L.: *Biotelemetry.* New York, Pergamon Press, 1965.
12. Mackay, R.S.: *Bio-Medical Telemetry.* New York, Wiley, 1968.
13. Winget, C.M., Averkin, E.C., and Fryer, T.B.: Quantitative Measurement by telemetry of ovulation and oviposition in the fowl. *Amer J Physiol, 209*:853–858, 1965.
14. Delgado, J.M.R.: Sequential behavior induced repeatedly by stimulation of red nucleus in tree monkeys. *Science, 148*:1361–1361, 1965.
15. Eisenberg, L. et al.: Radio frequency stimulation: A research and clinical tool. *Science, 147*:578–582, 1965.
16. Vodovnik, L., et al.: Myo-electric control of paralyzed muscles. *Trans IEEE BME-12*:169–172, 1965.
17. Reswick, J.B., and Vodovnick, L.: Topics on man-machine communication in orthotic and prosthetic systems in *Digest 7th Int Conf Med Bio-Engin,* Stockholm, Sweden, August, 1967.
18. Brindley, G.S., and Lewin, W.S.: The sensations produced by electrical stimulation of the visual cortex. *J Physiol, 196*:479–493, 1968.
19. Ko, W.H., and Yon, E.: Miniature FM implant biotelemetry transmitters and RF induction power supply for implant circuits, In *Proc 6th Int Conf Med Electr & Bio Engin,* Tokyo, August, 1965.
20. Ko, W.H.: Piezoelectric energy converter for electronic implants In *Proc 19th Conf Engin in Med & Biol,* San Francisco, November, 1966.
21. Lin, W.C., and Ko, W.H.: A study of microwatt-power pulsed carrier transmitter circuits. *Med Biol Engin, 6*:309–317.
22. Lin, W.C., and Garg, B.: An implantable pulsed microwatt-power transmitter circuit insensitive to battery voltage variation. In *21st ACEMB,* Houston, Texas, November, 1968.
23. Ko, W.H., and Robrock, R.B. II: A six channel physiological telemetering system. *Proc In Intern Telemet Conf,* Washington, D.C., May, 1965.
24. Ramseth D., Yon, E.T., and Ko, W.H.: A multiple multiplex channel integrated circuit biomedical telemetry system. In *Proc, 8th ICMBE,* July 20, 1969.
25. Starbuck, D.L., Mortimer, J.T., Shealy, C.N., and Reswick, J.B.: An implantable electrode system for nerve stimulation. In *Proc 19th Conf Eng Med Biol,* San Francisco, November, 1966.

DISCUSSION: BIOENGINEERING TECHNOLOGY (B)

Denis J. Prager, *Moderator*

Dr. Prager opened the discussion by asking for questions on Mr. Innis's paper concerning the use of fiber optics for visualization and localization.

Dr. Shubeck wanted to know the nature of the clad material on the outside of the fiber.

Mr. Innis replied that the material is glass. He compared the structure to that of bifocal lenses, where a small lens is fused into the major portion of the glass to permit both near and distant vision. Optical fibers have a glass of one composition on the outside fused to one of another composition on the inside. If the glasses are selected properly, the fibers will stay together without exploding.

Dr. Shubeck asked the reason for the variations in fiber diameters.

Mr. Innis explained that, in the selection of a monofilament to transport light, flexibility is of paramount importance. Larger fibers transport more light, but are not very flexible; as the diameter is decreased, the fiber flexibility approached that of hair.

Dr. Shubeck inquired about the largest fiber made by Mr. Innis.

Mr. Innis said that he had used a fiber of 300 μ. It was still flexible, but quite fragile, and broke if bent too much.

Dr. Segal noted that one of the catheters was 27 mm in length and asked if it was possible to distribute the light along the entire catheter length rather than continuing it to the tip.

Mr. Innis explained that this is accomplished by having the distal ends of the individual fibers distributed along the length of the catheter.

Dr. Prager wanted to know the possibilities for the use of plastic fibers.

Mr. Innis explained that plastic fibers are in use. They are more durable than glass fibers, but their transmission capacity is not quite as high, especially near the infrared range, and they can be injured by heat.

Dr. Prager asked if plastic fibers were cheaper and if they would be appropriate for the types of problems under consideration.

Mr. Innis thought that the use of plastic fibers would not be considerably cheaper, since the actual price of the materials is not a major component of the total cost of the equipment. He went on to explain further that very high resolution fiber optic systems utilize glass multifibers. He gave as example a filament composed of 3 fibers, with each fiber being a composite of 36 smaller diameter fibers. This was made by assembling 36 rods into a bundle and then drawing the entire bundle to a small diameter composite fiber. Such composites have great resolving properties because the sizes of the individual fibers and the components of the object to be resolved are comparable. The cross-sectional diameter of the fiber is 60 μ but since it consists of 36 elements, the diameter of each element is between 8 and 10 μ. This cannot be done with plastic materials.

Dr. Segal inquired if the light source can be changed.

Mr. Innis said that the light source can be changed. In the ultraviolet range, this is related to the type of glass used for the fibers. Glasses in general use transmit ultraviolet light very poorly. The UK Series of glasses from Germany transmit better than the flint glasses that are used generally. Quartz gives excellent transmission, but methods of cladding quartz are not known, precluding the use of flexible quartz fibers for the transmission of ultraviolet light.

Mr. Pontarelli commented on work with ultraviolet-transmitting fibers. Illinois Institute of Technology is collaborating with the Signal Corps in the development of ultraviolet-transmitting fibers with a wide spectral range and about fifty percent transmission. Transmission of ultraviolet in the three hundred nanometer range is being made possible by the development of new glasses, or the modification of existing ones. It is very expensive to coat quartz, e.g. coating three to five mil fibers with glass resin costs three dollars per foot. Such fibers will transmit up to twenty-five hundred angstroms but would have effective transmission of only 10 to 30 percent in 3-foot lengths.

Mr. Innis stated that American Optical makes such an instrument that employs fiber optics in catheters. The catheter has both an afferent and an efferent fiber bundle. Light, transmitted through one bundle, illuminated the blood at the end of the catheter.

The blood reflects light back through the other bundle to be detected and quantified by a photomultiplier. Light is transitted at two wavelengths alternately; one wavelength shows the baseline in terms of hemoglobin content; the other wavelength shows the degree of oxygen saturation of the blood. An instantaneous readout of blood oxygen content at the tip of the catheter is obtained. The catheter tip can be introduced into an artery and advanced into the left heart, or placed in the right heart through a vein.

Dr. Prager commented that this was an example of the complexity and versatility possible by mixing bundles and using different wavelengths.

Miss Randall (N.Y. Times) noted that it has been suggested that a flexible fiber optics proctoscope could increase the efficiency of screening for colonic cancer. She pointed out that the instrument costs about 1,000 dollars and wondered how long the price would be that high.

Dr. Brueschke explained that a proctoscope, with a plastic fiber bundle, was presently in production and could be expected to sell for about 300 dollars to 400 dollars. The tip is capable of being moved and there are other desirable features; it is being developed in cooperation with the National Institutes of Health.

Dr. Prager wanted to know the smallest tip size.

Mr. Pontarelli thought it was about 2 mm.

Dr. Lee noted that locating small stones in the kidney and urinary tract is difficult and wanted to know if there are plans to make a kidney-pelvic scope.

Mr. Innis admitted he had no plans for such an instrument; and asked what the maximum catheter size could be.

Dr. Zinsser replied that an instrument of up to 2 mm could be used.

Mr. Innis said that a Japanese firm has developed a bundle about two millimeters in diameter with tips that can be articulated. It may be possible to insert such an instrument through the bladder into the ureter to look for stones.

Dr. Prager asked Dr. Clyman and Dr. Cohen if they saw any need for improving gastroscopes.

Dr. Clyman stated that a flexible gastroscope was desired. Image resolution is a problem in gastroscopy; clarity is not up to desirable levels. He thought that, at present, rigid fiber optics were used only to transmit light to the end of the instrument.

Dr. Zinsser wanted to know how the cardioscope was sterilized.

Mr. Innis said they used ethylene-oxide gas. The light guides could be sterilized at 275° C at 15 pounds of pressure.

Dr. Segal asked if the quality of transillumination with the ureteral catheter was such that the blood vessels around the ureter could be seen.

Mr. Innis said that if there were vessels which were very close, they might be seen as dark streaks in the field.

Dr. Clyman said he had done such work and definitely had observed vessels in the wall.

Dr. Prager opened Mr. Swope's paper on a fiber optics laser probe for discussion.

Dr. Brueschke asked Mr. Swope if Dr. Goldman in Cincinnati was aware of his work.

Mr. Swope said that some of the work was done with Dr. Goldman's group. The work was not successful since neither the hair nor its roots were destroyed; this probably was due to ignorance of the absorption characteristics of the material. On the other hand, it was successful in that the device was built, it was introduced into the hair follicle, and the fiber produced about a thousandth of a joule. This corresponds to an energy density of about two hundred joules per square centimeter at the tip.

Dr. Brueschke suggested that they might have been more successful if they had used a carbon dioxide laser.

Mr. Swope was not aware of a material that could be used to conduct carbon dioxide energy.

Dr. Brueschke suggested arsenic trisulfide, if it was capable of sustaining sufficient transmission.

Dr. Prager asked if Mr. Swope knew of anyone who had experience in producing tissue lesions similar to those of interest to this conference.

Mr. Swope commented on some cancer destruction work at the National Institutes of Health, but noted that this work was confined to pigmented tumors which absorb laser energy very readily. The tissues under consideration at this conference appear to be quite translucent, even white. This problem might be circumvented by the introduction of a stain, but care would have to be exercised. For example, if carbon black were painted on the skin, it is possible that the carbon black could be removed without any skin damage at all.

This principle has been used in tattoo removal.

Dr. Prager noted that, when he first heard of this work, he was thinking of the possibility of using a bundle to conduct energy to the uterotubal junction, as a means of producing a lesion which would occlude the end of the oviducts.

Mr. Swope thought it was entirely problematical until more was known about the optical characteristics of the tissue. He suggested that rather than producing a lesion, which he considered a thermoreaction, it might be possible to induce a short-term photochemical reaction. It also might be possible for the carbon dioxide laser to occlude the fallopian tubes in a matter similar to that in which they were pinched. If the path were not tortuous, the carbon dioxide laser could be introduced and would undoubtedly produce a lesion.

Dr. Thompson noted that light energy was absorbed by a darkened lesion caused by placing carbon particles on the skin. He asked about the possibility of placing particles within the tubal lumen, staining the tissues with carbon (e.g. India ink), and producing a beam that might destroy the epithelium.

Mr. Swope admitted that the possibility existed, but that the light would have to reach the particles and be absorbed.

Dr. Neuwirth suggested coating the interior of the fallopian tube.

Dr. Thompson said that the portion of the oviduct which went through the uterine musculature was relatively straight.

Dr. Taylor said the discussion had been concerned with the

relative ease with which various devices could reach the oviducts. He thought that the chemical reaction should be considered also. When cryosurgery and electrocautery were being considered, the speed at which tissue damage decreased was of interest. Minimum destruction of the outer surface of the tube is desired. He thought that, in addition to considering how to get to the site, the nature of the tissue reaction and the rate of tissue damage fall-off should be matters of concern. He wanted to know what was known about the effects of lasers on tissues; in particular, the range between complete destruction and complete health of the tissues.

Mr. Swope said that he would have to discuss this in relation to the eye. Here, absorption occurs in a very thin layer of tissue, the pigmented epithelium; the interaction between laser energy and the tissue occurs in this very thin layer of the eye. He did not know the subsequent reaction of the entire retina to this process. He thought that experimenting with specific tissues would be necessary. The depth of penetration of the reaction into the tissue is determined by its homogeneity. In a homogenous material, penetration can be predicted from the absorption characteristics of the tissue.

Dr. Taylor asked if the effect on the epithelium decreased rapidly, would penetration go through the epithelium to the muscle.

Mr. Swope explained that epithelium is highly absorbent and muscle is nonabsorbent. If the laser energy could be delivered in a very short pulse, the thermal effects are of little concern. If the energy is delivered slowly, over a period of seconds, thermal conductivity becomes an important factor.

Dr. Brueschke suggested that one way to circumvent the problem would be to have an intermediate structure between the laser and the wall. The laser energy would be converted directly into heat, creating a local burn. This would not require particles, for the end of the catheter could serve as a particle. He wanted to know if a laser was capable of delivering sufficient energy of this type and if the end of the catheter could be heated very quickly.

Mr. Swope said yes.

Dr. Brueschke then wanted to know if the high-frequency sound reception capability of the squirrel monkey ear was destroyed because the tissues destroyed were in the proximal portion of the cochlea.

Mr. Innis stated that when the inner ear was irradiated, the portion of the cochlea considered to be responsible for the reception of high frequencies was destroyed. To that extent, it was the proximal part of the cochlea that was being irradiated. At the Jefferson Medical College, attempts to produce clinical lesions to alleviate tinnitus have not been successful. However, the laser lesions were highly specific to the cochlea and did not affect other organs of the inner ear. These results differ from those obtained by ultrasound and cryosurgery where everything is destroyed.

Dr. Corfman wanted to know how large an area could be destroyed with a laser.

Mr. Swope explained that it depended on many things, including the method of delivering the laser energy and the size of the laser needed. In terms of lesion size, the type of laser is the determining factor: with a little helium neon laser the lesion is limited to a very small area; whereas, carbon dioxide lasers can burn holes in doors.

Dr. Corfman asked if they were round holes.

Mr. Swope said the shape could be changed. If the lesion were to be made by a single application, then pains should be taken to configure the system to give the desired shape. If many applications were used, painting could be done and numerous small lesions could be produced. This is the method used in the eye; in photocoagulation of the retina, two or three hundred irradiations are used in a given session.

Dr. Corfman speculated about introducing a material into the oviduct. He asked if the operator would be confined to the production of point lesions or if the method could be modified to destroy segments of the organ.

Mr. Swope expained that with the pulse laser, lesion production would have to be point by point. On the other hand, if a continuously operating laser were used, it would be operating all the time and painting would have to be done. The procedure could not be accomplished all at once; it would be necessary to move the ends of the fibers and irradiate simultaneously.

Mr. Pontarelli wanted to know if a fiber could transmit sufficient energy to perform the jobs under discussion.

Mr. Swope thought that the question is the amount of energy required, since there is indeed a limit to the amount of energy that can be transmitted by a fiber. This is due to a number of factors. If the energy is introduced into the fiber from an external laser, then the ends of the fiber are subject to damage. If the output end of the fiber (the part of the fiber that is in contact with the tissue) becomes optically contaminated, high temperatures may result at the end of the fibers. Precautions to prevent this must be taken; by and large this is an engineering problem. Using a fiber optic with fused ends from a continuously operating laser, several watts have been conducted to a bundle of a few millimeters. In Mr. Innis's work with the eye the pulse energy was normally one joule. Mr. Swope said that he had produced about one joule in a diameter of about 1 mm.

Dr. Prager started the discussion of Dr. Ko's paper on microelectronics and telemetry by explaining that many of the things mentioned have been done. Dr. Ko demonstrated what he is doing now. He showed that the limitation on the size of the implant is the size of the batteries; the electronic circuits themselves can be made as small as desired.

Dr. Ko stated that the question of how long a battery will last depends on how the circuit was designed. The transmitter that was demonstrated will last for forty continuous hours; with the remote switch, this can be extended to six months. Circuits are being designed to reduce power consumption to about a tenth of the power now consumed, so that forty hours will become four hundred hours. Work is being done on so-called solid electrolyte batteries; these are supposed to have a life-time of ten to twenty years. A telemetry unit has been designed to consume a single microwatt of power. There is the potential of producing circuits that work at about one-thousandth of the power now required; this would make a complex implant computer feasible.

Dr. Hulka noted that the uterus was a pump that contracts

about every five minutes. He wanted to know if it could be used as an energy source in any way.

Dr. Ko explained that the subject would have to be studied. More reliable physiologic movements were available as power sources: the action of the heart, the process of respiration, and intestinal motility, for example.

Mr. Swope asked if batteries could be recharged by means of an external energy field.

Dr. Ko said that they could. One of the batteries could be charged by an external oscillator.

Dr. Prager commented that this had been done with pacemakers.

VI NONSURGICAL STERILIZATION

Sheldon Segal, *Moderator*

Chapter 26

ATTEMPTED CYROSURGICAL CLOSURE OF THE FALLOPIAN TUBES

Frederick W. Martens, Jr.

When Dr. Irving Cooper demonstrated the value of cryosurgery in successfully dealing with Parkinsonism, it was only natural that other uses for this new technique should be sought. Dr. William Cahan has reported on several facets of his work at Memorial Hospital. It was mainly through his efforts and the generous financial support of the New York Foundation that an experimental approach to human female sterilization was undertaken. The reasearch attempted to produce extensive cornual agglutination by cryosurgery in order to block the fallopian tubes and produce permanent sterilization.

METHOD AND PATIENTS

The freezing unit used is identical to the one first employed by Cooper and is shown in Figures 26–1 and 26–2. Liquid nitrogen at a temperature of approximately −190 C is stored in a stainless steel Dewar flask contained in the cabinet. The liquid nitrogen flows from the Dewar flask through a flexible hose to the probe (Fig. 26–3), which was designed by Union Carbide specifically for the purpose of cornual agglutination. The liquid nitrogen is delivered to the end of the probe; the temperature of the tip is monitored by a thermocouple, and is recorded on the small kymograph.

A warming device was added to the original unit. This permitted the temperature of the tip of the probe to be returned to a normal level quickly without waiting for a normal thawing period.

Since no previous uterine cryosurgical experimentation had been reported, autopsy specimens were first used in order to

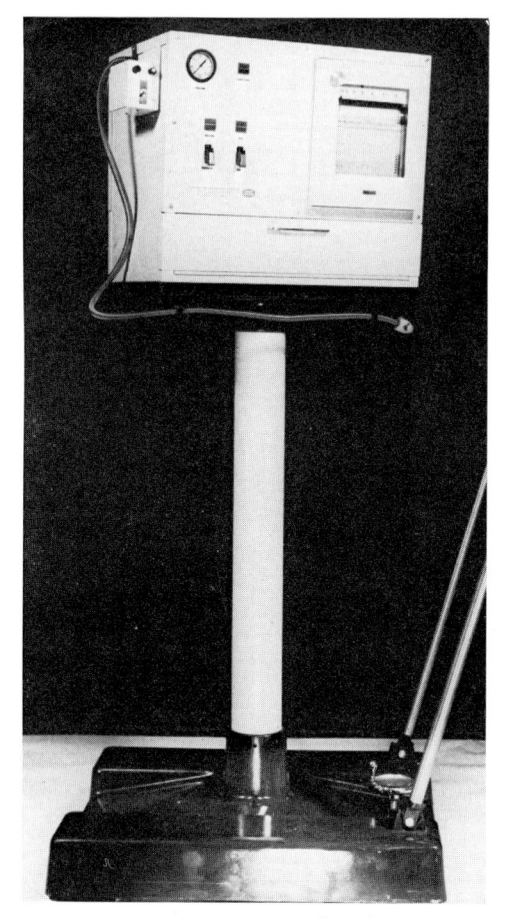

Figure 26-1. Freezing unit employed in experiment.

determine if the uterus would respond in a predictable manner to the freezing technique.

Multiple thermocouples were placed at varying distances from the freezing site, and accurate temperature readings were taken. When it was established that a predictable temperature response could be obtained from the autopsy specimen, it was considered practical to try it in the intact uterus, with its normal blood supply.

This was first done at the time of routine abdominal hysterectomy. With the abdomen open and the operator's hand on the

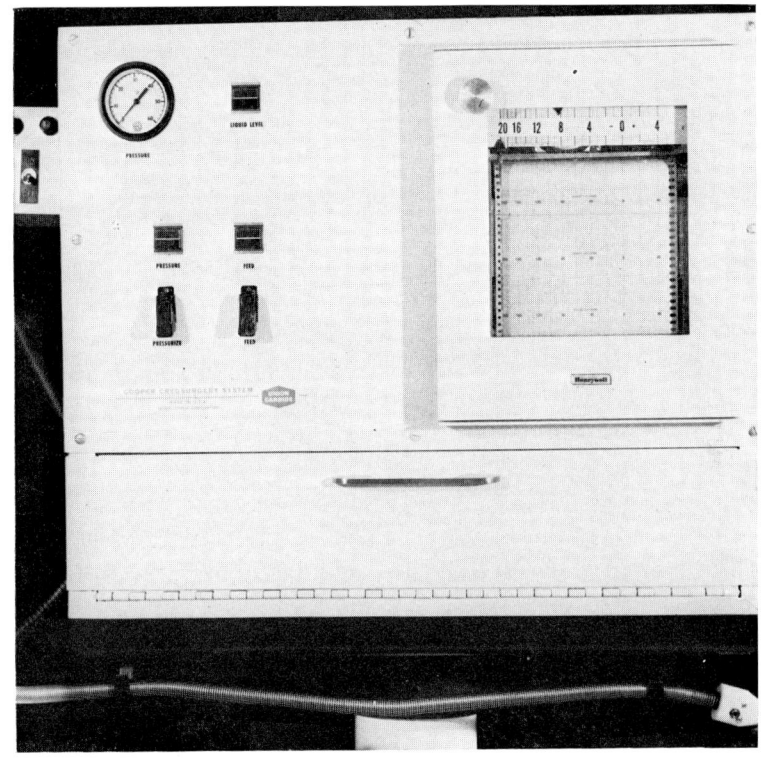

Figure 26-2. Freezing unit employed in experiment—close-up view.

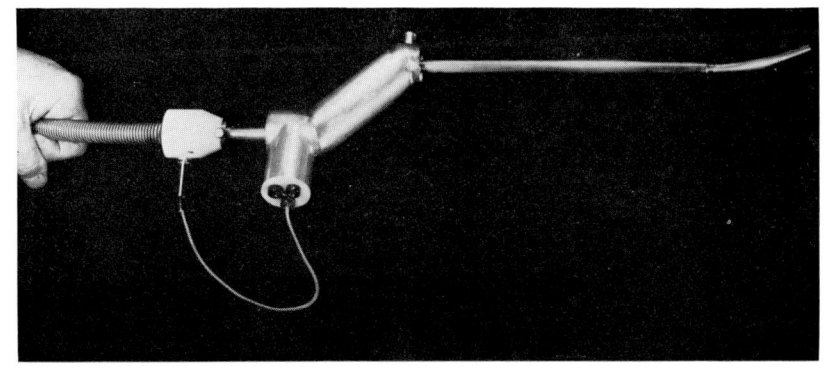

Figure 26-3. Flexible hose and probe.

uterus, the probe was inserted vaginally, through the dilated cervical canal, into the endometrial cavity. The temperature of the probe then was lowered to levels varying from −30 to −190 C. The operator's hand on the uterus prevented complete freezing of the entire uterine wall to the serosal surface as this might have endangered nearby pelvic organs. A satisfactory knowledge of safe working temperatures and duration of freezing was obtained in this manner.

The patients were selected in the immediate postpartum period. They had undergone an uneventful delivery; had a benign postpartum course; and, in most instances, were approved for sterilization because of their multiparity. Usually they returned to the hospital for sterilization between the sixth and eighth postpartum week.

A dilatation and curettage was performed, and the sterilization procedure was undertaken. In those patients who were being sterilized because of severe heart disease, diabetes, or other medical indication, a tubal ligation was performed in conjunction with the cryosurgical technique.

The uterine probe was inserted into the uterine cavity, and the tip of the probe was directed into one of the cornual regions. The temperature of the probe tip was lowered to levels of −60 to −160 C; it was maintained at these levels for two to six minutes. The probe was freed from the uterine wall after a short period and reinserted into the opposite wall, where the process was repeated.

If either an abdominal or vaginal tubal ligation was performed in conjunction with the cryosurgical procedures, the ligation was performed first. The cryosurgery then was done with either the abdomen or the cul-de-sac open so that direct vision or palpation of the cornual areas could be accomplished.

Patients in whom the cryosurgical technique was employed as the only sterilization method left the hospital within two days.

Hysterosalpingograms were taken after approximately two months.

RESULTS

The hysterogram in Figure 26–4 shows a satisfactory response to cryosurgical sterilization. Each cornual region is occluded and

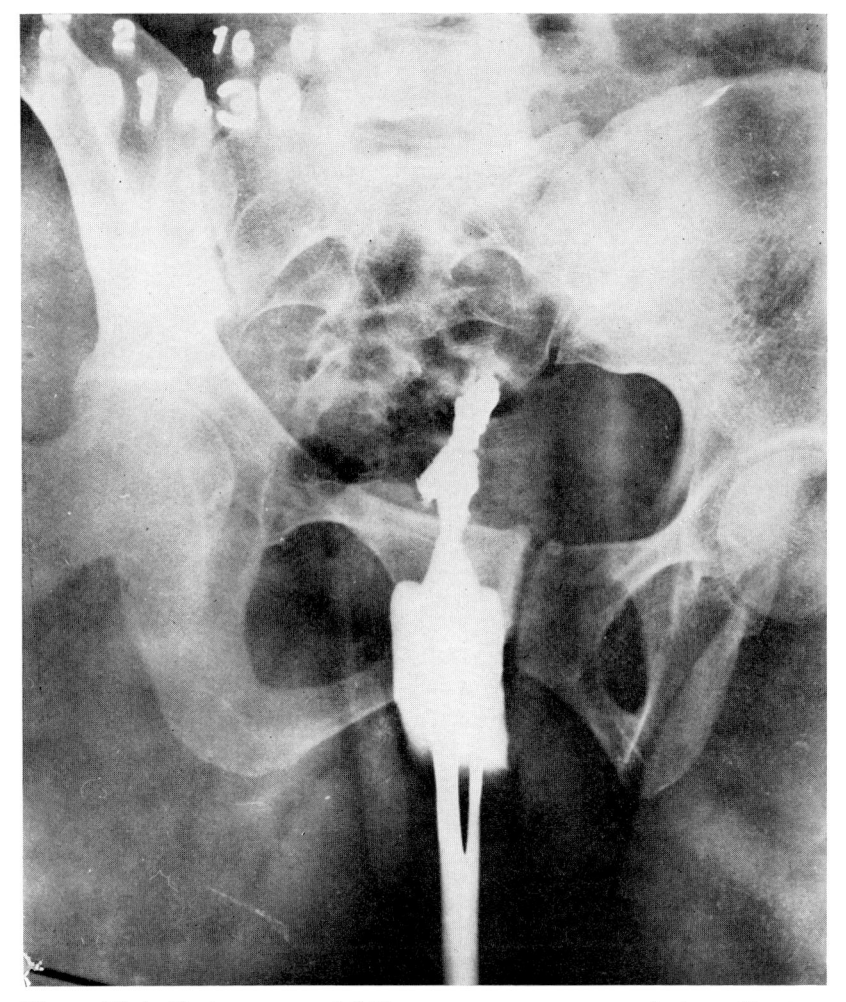

Figure 26–4. Hysterogram exhibiting response to cryosurgical sterilization: Tubal occlusion of both tubes.

no dye passed into the intramural portion of the tube. Of the 32 cases, only 11 oviducts were closed successfully by cryosurgery alone.

Figure 26–5 shows 1 patent oviduct and 1 occluded one; this occurred in 5 cases.

Cryosurgery was done on 32 oviducts: 11 were closed satis-

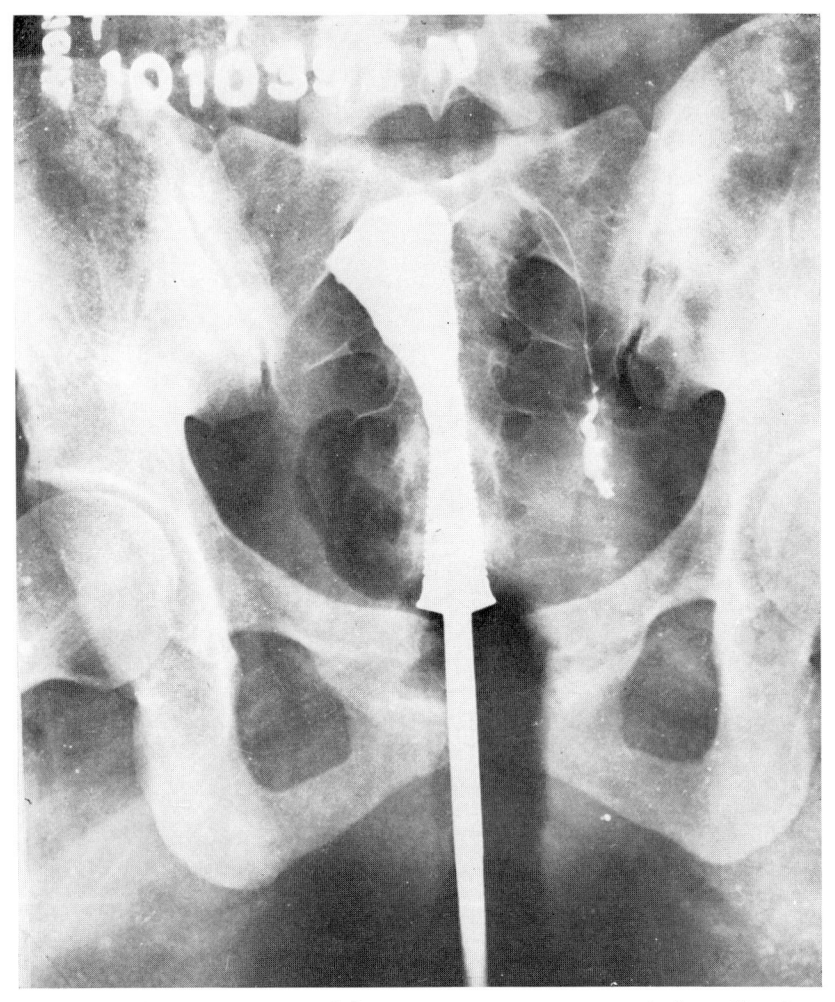

Figure 26–5. Hysterogram exhibiting response to cryosurgical sterilization: One tube is closed, the other open.

factorily; 13 remained open, 2 of these in spite of vaginal tubal ligation; and 8 tubes were not tested.

DISCUSSION

Obviously, this method has not proved to be a successful sterilization procedure. The reasons for failure, however, are not clear.

Is the probe positioned in the proper place? Since the probe cannot be directed to the tubal opening under direct vision, it certainly is possible that the tip of the probe does not come into contact with the ostia. However, the section of freeze or ice ball which is produced by the probe encompasses an area of several centimeters; this would include the tubal opening.

Are satisfactory temperatures being maintained for a sufficient length of time? If the temperature of the tip of the probe is taken in degrees centigrade and multiplied by the number of minutes that the temperature was maintained at this level, the unit of measurement designated as *degree minutes* is determined. Table 26-I shows each procedure arranged in order of degree minutes. In the first patient, the temperature of the probe was −160 C for 5 minutes or 800 degree minutes. It would appear from this table that the temperatures and times are not the critical factors.

Several uteri have been removed for various reasons following

TABLE 26-I

Patient	Degree Minutes	Tube
Ap	800	open
Ap	800	open
Co	800	open
Ri	700	closed
Ca	640	?
Ri	560	closed
Co	500	open
Gr	480	?
Gr	480	?
Ba	360	open
Go	360	?
Go	360	?
Di	360	open
Di	300	open
Ua	300	closed
Ve	270	open
Ve	270	closed
Ob	240	closed
Ob	240	closed
Ja	240	open
Ja	240	closed
Ba	240	closed
Ya	250	open
Cs	210	open
Cs	210	closed
Wi	240	open
Wi	240	open
St		?
St		?

the cryosurgical sterilization attempt, and in one of these essentially no fibrosis or scarring could be demonstrated in the cornual areas. There has been no opportunity to explore the reasons for this further.

Six to eight weeks postpartum may not be the optimum time to perform this procedure; perhaps a different time in relation to the menstrual cycle may give more predictable results.

The cryosurgical approach is a safe and easy one and has been performed without general anesthesia on several occasions. Reasons for failure should continue to be explored. If satisfactory results could be obtained, a sterilization procedure for large masses of people would be available.

Chapter 27

CAUTERIZATION FOR TUBAL STERILIZATION

J.F. Hulka and K.F. Omran

The use of cautery has been a historic method in healing attempts. With the origin of the germ theory, its use for the management of war wounds was discontinued. The development of electricity refined cautery so that it is a limited, but useful, surgical tool. The term *cautery* has changed in meaning from the concept of placing a red-hot poker to sear flesh to the modern definition of causing tissue death by the heat generated by an electric current. The concept of cautery also included tissue necrosis generated by chemicals or freezing techniques.

The human uterotubal junction is a tempting target for tissue destruction; it is microscopic in size, is buried in a mass of protective myometrium, and is surgically accessible without the necessity for either anesthesia or incision through the cervical canal.

These factors were appreciated first by Dickinson in 1912; (Figures 27–1 – 27–3) he devised an instrument to bring heat to the uterotubal junction and published his findings in 1916.[3] It is interesting to note that Dickinson had to travel to the Chicago Medical Society on February 16, 1916 to partake in what appears to be the first symposium on methods of birth control and sterilization. Dr. Dickinson noted that the Chicago Gynecologic Society had "started . . . a frank discussion of the subject that we in the East have not undertaken."[4] He gave a scholarly description of the anatomy of the approach to the uterotubal junction from below; this still deserves careful reading today. It is a curious fact that in his last publication on the subject[5] he reviewed the world literature on the subject of sterilization, described tubal cauterization as a promising method, but acknowledged that he had performed only 40 such procedures

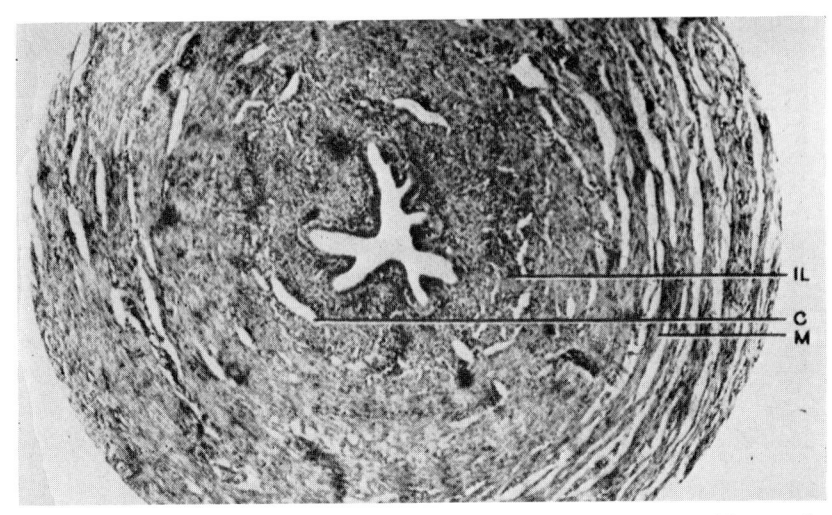

Figure 27-1. Histology of the uterotubal junction (from Lisa, J.R. et al.: Observations on the interstitial portion of the fallopian tube. *Surg Gynec Obstet*, 99:159, 1954).

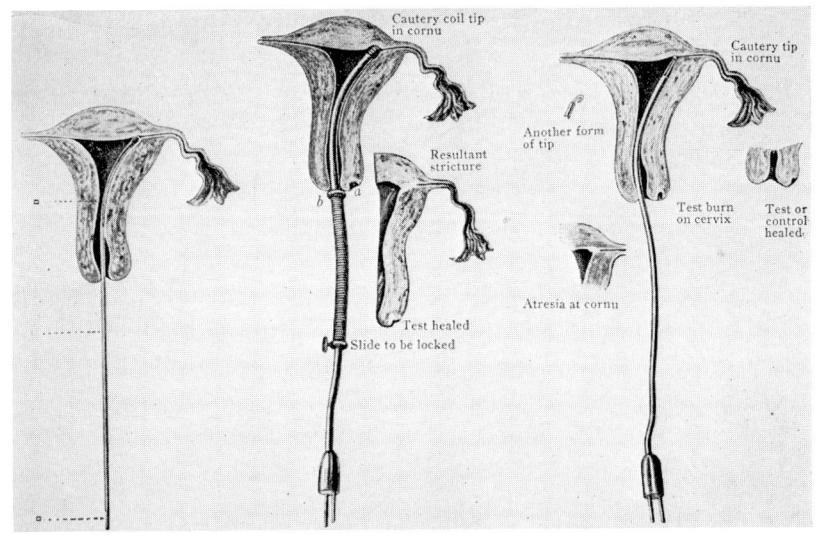

Figure 27-2. Original description of cautery probe for tubal occlusion (from Dickinson, R.L.: Simple sterilization of women by cautery stricture at the intrauterine tubal openings, compared with other methods. *Surg Gynec Obstet*, 23:234, 1916).

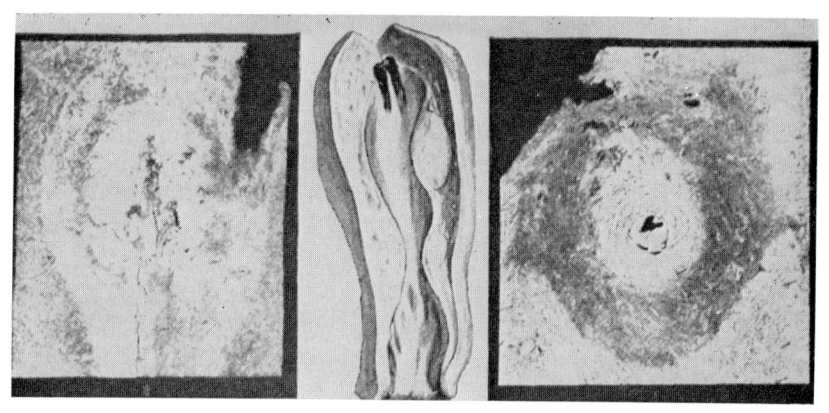

Figure 27-3. The first published human trial of uterotubal occlusion by cautery (from Dickinson, R.L., *ibid.*).

between 1916 to 1950 without complication. His results were never published otherwise. The method he used was a loop of wire heated by an electric current; this created a burn in the adjacent tissue.

In 1934, Hyams, also of New York City, described an instrument similar in shape to Dickinson's. It differed in that an insulated sheath allowed an electrode to protrude into the uterotubal junction and served as an electrode for high-frequency electrocoagulation.[6] His paper describes the instrument and the technique in detail, but again gives no detailed clinical results. It is a curious note that there were no subsequent publications by Hyams reporting the results of his technique in human patients. In a footnote, Dickinson[5] mentioned that Hyams evidently had performed over two hundred such procedures.

ANALYSIS OF HUMAN TRIALS

Since these two basic techniques were described, there have been 6 reports of uterotubal cautery techniques in humans analyzing results (De Vilbiss, 1935; Bowers, 1938; Yasui, 1953; Porter, 1957; Sheares, 1958; and Pasricha, 1968). For a comprehensive review of the literature concerning uterotubal occlusion by cautery, it is advisable to read Dickinson[5] and Tietze.[11]

In 1935, De Vilbiss[2] tried the Dickinson technique on 30

patients; and Bowers reported its use on 12 patients in 1938.[1] All the other reports described the use of the Hyams technique of electrocoagulation. In 1953, Yasui[13] reported on the largest series in the literature. He used a careful modification of the strength, duration, and frequency of the electric current, and performed the majority of the procedures (244) at the time of induced abortion. Yasui reported no serious complications in his series.

Since then, Porter[9] (in the United States) attempted this procedure on 45 patients and noted a 40 percent pregnancy rate. He concluded that the technique "does not present a reliable means of sterilization." At about the same time, Sheares,[10] in Malaya, reported a total of 128 patients subjected to the Hyams technique with a modification of the electrocautery tip by Sheares. The modification followed a fatality: "there were definite signs of severe general peritonitis, such as occurs with gut perforation." This is the only fatality in the world literature.

Most recently, Pasricha[8] (in New Delhi, India) reported her experience with 89 patients; there were 5 pregnancies and 4 cases with significant complications. The summary of all these human studies appears in Table 27-I.

A total of 603 patients in analyzed series have undergone cauterization of the cornual tip, with an overall pregnancy rate of about 8.4 percent. In all these studies, an attempt to ascertain whether or not the technique had been successful had been made by performing either a Rubin's test or hysterosalpingography after the procedures. The results listed in the table indicate the author's first observation after the initial attempt at occlusion of the uterotubal junction. Many authors recommend repeated attempts if subsequent hysterosalpingograms or Rubin's test revealed persistently patent tubes. The range of success as gauged by salpingography is between 40 and 80 percent; in general, about half of the patients were considered to have bilateral occlusion after the first attempt.

The pregnancy rate reported in the literature varies between 0 and 40 percent. The three larger series have a pregnancy rate between 4 and 6 percent. These pregnancies, however, are usually within the first year of the author's experience with the technique;

TABLE 27-I
SUMMARY OF REPORTED ATTEMPTS AT STERILIZATION WITH CAUTERY IN HUMANS

Author	Technique	Number of Patients	Percent Occluded	Pregnancies Number	Pregnancies Percent	Complications
De Vilbiss Florida, 1935	Dickinson	30	56	7	23.0	1 hemorrhage
Bowers Tennessee, 1938	Dickinson	12	41	0	0.0	0
Yasui Tokyo, 1953	Hyams	299	80	13	4.4	0
Porter Arkansas, 1957	Hyams	45	51	18	40.0	1 peritonitis
Sheares Malaya, 1958	Hyams	128	50	8	6.2	4 hemorrhage, 5 peritonitis, (1 death)
Pasricha New Delhi, 1968	Hyams	89	47	5	5.6	1 hemorrhage 3 peritonitis
Totals		603		51		15 (2.5%)
Dickinson New York, 1950		40				
Hyams New York, 1950		200				
Total Number of Humans Reported		843				

no publication has appeared analyzing pregnancies over a period much longer than a year or two. It can be suspected that subsequent pregnancies also would occur.

It is of interest to note the complications which were severe enough to warrant hospitalization. Uterine hemorrhage appearing after cauterization, usually at the time of the slough of the lesion, was noted in 6 cases; peritonitis suggesting uterine perforation and bowel damage was noted in 9 cases. This gives an overall serious complication rate of about 2.5 percent. There was one death reported from peritonitis. It is important to note that the Japanese workers,[12,13] found no significant complications in cornual cauterization performed after therapeutic abortion.

SAFETY OF THE TECHNIQUE

The major complication rate of 2.5 percent and the death rate of 1 per 844 cases seems to make uterotubal cautery too dangerous for general use, regardless of the ease with which it can be accomplished. These complications appear to arise from two difficulties: assurance of the intra-uterine location of the cautery, and control of the size of the lesion produced. The exact location of the tip can be determined with fluoroscopy by injecting a radio-opaque dye through a tube; this evidently had been part of the design in the Hyams applicator. In the experience of both Yasui, and Dickinson, it is not very difficult to find the intrauterine opening of the tube by feel alone. In a population control tool, more assurance than clinical *feel* that the cauterizing tip is at the uterotubal junction is needed. Perhaps a colored dye injected at the tip of the cautery instrument prior to the application of the current would flow back through the cervical canal into the vagina and provide evidence that the tip is intrauterine. This possibility is illustrated in Figure 27-4, which shows radio-opaque dye flowing freely out of the cervix of a hysterectomy specimen after having been injected through a cryoprobe designed for uterotubal occlusion. If the tip had already perforated the uterus, the dye would flow harmlessly into the peritoneal cavity and not be visible at the cervix.

Assuming the tip is at the junction, the techniques devised for determining the degree of tissue damage caused by cautery are horrifying. Dickinson recommended applying the heat cautery to an area of the visible cervical mucosa, and timing the electric current to that required to produce a shallow crater. Yasui described a "vibrational sound" which occurred after twenty to thirty seconds of electrocautery. This sound is described by Sheares more vividly as "sizzling," "cracking," or "bubbling." It was recommended that these noises be permitted to continue for 15 seconds. It is obvious that the sounds represent the boiling and burning of uterine tissue; there is a very real possibility that the tip might be able to burn its way through the uterus and damage the peritoneal contents.

It is quite probable that conditions of electrocoagulation of the uterotubal junction could be found which would *cook* the tissue without actually destroying it, allowing for tissue coagulation without the danger of uterine perforation. In the case of the Dickinson technique of heating a metal tip with electric current, it is important to note that the temperature of such a probe varies as a function of the conductivity of the surrounding tissue,

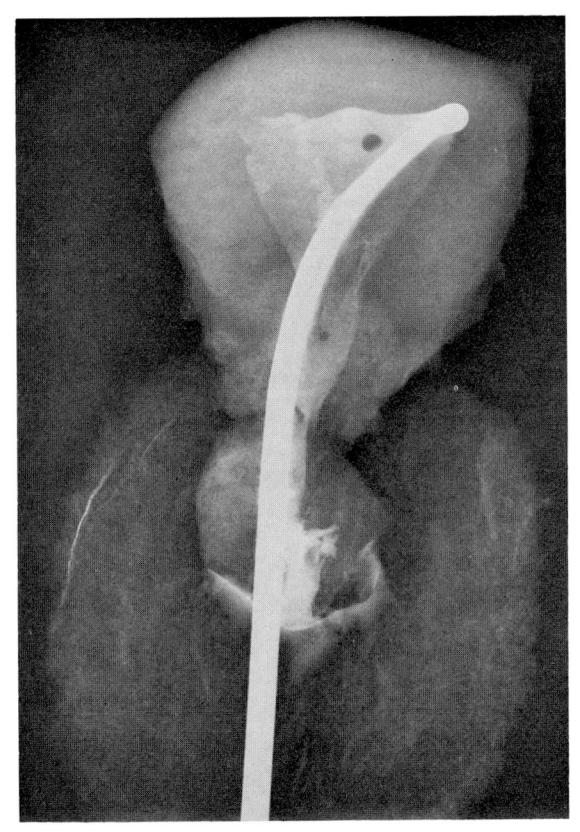

Figure 27–4. X-ray of a cryoprobe at the uterotubal junction in a hysterectomy specimen. Radio-opaque dye has been injected through a special channel of the instrument. Note the location of the tip of the probe in relation to the uterine cavity; the thickness of myometrium surrounding the tip; and spillage of the dye in a retrograde manner back through the cervix.

which varies as that tissue is charred. The temperature can be regulated by means of an electronic mechanism devised in our laboratories (Fig. 27–5) to see if a controlled coagulation lesion can be induced with heat.

EFFECTIVENESS OF CAUTERY IN OCCLUDING THE UTEROTUBAL JUNCTION

Efforts to determine the healing process in human uteri after coagulation were reported by Yasui,[13] who noted that "even

CONTROLLED HEAT SOURCE FOR CAUTERY STUDIES

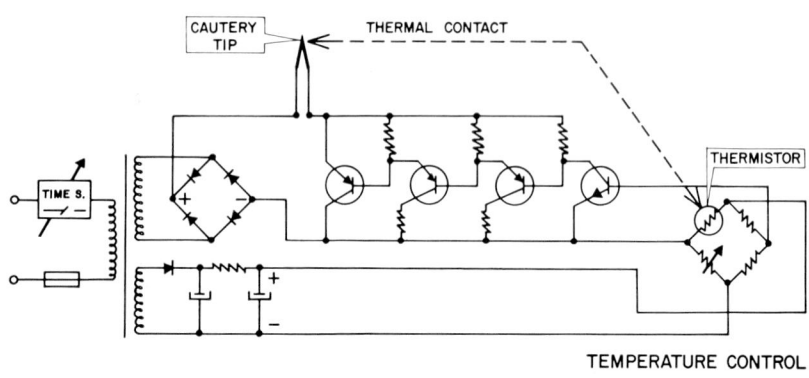

TEMPERATURE CONTROL

AFTER ANTONIN DOCKALEK
CHAPEL HILL, N.C.

Figure 27-5. A circuit to regulate the temperature of a cautery tip. A thermistor is embedded in the tip and regulates the current through the cautery element as a function of the thermistor temperature.

three weeks after cauterization it seemed that changes had not reached the end but were still continuing." Sheares'[10] histological study demonstrating obstruction at the uterotubal junction also can be interpreted to be tangential sections between the uterus and the tube (Fig. 27-6). The average reported success rates of about fifty percent demonstrated with hysterosalpingography or Rubin's test also may be overestimates of actual occlusion; the edema of the healing process may be prolonged, but gradually could resolve and restore functional patency of the area.

Cryoprobe freezing of the rabbit uterotubal junction was not successful (Fig. 27-7). The tissue was frozen white for a diameter of about 6 mm.

Figure 27-8 illustrates the uterotubal junction of a rabbit 3 weeks after such treatment. Although this was interpreted as showing histologic occlusion, this section was obtained after noting that this junction was grossly patent at autopsy. That Rubin's insufflation or hysterosalpingography also may be misleading is illustrated by Figure 27-9, which shows a rabbit uterus that had undergone cryosurgery at the uterotubal junction. In

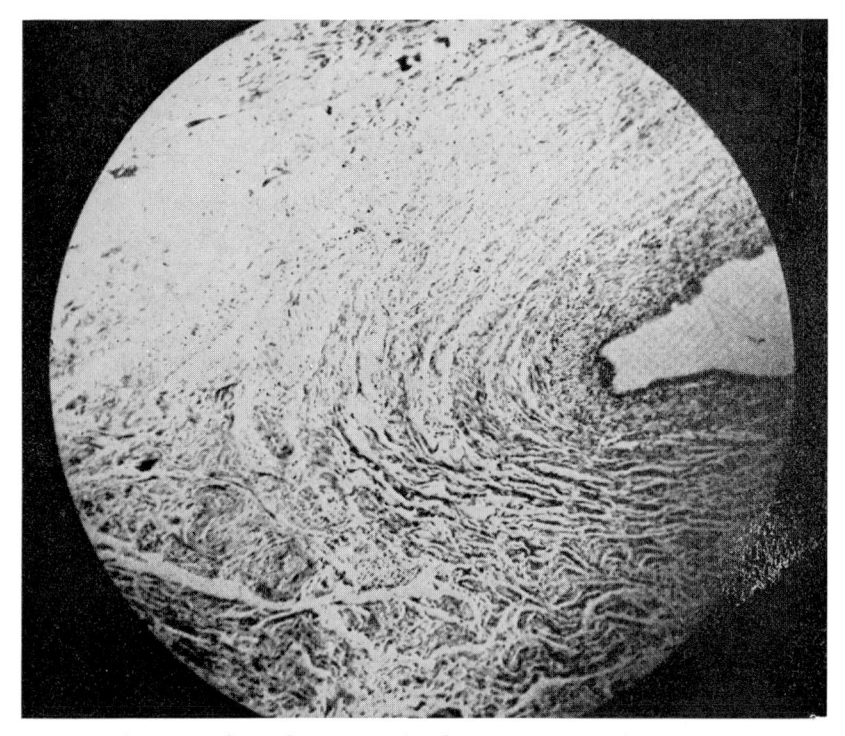

Figure 27-6. Histological section of a human uterus subject to cautery at the uterotubal junction. Integrity of myometrium around the endometrium suggests this is a tangential section rather than one through an area of blockage (from Sheares, B.H.: Sterilization of women by intrauterine electro-cautery of the uterine cornu. *J Obstet Gynec Brit Emp*, 65:419, 1958).

jection of saline after tying off the cervical end of the uterus resulted in bilateral distension. The tubes were judged to be so grossly obstructed as to make photographing them worthwhile. Histological serial sections revealed one tube to be patent throughout the uterotubal junction; the other tube was occluded.

The author has made efforts to occlude the uterotubal junction by various means in 33 rabbits to date. In 12 animals cryosurgery reaching a probe temperature of —35 C was applied to the junction for 2 minutes. In 12 rabbits, a silver nitrate applicator was held at the uterotubal junction for 2 minutes. Serial sections throughout all of these junctions revealed that silver nitrate

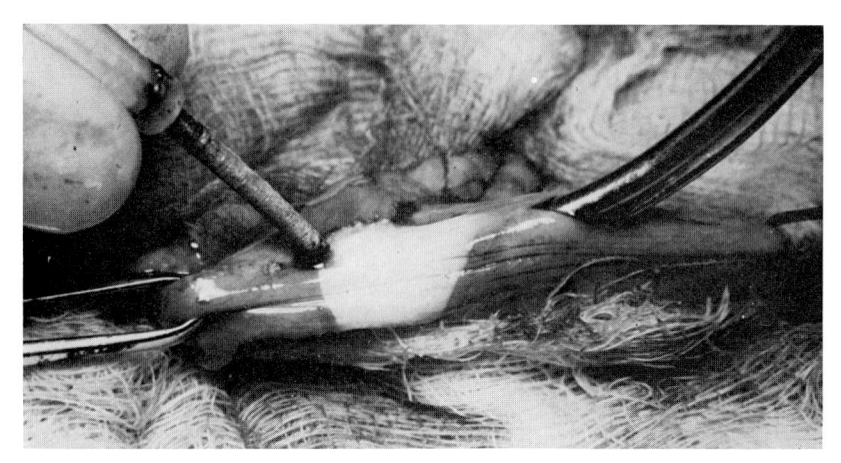

Figure 27–7. Cryoprobe freezing a rabbit uterotubal junction. Despite the large area of frosting seen grossly, thermocouples (in the probe at the right) indicated that destructive temperatures did not extend beyond 1 mm from the cryoprobe; and healing was complete.

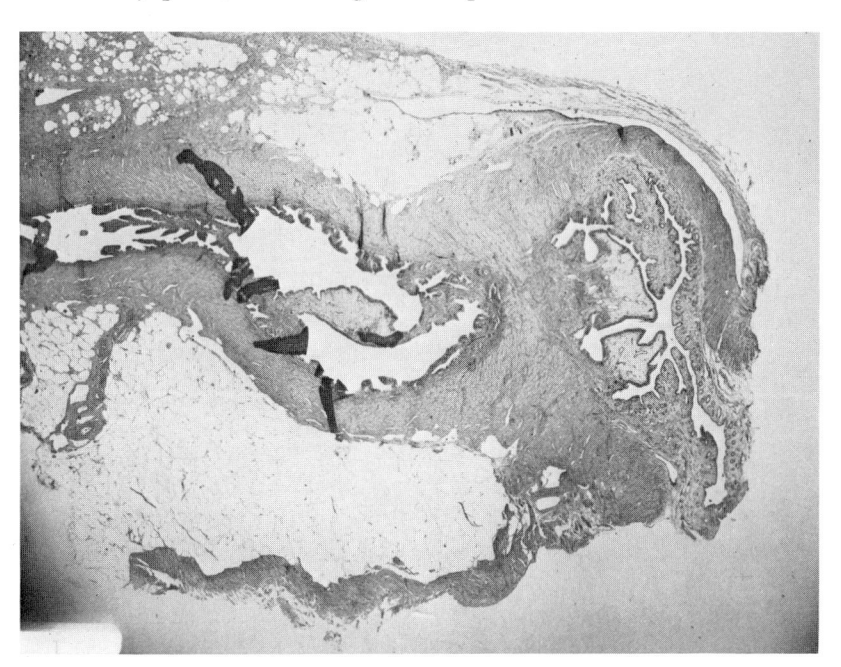

Figure 27–8. Healing at uterotubal junction in a rabbit cryosurgery. Normal tubal epithelium at left; uterine epithelium at right, with a band of scar tissue between. Although no patency was demonstrated with serial sections through this specimen, the junction had been judged to be grossly patent at autopsy and allowed saline under pressure to pass from the uterus through the tube.

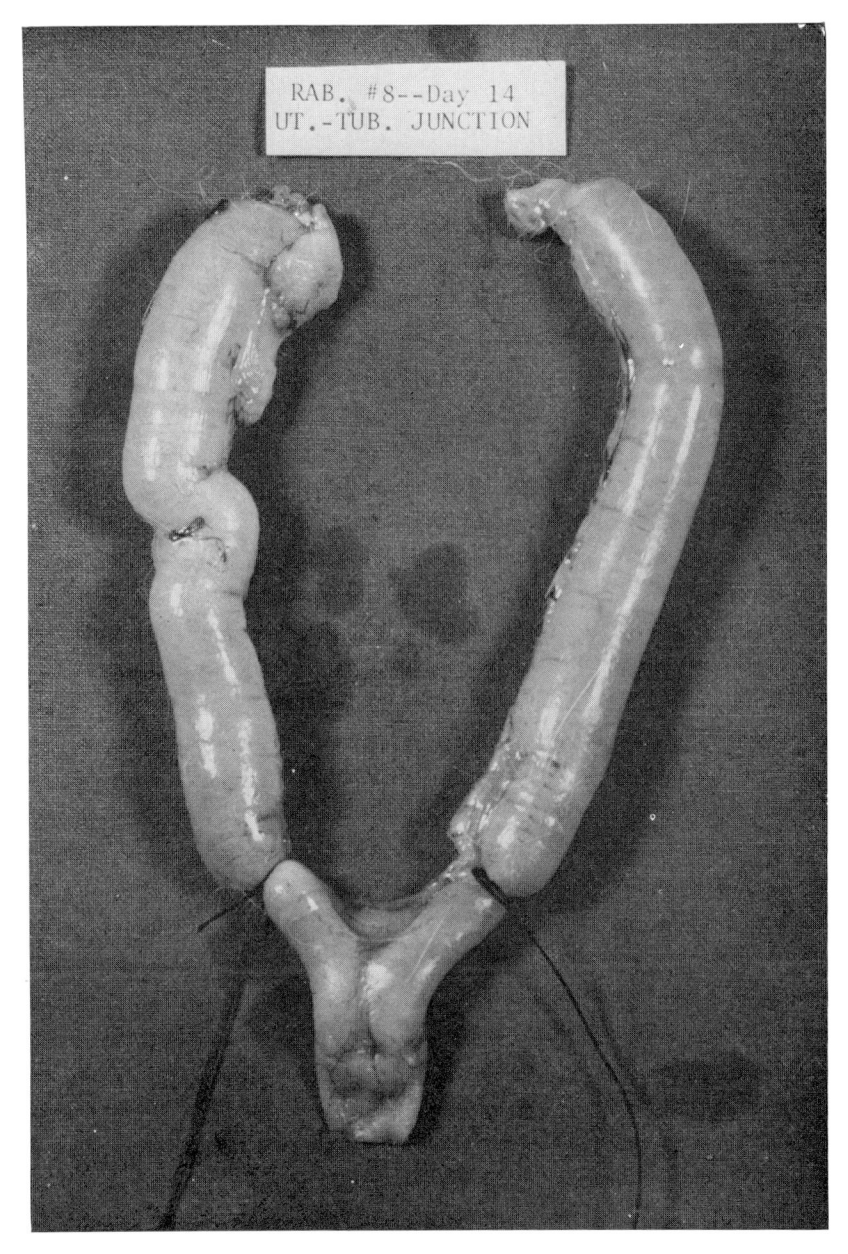

Figure 27–9. Cross-section of uterotubal obstruction 2 days after cryosurgery. Saline was injected under pressure in both uterine horns after the cervical end was tied off. Microscopically, one of the tubes was patent throughout.

induced a lesion of at least 3–10 mm in length and 5 mm in diameter. As was observed by Yasui, the healing process was still going on 3 weeks after chemical treatment. The photograph of a rabbit uterus 3 days after silver nitrate application. (Figure 27–10) illustrates the unquestionable degree of necrosis which

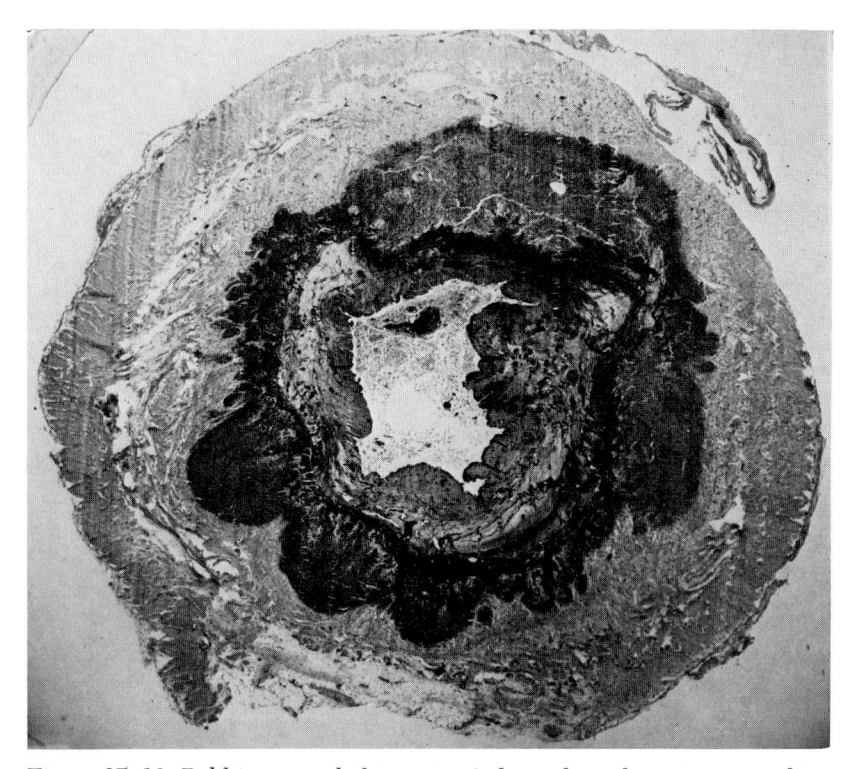

Figure 27–10. Rabbit uterotubal junction 3 days after silver nitrate application. Destruction of epithelium is complete, and inflammation process involves surrounding myometrium. The entire reaction is contained within the uterotubal lumen.

can be induced. In 9 rabbits, the uterotubal junction was treated with liquid nitrogen reaching temperatures of −160 C at the probe tip. In all but one tube of the above rabbits, histological obstruction could not be demonstrated. The one successfully occluded tube had been frozen at −160 C (Fig. 27–11).

A scheme to evaluate the effects of these techniques on subsequent fertility (Fig. 27–12) was devised. To date, a total of 40 pigs of proven fertility have undergone cryosurgery or silver nitrate destruction of the uterotubal junction, and were sacrificed

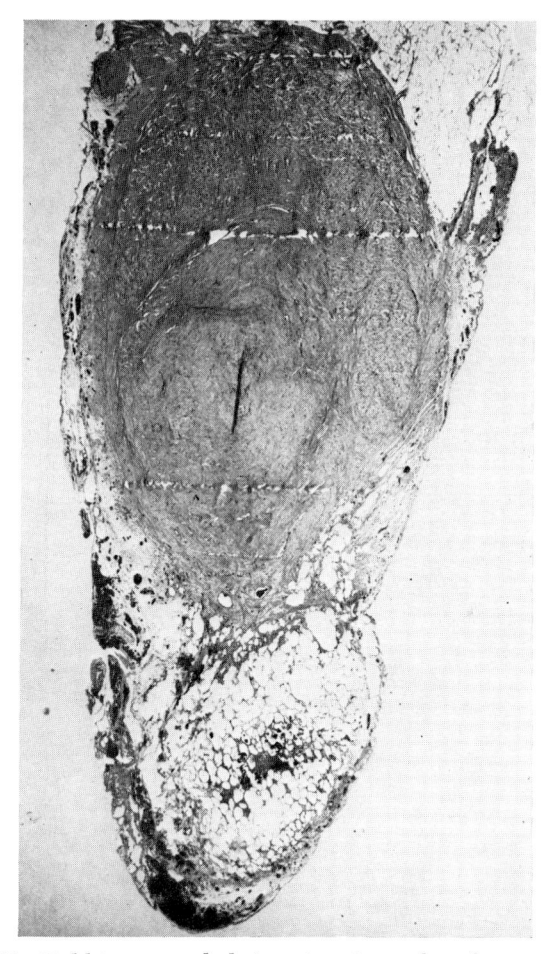

Figure 27–11. Rabbit uterotubal junction 3 weeks after cryosurgery at −160 C. The only serial section to date convincingly demonstrating obliteration of the lumen at the uterotubal junction.

after subsequent mating. All of the uterotubal junctions treated by these physical agents were subject to serial sectioning at 1 mm intervals at autopsy three to ten weeks after treatment. In the 36 animals studied to date, no occlusion of the uterotubal

FERTILITY TEST SYSTEM

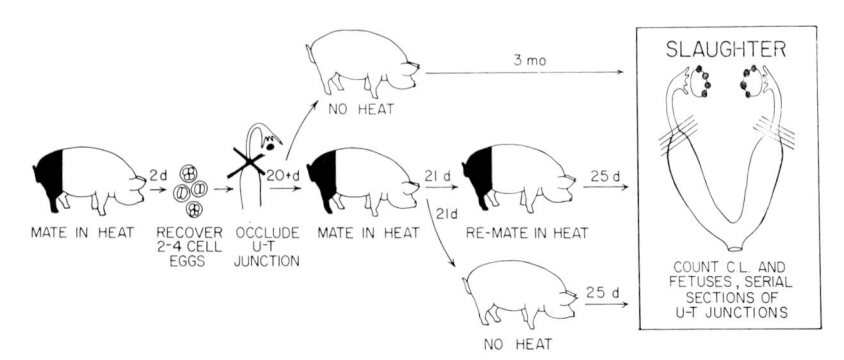

Figure 27–12. Experimental design to evaluate the effect of uterotubal injury on subsequent fertility in pigs. All uterotubal junctions subject to these studies were serially sectioned at slaughter.

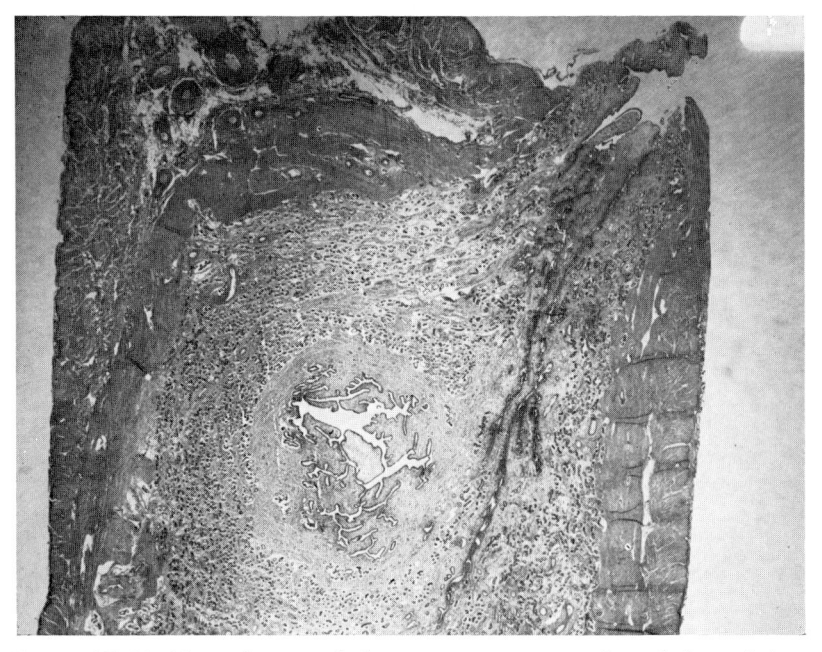

Figure 27–13. Normal uterotubal junction in a pig. The tubal epithelium protrudes into the uterine lumen surrounded by a muscular sheath for a distance of 1 to 2 mm. This pig was 26-days pregnant.

junction could be found histologically. Figure 27–13 shows the peculiar papillary formation of the normal uterotubal junction of the pig, with protrusion of tubal epithelium into the lumen of the uterus surrounded by uterine glandular tissue. Figure 27–14 was taken from an animal 6 weeks after silver nitrate destruction of the uterotubal junction. Although the area is scarred, the epithelium reformed, and there was continuity throughout the tubal and the uterine lumen. This is remarkable in view of the extensiveness of the destruction illustrated in Figure 27–10.

Thus, in animal studies to date in our laboratory, the uterotubal junction appears to be remarkably resistant to occlusion by physical or chemical agents inducing destructive lesions. This may very well be due to the fact that both the uterus and the tube are secreting fluids which flow through this junction, creating the condition of healing in the presence of a fluid flow. Fistula formation results under these conditions, and a fistulous

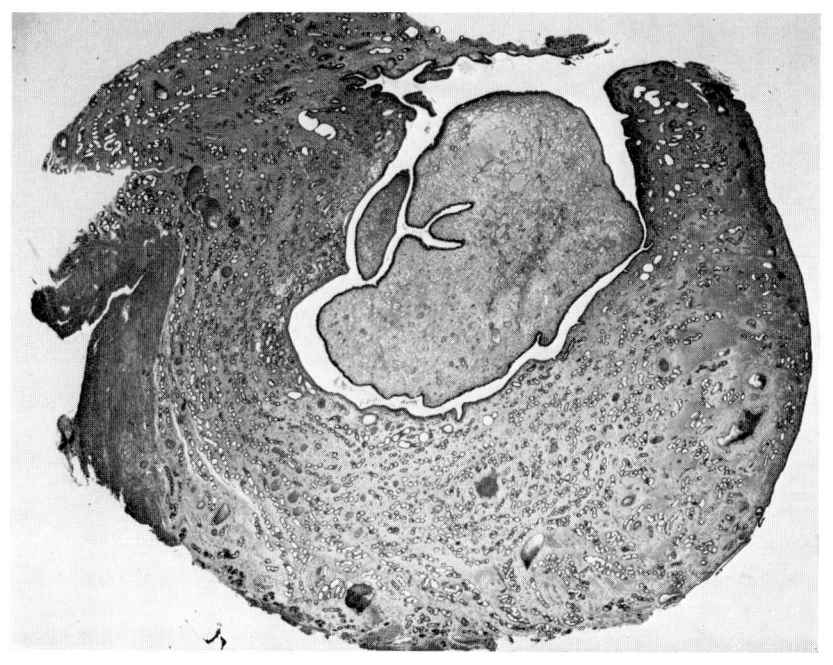

Figure 27–14. Restoration of lumen at uterotubal junction 6 weeks after silver nitrate destruction in a pig. Compare this with Figure 27–10; note the regenerative power of these structures.

tract then can be epithelialized to restore continuity between the tubes and uterus. The use of progestational agents as adjuncts to uterotubal occlusion to inhibit secretory activity of the uterus and the tube currently is under study in our laboratory. Such agents also should inhibit epithelial proliferation. No results are available as of this date. Mechanical obstruction of the junction during the healing process also deserves exploration as a method of avoiding a fistulous healing tract.

EFFECTS OF CRYOPROBE ON UTEROTUBAL HISTOLOGY AND SUBSEQUENT FERTILITY

In an effort to explore the technique of cryosurgery as a method of occluding the uterotubal junction to induce sterilization, a probe of the general dimensions of the uterine sound was constructed by the Frigitronics Corporation. Using Freon®, the tip of this probe was capable of reaching between —35 C to —40 C in myometrial tissue. Figure 27–15 shows the probe configuration compared to an ordinary uterine sound.

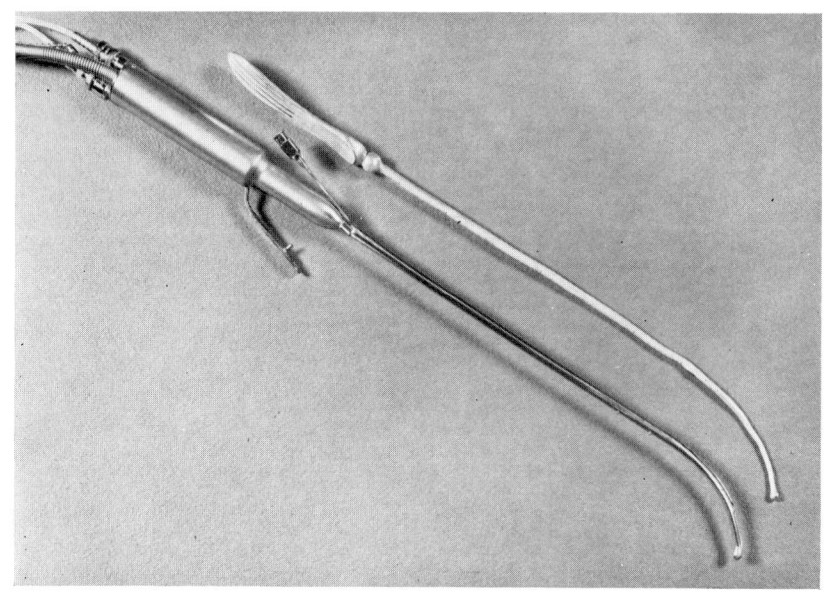

Figure 27–15. Cryosurgery probe modeled after a uterine sound (shown for comparison).

Preliminary studies in dog myometrium, rabbit skeletal muscle, and human myometrium held in 37 C waterbaths led to the construction of the isotherms shown in Figure 27–16. They revealed that temperatures of −5 C, barely adequate to kill tissues, were reached a distance of about 1 mm from the probe.

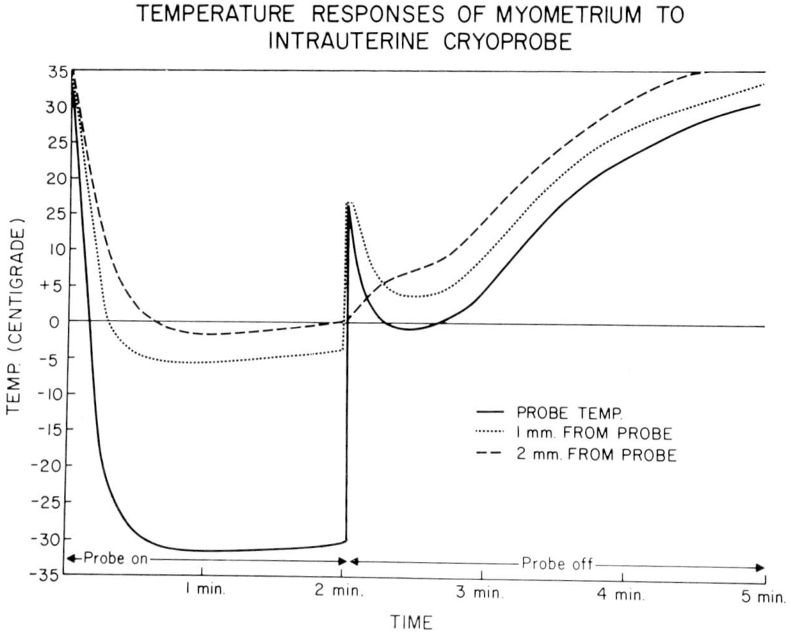

Figure 27–16. Temperatures reached in living myometrium at the tip of a cryoprobe, and 1 mm and 2 mm away. Permanent tissue destruction rarely occurs above −5 C. The sudden jump at the end of 2 minutes is induced by rapidly thawing the instrument to remove it from the uterus.

Healing of the lesions induced by such a probe was studied by sacrificing 12 rabbits at periods of up to three weeks. The damage caused by the cryosurgery generally was superficial and was limited to hemorrhage in the mucosal area. Healing by the end of three weeks generally was complete; tubal patency was demonstrated histologically. All rabbits received medroxy progesterone weekly after treatment.

As part of the study, an effort was made to see if the probe would be dangerous if it accidentally perforated the uterus and froze the bowel, blood vessels, or nerves of the abdominal cavity. This was studied experimentally by deliberately placing a cryoprobe on the bowel of all the rabbits undergoing uterotubal blockage as well as on the artery, vein and nerve of the femoral region of the leg. There were no deaths from peritonitis or any other cause; there was no limping noted, nor was there atrophy in the legs subject to cryosurgery. At autopsy, there were occasional adhesions at the site of bowel freezing, but no obstruction. However, histologically the cryoprobe caused complete slough of the mucosa of the bowel at about the third day of healing. (Figure 27–17). Although no deaths were recorded, this degree of slough would be sufficiently dangerous to make such accidental perforation hazardous in human use. It also would make the positive identification of the tip of a cryoprobe inside the uterine cavity absolutely necessary if such an instrument were to be used as a population control tool.

In an effort to see if this probe could affect fertility, a total of 31 pigs underwent cryosurgery according to the technique shown in Figure 27–12. The results are seen in Table 27–II. Twenty animals served as controls. These studies were carried out in conjunction with Dr. Ulberg of the North Carolina State Division of Animal Sciences at the Reproductive Physiology Laboratory in Raleigh, North Carolina. Although there was a slight decrease in the average number of fetuses per animal after subsequent mating (7.7 in the controls compared to 4.5 in the pigs undergoing cryosurgery), most of the difference could be accounted for by 9 animals who had undergone cryosurgery and were found to have normal corpora lutea—*but no* embryos after mating. Histological studies of serial sections of all of the uterotubal junction revealed that all were patent.

TABLE 27-II
CRYOSURGERY OF PIG UTEROTUBAL JUNCTION

	Control	Cryosurgery
Number of Animals	20	31
Total Number of Corpora Lutea	213	328
Total Number of Fetuses	155	141
Average Number Fetuses Per Animal	7.7	4.5
Percent Corpus Luteum *with* Fetus	72.7%	42.7%
Number of Animals with Corpus Luteum and *No* Embryos	0	9

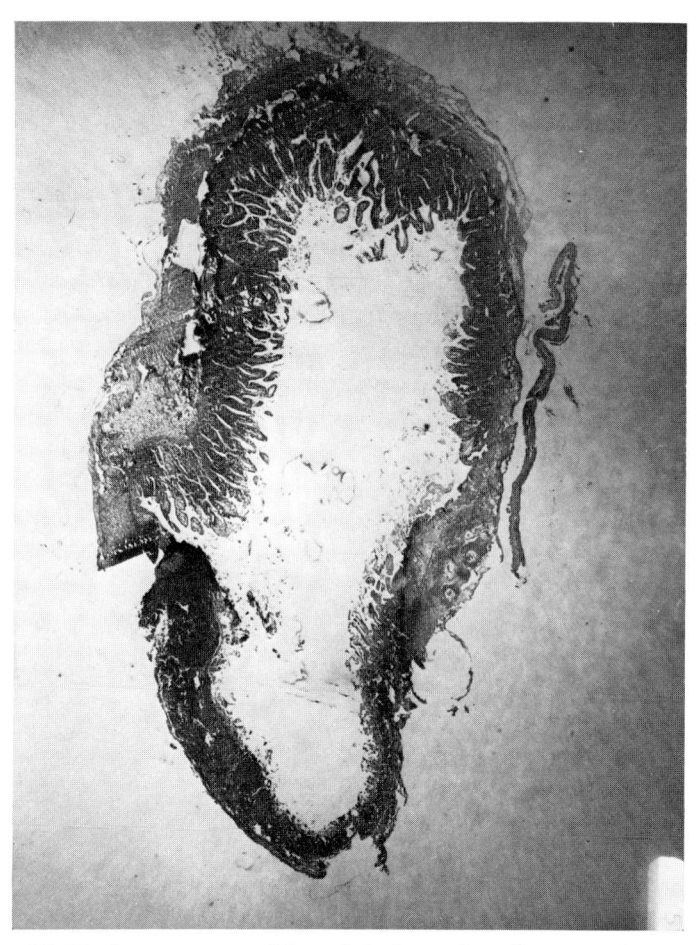

Figure 27–17. Cross-section of bowel 3 days after direct application of a cryoprobe for 2 minutes at −35 C. Although mucosa has sloughed and the muscularis is damaged, none of these bowel lesions perforated.

Thus, the hypothesis that freezing the uterotubal junction by means of a Freon cryoprobe can induce uterotubal blockage was not sustained. There was some interference with the fertility of the treated animals; some failed to get pregnant after ovulation and mating despite the patency of tubes. This interference may be related to functional damage of the uterotubal junction not evident histologically.

It was evidence that a Freon cryoprobe would not be adequate to induce the amount of damage necessary to occlude a tube. Nine rabbits, therefore, underwent treatment with a 5 mm diameter cryoprobe utilizing liquid nitrogen in the laboratories of Dr. Sydney Shulman of the New York Medical College. These tubes also were serially sectioned and studied histologically. Of the 18 oviducts, only 1 revealed satisfactory occlusion. (Fig. 27-11). It was also noted that there was a high incidence of adhesions around the uterotubal junction in the animals. The instrumentation and need for liquid nitrogen with the technique make it seem unlikely that this approach can be developed into a population control tool.

Experiments are currently underway evaluating the use of nitrous oxide as a method of inducing freezing lesions. Preliminary tests indicate that the nonelectric, rugged, portable system developed by the Frigitronics Corporation is capable of reaching temperatures of between -65 and -70 C at the tip when inserted in rabbit skeletal muscle. If studies indicate that sufficient damage to the uterotubal junction can be induced to affect fertility, this instrument might be more advantagous as a population control tool than liquid nitrogen because it is simple and requires only an adequate supply of nitrous oxide.

Mr. Frank Reynolds of the Frigitronics Corporation indicated that problems similar to the inadequate uterotubal lesions caused by cryosurgery also had been encountered in other areas of the body. The double freezing of tonsillar tissue (putting the tissue through a freeze-thaw-freeze-thaw cycle rather than a single freeze-thaw cycle) results in much greater tissue destruction than the single application of the probe. This possibility also is being evaluated in the authors' laboratories.

REFERENCES

1. Bowers, C.J., and Bowers, M.K.: Sterilization of female by cauterization of uterine cornu. *J Tenn Med Ass*, 38:381, 1938.
2. De Vilbiss, L.A.: Preliminary report on sterilization of women by intrauterine coagulation of tubal orifices. *Amer J Obstet Gynec*, 29:563, 1935.
3. Dickinson, R.L.: Simple sterilization of women by cautery stricture at

the uterine tubal openings, compared with other methods. *Surg Gynec Obstet*, 23:203, 1916.
4. Dickinson, R.L.: Transactions of Societies: Joint Meetings of the Chicago Medical and Chicago Gynecological Societies, Held February 16, 1916. *Surg Gynec Obstet*, 23:234, 1916.
5. Dickinson, R.L., and Gamble, C.J.: *Human Sterilization: Techniques of Permanent Conception Control.* Waverly Press, Inc. Baltimore, Waverly Press, 1950.
6. Hyams, M.N.: Sterilization of the female by coagulation of the uterine cornu. *Amer J Obstet Gynec*, 28:96, 1934.
7. Lisa, J.R., Gioia, J.D., and Rubin, I.C.: Observations on the Interstitial portion of the fallopian tube. *Surg Gynec Obstet*, 99:159, 1954.
8. Pasricha, K.: Sterilization by cornual cautery. *Amer J Obstet Gynec*, 100:877, 1968.
9. Porter, J.O., Sutherland, C.G., and Brown, W.E.: Transuterine tubal cautery for sterilization. *Amer J Obstet Gynec*, 74:341, 1957.
10. Sheares, B.H.: Sterilization of women by intrauterine electrocautery of the uterine cornu. *J Obstet Gynec Brit Emp*, 65:419, 1958.
11. Tietze, C.: *Bibliography of Fertility Control 1950–1965.* New York National Committee on Maternal Health, Inc., 1965.
12. Yasui, S., Kusumoto, M., Shimodaira, K., and Koya, T.: Sterilization method by cauterization of the cornu. *Arch Pop Ass Japan*, 2:76, 1953.
13. Yasui, S.: Sterilization of the female by electrocoagulation of the uterine cornu. *Japan Med J*, #1475, 1952.

Chapter 28

TUBAL STERILIZATION BY CORNUAL COAGULATION UNDER HYSTEROSCOPY

MOTOYUKI HAYASHI

From 1952 through 1957, permanent sterilization by cornual coagulation was performed on many patients. Currently, however, many Japanese gynecologists have abandoned the method because of poor clinical results.

PREVIOUS CLINICAL STUDIES

The studies were done on 568 patients who were subjected to the Hyams method. Among 358 nonpregnant cases, there were 225 (63%) cases of tubal occlusion. In pregnant patients (210 cases), 103 (49%) showed lack of patency. These results were obtained from a single coagulation.

With two coagulations, success was achieved in 243 out of 358 nonpregnant patients (68%) and in 120 out of 210 (57%) of the pregnant patients.

Hysterosalpingography was performed after coagulation in

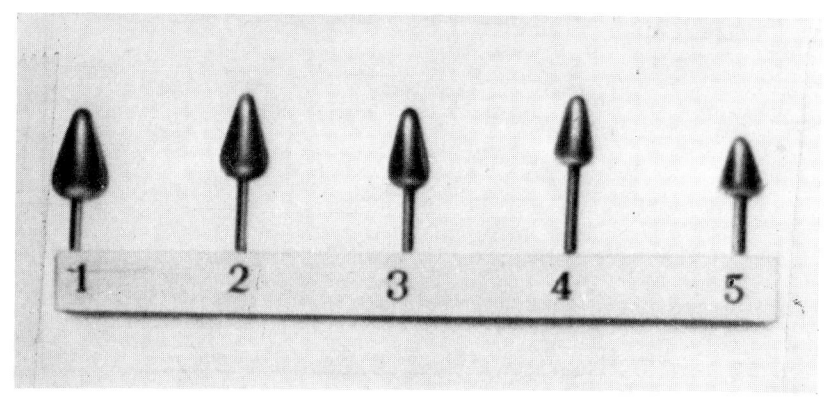

Figure 28–1. Hyams cone electrodes.

219 cases; the success rates were 72 percent for the nonpregnant patients and 46 percent for the pregnant women. Pregnancy ensued in 17 of the 130 cases in which both cornua were closed.

Disturbances in menstruation were seen in about 10 percent of the postcoagulation cases, and some patients complained of lumbago. Serious complications included tubal pregnancy (3 cases), malignant chorioepithelioma (2 cases), and perforation (1 case). There were no fatalities in this series.

The results of these procedures were not considered favorable.

Hayashi-Ishikawa Experiments (1953–1969)

Dr. Ishikawa designed electrodes capable of producing better coagulation under the control of hysteroscopy or fluoroscopy.

Precautions must be taken when using these instruments. The shape of the apparatus should be that of a parabola. The diameter should be 10 mm; the length 15 mm; and the diameter of each

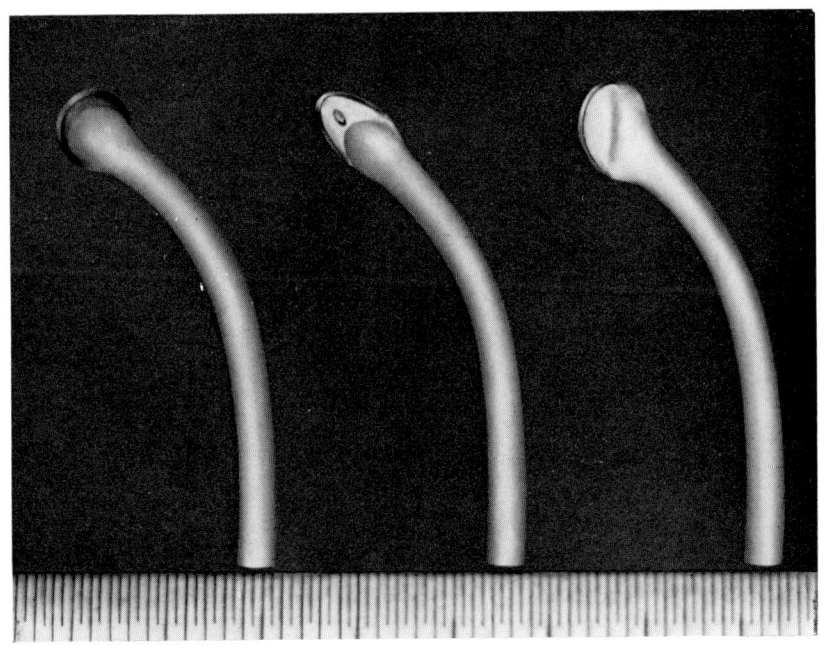

Figure 28–2. Ishikawa and Hayashi parabola electrodes.

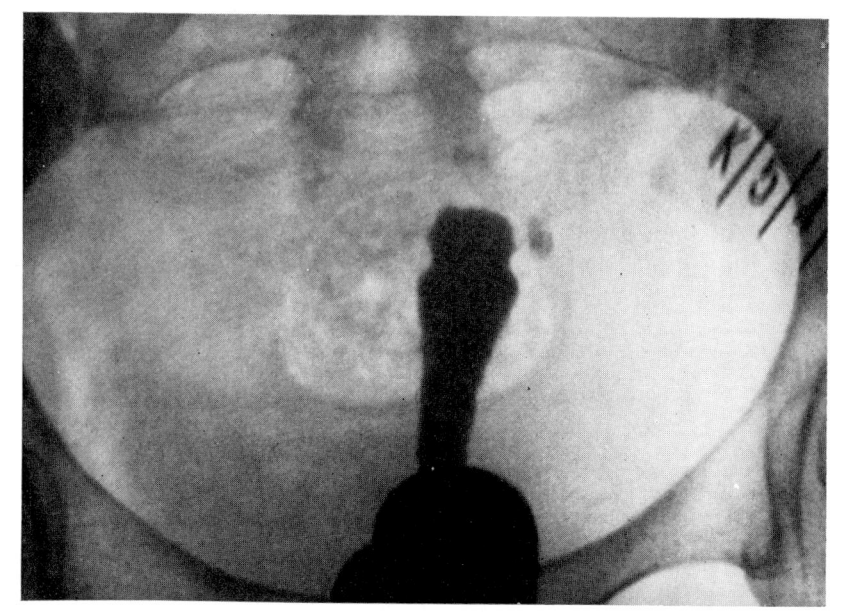

Figure 28–3. Hysterosalpingography 2 months after cornual coagulation.

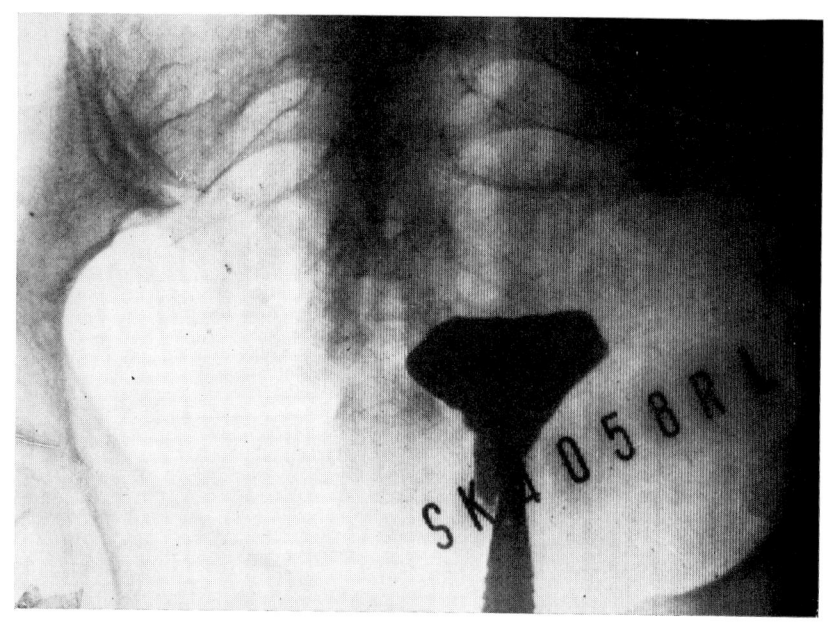

Figure 28–4. Hysterosalpingography 1 year after cornual coagulation.

edge should range between 8–10 mm. The depth of coagulation possible ranges from 6–10 mm. The electrode must be applied firmly to the uterine ostium of the oviduct. A special thermometer should be used to give a direct measurement of the temperature of the electrode.

In most cases intravenous anesthesia was used, although it is not strictly required for the procedure. Hysteroscopic observation is done after dilation of the external cervical os. The electrode is inserted slowly; the temperature is between 110 and 120C, and the maximum electric current should be 520 milliamperes. It takes from thirty-four to forty-six seconds to spark an electrical discharge. The time for the entire coagulation procedure ranges between fifty-four and seventy seconds.

Among 106 cases in which the cone electrode was used (1953–1957), 88 (83%) became pregnant. When a round electrode was

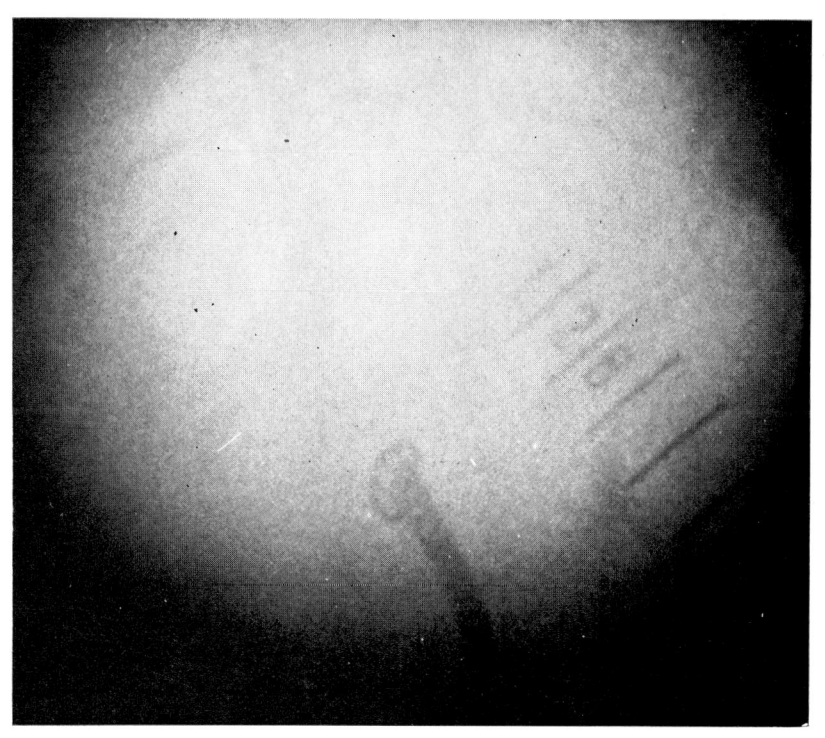

Figure 28–5. Fluoroscopic visualization of parabola electrode in uterine cavity.

employed (1858–1966), there were 157 pregnancies among 402 cases (39%). From 1967 through 1969 a curved (ellipsoid) electrode was employed; 5 pregnancies ensued among 98 cases (5%).

There were no serious side effects, although some of the patients complained of abdominal pain.

Possible improvements of the method include improvement of the coagulation procedure with better hysteroscopic and fluoroscopic control. Special materials to occlude the internal ostium also should be considered.

REFERENCES

1. Hyams, M.N.: Sterilization of the female by coagulation of the uterine cornu. *Trans Amer Ass Obstet Gynec Abdom Surg, 47:*263, 1934.
2. Ishikawa, H.: Studies on the electronic pole of the coagulation apparatus of the uterine horn with high-frequency electronics. *Jap J Fertil Steril, 9:*280, 1964.
3. Ishikawa, H.: The result of tubal sterilization by cornual coagulation. *Jap J Fertil Steril, 10:*209, 1965.
4. Ishikawa, H.: The coagulation grade. Sterilizing effect and pregnancy rates after sterilization with uterine cornual coagulation. *Jap J Fertil Steril, 11:*151, 1966.
5. Nishizaki, S.: Tubal sterilization by cauterization. *Jap J Obstet Gynec, 13:*204, 1930.
6. Yasui, S.: Clinical study on sterilization by cornual coagulation. *Jap J Fertil Steril, 8:*63, 1963.

Chapter 29

CHEMICAL AGENTS FOR TRANSVAGINAL STERILIZATION*

Jaime Zipper, M. Medel, E. Stachetti, L. Pastene, M. Rivera, and R. Prager

The use of chemical agents to produce obstruction in the human oviduct was proposed more than a century ago.[1] In 1967, Corfman did a historical review of the problem.[2] The injection of caustic agents into the uterine cavity for contraception and sterilization is a technique that actually is in use in some countries.[3] No clinical evaluation of these methods has been done, with the exception of a preliminary communication[4] to the Fifth World Congress on Fertility and Sterility held in Tel Aviv in 1968.

The importance of the development of a nonsurgical sterilization method using cytotoxics or antimetabolites has led to a systematic study of the action of chemical agents on the uterine epithelium of the rat[5] and on the tubal epithelium of the rabbit.[6] Research indicates that there are different groups of chemical agents that are capable of producing histological and functional changes which are potentially useful at different periods of time. Reversibility is not possible when there are intense cicatricial lesions that obstruct the treated cornua permanently.

This paper is an evaluation of the clinical use of two groups of chemical agents: nonspecific sclerosing agents which obstruct the oviducts with the production of nonspecific cicatricial lesions; and highly specific chemical agents capable of inducing changes in the tubal epithelium by modifying its morphophysiology.

Ethanol formalin, a nonspecific chemical agent, was used for three years of experimentation.

---

* Supported by Grant # M 67–69, Biomedical Division, the Population Council.

Quinacrine also was used in these studies. This is an antimetabolite that has a highly specific action on the tubal epithelium near the uterine ostium; it does not damage the rest of the tubal epithelium or the endometrial mucosa. The use of quinacrine in humans was proposed after extensive experience in rats,[7] where its capacity to produce changes in the uterine epithelium was demonstrated. In these rats, the epithelium proliferated to such an extent that it totally obscured the uterine cavity for prolonged periods; the duration of the obstruction was dependent upon the dosages employed. Reversal could be obtained by successive pregnancies in the untreated horn or through the administration of exogenous ovarian hormones. The studies of Gelhorn,[8,9,10] Reiner,[10] and Rochlin[11] show the possibilities of the use of quinacrine in this specific field.

Results were analyzed with the Life Table method of statistical interpretation to summarize the demographic projections of this technique.

ETHANOL FORMALIN (2%)

This study included 97 volunteer patients who were potential candidates for surgical sterilization. The women were informed that they would have to have at least six instillations of the chemical in consecutive menstrual cycles; two months tolerance after the last instillation would be given before they were regarded as *drop-outs*. These patients would be excluded from the study and would either be given contraceptive devices or surgical sterilization.

Instillation of the ethanol formalin was done after a gynecological examination. Then the cervix was observed with a speculum. A tenaculum was placed on the superior cervical lip, and the size of the uterus was measured with a uterine sound. Two milliliters of the cytotoxic substance (95 parts ethanol and 5 parts of 40% formalin—final concentration 2% ethanol formalin) was introduced slowly into the uterine cavity with a 5 ml syringe attached to a biopsy cannula capable of reaching the uterine fundus. The cannula was withdrawn after one to two minutes to avoid reflux. Instillations were done following menstrual periods.

Wherever possible, insufflation to evaluate tubal patency was performed after each instillation. Once nonpatency was obtained, instillations were suspended. To follow the evolution of tubal patency as many tubal insufflations or hysterosalpingographies as possible were performed.

Menstrual cycles were followed regularly. Endometrial biopsies were obtained during instillation and in later cycles. Two patients had hysterectomies 48 hours after the first instillation to study the effects on the endometrium and the oviducts. Total tubal resection was done on 5 patients to follow up the evolution of obstruction for periods that lasted up to eighteen months.

The Life Table Method was used to evaluate the effectiveness and acceptability of the technique (Table 29-I). Patients who did not have 6 consecutive instillations appear as *drop-outs*, and

TABLE 29-I
CUMULATIVE RATES OF EVENTS AND CLOSURES FOR 100 WOMEN TREATED WITH 2 PERCENT ETHANOL FORMALIN: 3, 6, 9, 12, 24, AND 30 MONTH FOLLOW-UP

	\multicolumn{6}{c}{Months Following Treatment}
	3	6	9	12	24	30
Events						
Pregnancies						
After tubal obstruction	0.0	3.1	4.1	6.4	8.7	8.7
During treatment	1.0	4.1	8.4	8.4	8.4	8.4
Spontaneous recovery of tubal patency	0.0	0.0	1.0	1.0	8.9	8.9
Bleeding	0.0	0.0	1.0	1.0	1.0	1.0
Oligo and/or Hypomenorrhea	1.0	3.4	5.6	7.8	10.2	10.2
Amenorrhea	0.0	1.4	3.5	6.8	10.5	10.5
Pelvic inflammatory disease	0.0	0.0	0.0	1.1	2.2	2.2
Medical relevant	1.0	1.0	1.0	1.0	1.0	1.0
Other medical (nonrelevant)	0.0	0.0	0.0	1.1	3.7	3.7
Personal relevant	2.0	2.0	2.0	2.0	2.0	2.0
Drop-out	10.3	20.7	24.9	26.0	26.0	26.0
Failure of treatment	0.0	0.0	2.1	3.2	3.2	3.2
Relevant Closures						
Total pregnancies	1.0	7.2	12.5	14.8	17.1	17.1
Spontaneous recovery of tubal patency	0.0	0.0	0.0	0.0	5.3	5.3
Bleeding	0.0	0.0	0.0	0.0	0.0	0.0
Oligo and/or hypomenorrhea	0.0	0.0	0.0	0.0	0.0	0.0
Amenorrhea	0.0	0.0	0.0	0.0	0.0	0.0
Pelvic inflammatory disease	0.0	0.0	0.0	0.0	0.0	0.0
Medical relevant	1.0	1.0	1.0	1.0	1.0	1.0
Personal relevant	2.0	2.0	2.0	2.0	2.0	2.0
Drop-out	10.3	20.7	24.9	26.0	26.0	26.0
Failure of treatment	0.0	0.0	2.1	3.2	3.2	3.2
Total relevant closures	14.3	30.9	42.5	47.0	54.6	54.6
Continuation rate	85.5	68.8	57.2	52.7	45.0	45.0
Woman months	265.5	483.5	660.0	805.0	1275.0	1336.5

those who were not obstructed after 6 instillations are termed *failure of treatment.*

Nonpatency was obtained in only 54 (55.6%) of the 97 patients who were treated with ethanol formalin. Tubal insufflation after each instillation was possible in 57 patients.

TABLE 29-II
EFFECT OF NUMBER OF INSTILLATIONS OF 2 PERCENT ETHANOL FORMALIN ON TUBAL PATENCY

Number of Instillations	Number of Patients	Nonpatent Number	Patients Percent	Number of Patent Patients	Cumulative Obstruction Rates*
1	8	0	0.0	8	0.0
2	18	7	38.8	77	12.2
3	21	13	61.9	8	35.0
4	30	23	76.6	7	75.6
5	12	10	83.3	2	92.9
6	4	1	25.0	3	94.7

* Cumulative obstruction rates were calculated from 57 patients studied: 54 were nonpatent and 3 were patent.

Table 29-II shows tubal patency and nonpatency after successive instillations and insufflations; cumulative rates of obstructions also were calculated. There were no obstructions after one instillation; but cumulative rates of obstruction after six instillations were 94.7 percent.

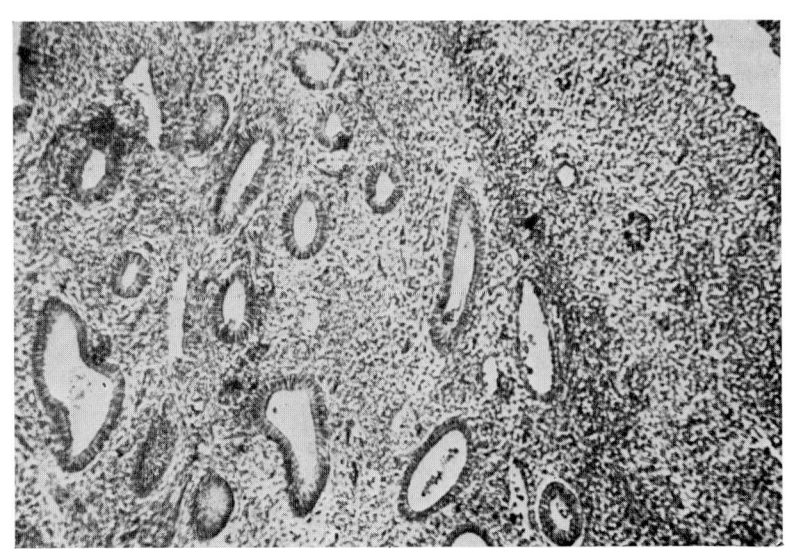

Figure 29–1. Section of a uterus after hysterectomy 48 hours after instillation of ethanol formalin (2%).

Data analyzed at the end of two years (Table 29-I) reveal that the rate of accidental pregnancies after diagnosed tubal obstruction was 8.7 percent; during the treatment period, the rate of accidental pregnancies in women with patent tubes was 8.4 percent. The *drop-out* rate was 26.0 percent, and continuation after the second year was 45.0 percent.

A year following treatment 78 of 100 women demonstrated oligomenorrhea and/or hypomenorrhea; this phenomenon did not increase significantly as time passed. The incidence of amenorrhea was distributed unevenly; all patients recovered spontaneously.

Endometrial biopsies taken during the treatment cycle showed a chemical curettage that partially modified glandular development (Fig. 29-1). Biopsies taken in consecutive cycles did not demonstrate significant alterations.

Serial sections of the tubes showed that the lesions essentially were situated in the zone of insertion of the uterine tube. The histological picture is characterized by obstruction of the lumen with fibrous connective tissue; no epithelial tissue was observed (Fig. 29-2). The pattern remained unchanged in chronic cases.

If the ethanol formalin is instilled slowly, it does not produce

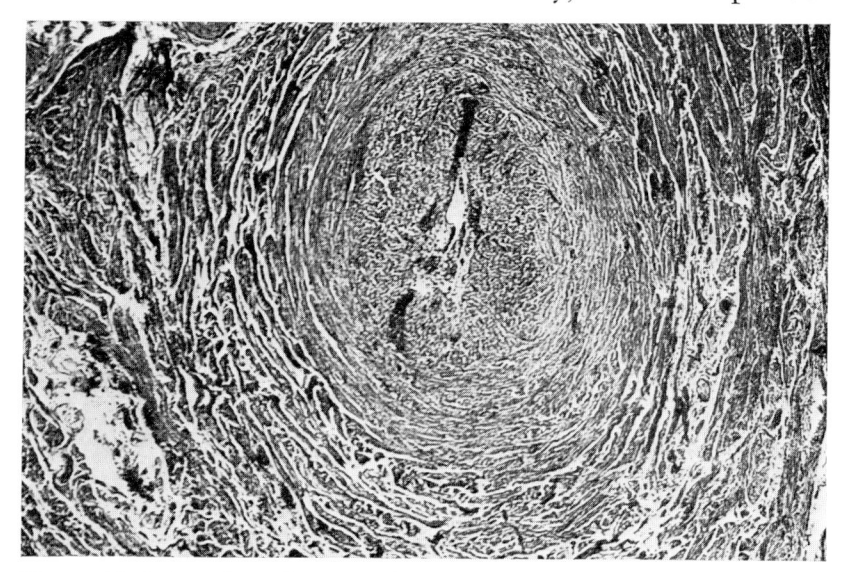

Figure 29-2. Histological aspect of the lesion induced by ethanol formalin in the human fallopian tube ($\times$ 100).

local or systemic effects. There have been neither complications nor tubal pregnancies to date.

QUINACRINE

Quinacrine chlorhydrate was used in two different concentrations and volumes, and two different treatment patterns were employed. In both instances, solutions were prepared immediately before use.

In the first group (Group A), a suspension of 125 mg of quinacrine per milliliter was injected into the uterine cavity (2 ml total volume). These instillations were done after a menstrual period. Wherever possible, a tubal insufflation was done following each instillation. When nonpatency was observed, treatment was suspended; periodic insufflations or hysterosalpingographies were performed to evaluate tubal obstruction. If the oviducts were still patent after 3 instillations, the patient was termed a *failure of treatment* and was given either a contraceptive device or surgical sterilization. Two months following the last instillation, the patient was considered a *drop-out* if she failed to reappear. Tubal resection was done on 4 patients to observe the histopathologic alterations produced in the oviduct by the quinacrine. The Life Table method was done to analyze this group of patients.

The second group of patients (Group B) had a suspension of 250 mg of quinacrine chlorhydrate injected into the uterine cavity (4 ml total volume.) Only 2 consecutive instillations were done.

Of the patients who had instillations of 125 mg of quinacrine (Group A), tubal obstruction was observed in 60 of the 85 women (70.5%). Tubal insufflation to diagnose patency in consecutive cycles was done in 68 patients.

Data analyzed by the Life Table method (Table 29-III) show that the pregnancy rate was 10.4 percent after diagnosed tubal obstruction. During the treatment period, the rate of accidental pregnancies in the women with patent tubes was 5.8 percent. The *drop-out* rate was 10.6 percent, and the continuation rate was 59.7 percent at the end of a year. No closures were recorded during the second year, although the figures are not completely significant.

TABLE 29-III
CUMULATIVE RATES OF EVENTS AND CLOSURES FOR WOMEN TREATED WITH 125 MG OF QUINACRINE CHLORHYDRATE: 3, 6, 9, 12, AND 24 MONTH FOLLOW-UP

	Months Following Treatment				
	3	6	9	12	24
Events					
Pregnancies					
After tubal obstruction	0.0	5.1	6.5	10.4	10.4
During treatment	5.8	5.8	5.8	5.8	5.8
Spontaneous recovery of tubal patency	0.0	0.1	1.3	5.2	5.2
Bleeding	1.1	2.4	3.9	3.9	3.9
Oligo and/or hypomenorrhea	0.0	0.0	1.5	1.5	1.5
Amenorrhea	0.0	0.0	0.0	0.0	0.0
Pelvic inflammatory disease	1.1	1.1	2.5	2.5	2.5
Medical relevant	0.0	0.0	0.0	0.0	0.0
Other medical	1.1	1.1	1.1	1.1	1.1
Personal relevant	0.0	0.0	0.0	0.0	0.0
Drop-out	9.4	10.6	10.6	10.6	10.6
Relevant Closures					
Total pregnancies	5.8	10.9	12.3	16.2	16.2
Spontaneous recovery of tubal patency	0.0	0.0	0.0	3.9	3.9
Bleeding	0.0	0.0	0.0	0.0	0.0
Oligo and/or hypomenorrhea	0.0	0.0	0.0	0.0	0.0
Amenorrhea	0.0	0.0	0.0	0.0	0.0
Pelvic inflammatory disease	0.0	0.0	0.0	0.0	0.0
Medical relevant	0.0	0.0	0.0	0.0	0.0
Personal relevant	0.0	0.0	0.0	0.0	0.0
Drop-out	9.4	10.6	10.6	10.6	10.6
Failure of treatment	9.4	9.4	9.4	9.4	9.4
Total closures	24.6	30.9	32.3	40.1	40.1
Continuation rate	75.3	68.9	67.5	59.7	59.7
Woman months	220.5	394.5	540.5	631.5	768.0

Table 29-IV shows the correlative rate of obstructions related to number of instillations. Three consecutive instillations of 125 mg of quinacrine hydrochloride produced 88.2 percent obstruction.

Table 29-V shows the rates of pregnancies after 2 years. In patients who had 1 instillation, there were 5.7 percent preg-

TABLE 29-IV
EFFECT OF NUMBER OF INSTILLATIONS OF 125 MG QUINACRINE CHLORHYDRATE ON TUBAL PATENCY

Number of Instillations	Number of Patients	Nonpatent Patients Number	Percent	Number of Patent Patients	Cumulative Obstruction Rates*
1	55	24	43.6	31	35.2
2	41	24	58.5	17	70.5
3	20	12	60.0	8	88.2

* Cumulative obstruction rates were calculated from 68 patients studied; 60 were nonpatent and 8 were patent.

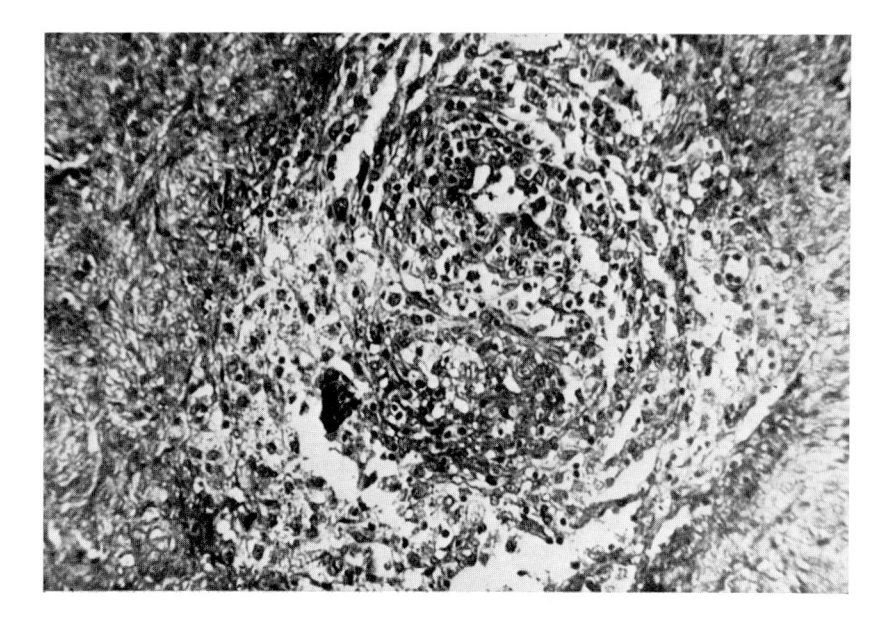

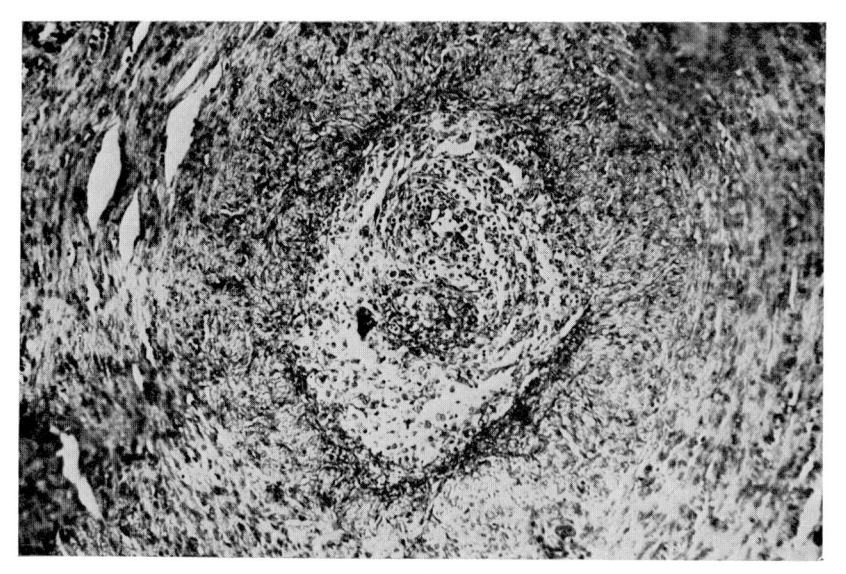

Figure 29–3A, 3B, 3C, and 3D. Serial sections of a human fallopian tube 60 days after a single instillation of quinacrine dose A ($\times$ 100 and $\times$ 200).

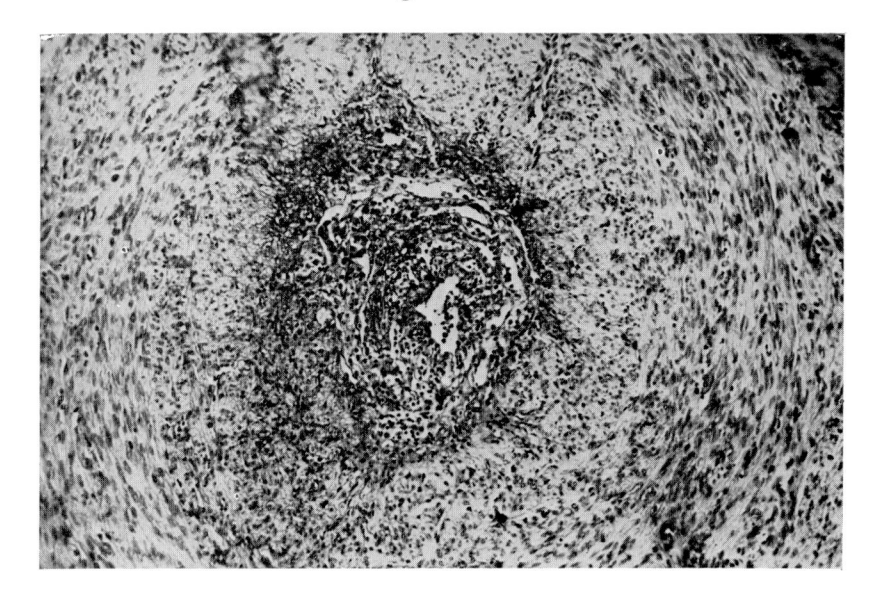

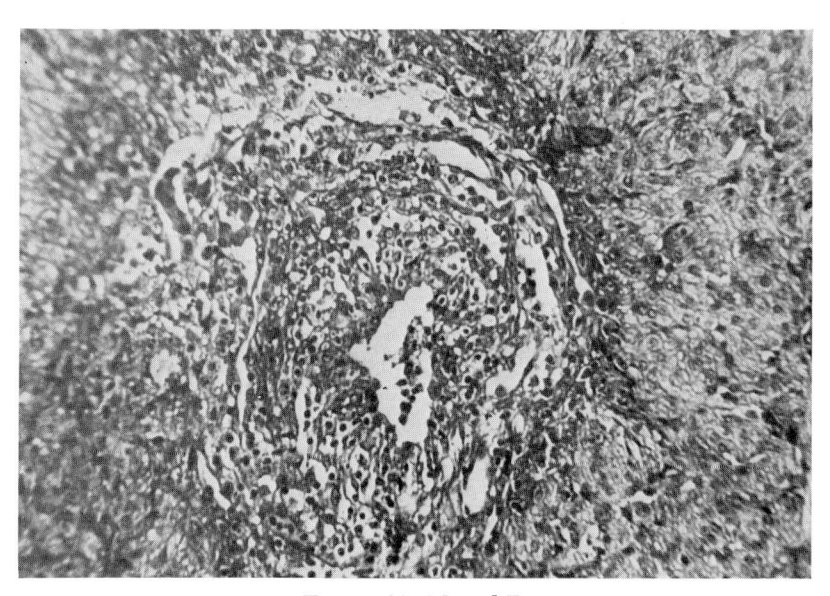

Figure 29–3C and D.

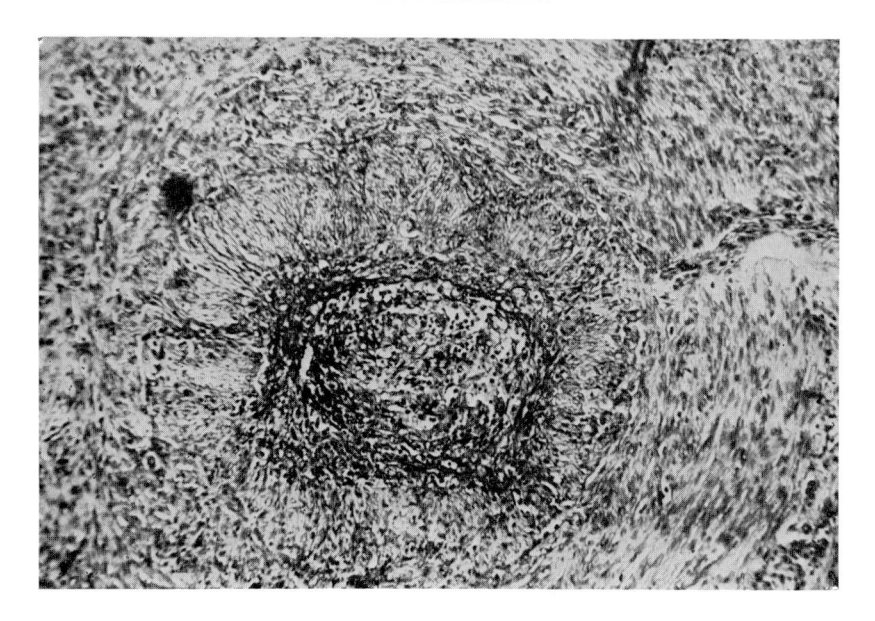

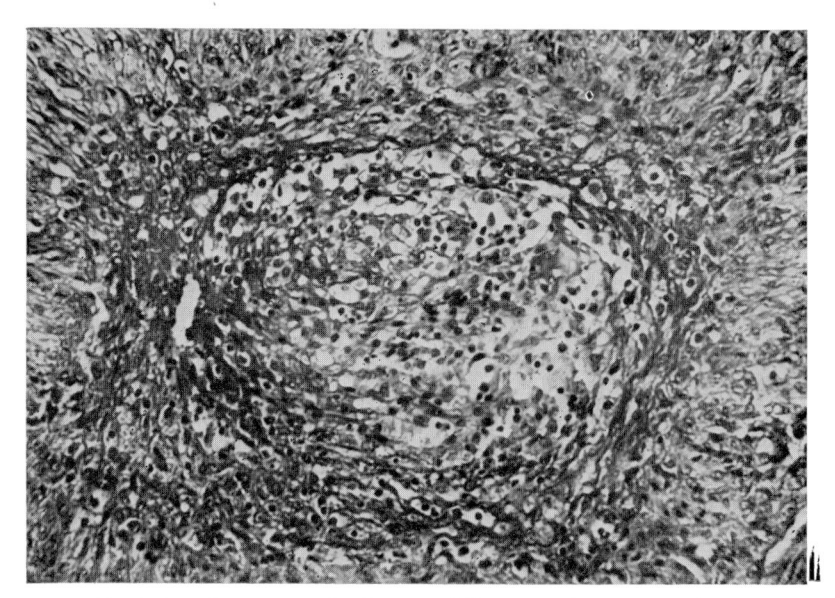

Figure 29–4. Serial sections of a human fallopian tube 1 year after a single instillation of quinacrine dose A ($\times$ 100 and $\times$ 200).

TABLE 29-V
PREGNANCIES TWO YEARS AFTER INSTILLATION OF 125 MG
QUINACRINE CHLORHYDRATE PRODUCING TUBAL OBSTRUCTION

Number of Instillations	Number of Patients	Number of Pregnancies	Percent of Pregnancies
1	24	4	5.7
2	24	2	3.4
3	12	1	1.3

nancies; those who had 3 installations, had a pregnancy rate of 1.3 percent.

Endometrial biopsies were performed and menstrual patterns were followed. No significant changes were observed in the menstrual cycle.

Serial sections of the oviducts of patients who had had instillations of 125 mg of quinacrine chlorhydrate showed that the lesion was located in the intramural portion of the tube and extended for about 2-3 mm. The obstruction of the tubal lumen occurred because of a cellular reaction of the granulomatous type; the cells were lightly colored with regular nuclei. Muscular layers did not show important alterations (Fig. 29-3 and 29-4). The pattern remained unchanged a year after treatment.

In the 20 patients who had been instilled with 250 mg of quinacrine chlorhydrate, insufflation was done after the first instillation. This revealed 13 nonpatent and 7 patent tubes, a nonpatency percentage of 65. Endometrial biopsies were done, and menstrual patterns were followed.

Only 1 complication ensued after the administration of more than 150 quinacrine instillations. One patient suffered immediate central nervous system excitation; this was similar to that induced by the injection of intravenous procaine. The condition was controlled by barbiturates and the injection of chlorpromazine. No serositis or abdominal pain was reported, and no ectopic pregnancies were observed.

SUMMARY AND CONCLUSIONS

Experimental[5,6,7] and clinical[4] experiences of the authors suggest the possibility of developing simple methods to occlude the human oviduct at the level of the ostium. The anatomical and physiological properties of this area permits action at this site, which is essential for the transport of sperm and blastocysts. The endometrial mucosa is not affected to a substantial degree because of its thickness and its capacity for periodical recovery; endometrial recovery is dependent upon glandular mechanisms which are not affected by cytotoxics. Since the ostial region of the tubal mucosa is thin, it is easy to produce changes in it by the injection of cytotoxics if they make contact in adequate concentrations.

Sclerosing agents probably would require many applications to obtain the desired effect, because a mass of coagulated material is formed rapidly in the uterine cavity; this mass prevents the entrance of the chemical agent. On the other hand, antimetabolites that have a specific action on the tubal epithelium, e.g. quinacrine, seem to be preferred for tubal occlusion because they can pass through the tubes to the peritoneum without coagulating proteins or causing important systemic or local reactions.[9,11]

The clinical and demographic effectiveness of a transvaginal sterilizing technique essentially depends on the number of applications necessary to obtain obstruction. Where more applications are needed, more patients are *drop-outs*: the 6 application ethanol formalin technique had a *drop-out* rate of 26 percent; the 3 application quinacrine method had a rate of 10.6 percent. Risk of pregnancy decreases significantly when the treatment period is shortened: 8.4 percent for ethanol formalin, and 5.8 percent for quinacrine. Pregnancy during treatment is also a cause of termination of therapy. Therefore, transient protection with an intra-uterine contraceptive device is essential to fulfill the aims of chemical transvaginal sterilization.

In the study with 125 mg instillations of quinacrine chlorhydrate, the rates of pregnancies after tubal obstruction are related to the number of instillations that caused obstruction. This suggests that the drug has a cumulative effect. The rates of postobstruction pregnancies decreased from 5.7 to 1.3 percent in the patient who was instilled for 3 consecutive cycles. Where ethanol formalin was used, most patients became nonpatent after 3 or 4 instillations. When a 250 mg dosage of quinacrine chlorhydrate was used, nonpatency was obtained after a single instillation in 65 percent of the patients. It is quite probable that the rate of 90 to 95 percent of nonpatency could be obtained with 2 consecutive instillations.

In some cases, the lesions produced by sclerosing agents seem to be spontaneously reversible. Experiments with rats have shown that histological alterations produced by quinacrine were reversible in epithelium that is responsive to exogenous ovarian hormones.[7] Increasing the dosage of quinacrine seems to make the alterations irreversible. Clinical studies of patients instilled in 3 cycles with doses of 125 mg of quinacrine chlorhydrate show a very low spontaneous recovery rate. Only a more prolonged observation would reveal the necessary data on the rate of spontaneous recovery.

The possibility of developing a nonsurgical sterilizing technique using a chemical agent of low toxicity that requires no sophisticated application apparatus, that can be employed by paramedical personnel, and requires only two applications, opens unexpected perspectives in human fertility control.

REFERENCES

1. Froriep, R.: Zur vorbeungung der nothwendigkeit des kaiserschnitts und der perforation. *Not Gebiete der Natur Heilkunde,* 211:9, 1849.
2. Corfman, P.A.: Advances in Planned Parenthood Proceedings of the Third and Fourth Annual Meeting of the American Association of Planned Parenthool Physicians International Congress, Series N138, Sobrero, A.J. and Lewit, S., Eds. *Exp Med Found,* (1967), p. 183.
3. Salgado, C.: Esterillivacao provocado pela ijeco intrauterina de causticos; documentos radiologicos. *Ann Brasil Ginecol,* 11:503, 1941.
4. Zipper, J., Medel, M., Pastene, L., and Rivera, M.: Intrauterine instillation of chemical cytotoxic agents for tubal sterilization and treatment of functional metrorrhagias. *Intern J Fertil,* 14:280, 1969.
5. Zipper, J., Medel, M., and Prager, R.: Alterations in fertility induced by unilateral intrauterine instillation of cytotoxic compounds in rats. *Amer J Obstet Gynec, 101:*971, 1968.
6. Zipper, J., *et al.* In preparation.
7. Zipper, J., Prager, R., and Medel, M.: Biological changes induced by unilateral intrauterine instillation of quinacrine in the rat. Reversion

through the use of estrogen and progesterone. Submitted for publication to *Fertility and Sterility*.
8. Gellhorn, A., et al.: *In vitro* and *in vivo* effects of chemical agents on human and mouse glioblastoma multiforme. *Proc 2nd Internat Congr Neuropathol Part 1*:265, 1955.
9. Gellhorn, A., et al.: The use of atabrine (quinacrine) in the control of recurrent neoplastic effusions. *Dis Chest, 39*:165, 1959.
10. Reiner, L., and Gellhorn, A.: Localization of drugs within cells. Binding of quinacrine by liver cell constituents. *J Pharmacol Exp Ther, 117*: 52, 1955.
11. Rochlin, D.B., et al.: The control of recurrent malignant effusions using quinacrine hydrochloride (atabrine). *Surg Gynec Obstet, 119*:991, 1964.

Chapter 30

TRANSVAGINAL DELIVERY OF STERILIZING CHEMICALS[*]

Horace E. Thompson, Thomas Moulding, Charles Dafoe and Dale L. Osterling

For more than a century, attempts have been made to accomplish tubal occlusion for sterilization by the transvaginal route. As early as 1849, Froriep attempted to apply silver nitrate to the uterine cornu by this approach. Several investigators in the past, including Kocks,[6] Dickinson,[2] Hyams,[5] Sheares,[10] Porter et al.[8] have reported varying success with electrocautery by the transvaginal route. Until recent years, however, only sporadic attempts were made to accomplish sterilization by this approach, and none were adequately successful or sufficiently without danger to warrant their generalized acceptance.

The population explosion has made the need for a new and more easily performed sterilization procedure most urgent. Therefore, renewed and more intensive studies in this area have been instituted. In the past, tubal ligation and hysterectomy, necessitating the invasion of the abdominal cavity, with all of its implications, have been the only generally accepted methods of human female surgical sterilization. These techniques have been undesirable for large-scale sterilization because they are time-consuming and adequate surgical facilities may not be available. Therefore, the need for a transcervical approach which can eliminate the need for hospitalization, general anesthesia, and highly skilled personnel has provided the impetus for new research on the procedures.

Investigative work (Hefnawi et al.[4] Nishizaki,[7] Corfman and Taylor,[1] Rakshit,[9] and our experimentation) has demonstrated that the fallopian tube orifice can be approached with considerable accuracy through the cervical canal in most instances. This

---

[*] Supported in part by Grant No. M 68216 from the Population Council.

has been done blindly with a curved, blunt instrument locating the cornual recess at which point the fallopian tube enters the uterine cavity, and by direct visualization of the uterine cavity through the hysteroscope. The introduction of sterilizing agents by the latter technique, however, has been limited.

Corfman and Taylor have devised an ingenious instrument for the delivery of chemicals to the cornual region.[1] The device consists of a small, narrow syringe mounted at the tip of a curved cannula which is filled with a known amount of the sterilizing solution. Filling and discharge of the syringe can be accomplished after it has been introduced into the uterine cavity and placed in the cornual recess. A small balloon at the tip of the cannula helps guide the instrument into the cornu. These investigators attempted to fill the oviduct with various solutions with only partial success.

Rakshit[9] has attempted to fill the oviduct with various foreign-body materials filling the uterine cavity under pressure with the desired chemical agent, thereby forcing the material into the oviducts. The excess material is irrigated from the uterine cavity.

Various tissue adhesives and sclerosing agents have been considered for the permanent occlusion of the fallopian tubes. Attempts have been made to introduce these agents into the tubes by the abdominal as well as by the transcervical approach. Success to date has not been very great. In some instances, the chemical has been difficult to insert. When the agent has been inserted, the tubal occlusion is not always complete. Temporary sterilization by the introduction of plastics into the rabbit fallopian tubes has met with approximately fifty percent success (Hefnawi *et al.*).[4]

A review of the literature, as well as the production of casts of the endometrial cavity, has demonstrated a wide variation in the contour of the uterine cavity and the appearance of the uterine cornua. However, in a large percentage of cases, this variation is slight enough so that identification of the cornual area is possible by the blind as well as the direct-vision technique.

In addition to the production of uterine casts, the authors have explored the uterine cavity by the blind technique with a curved, blunt cannula, and by direct visualization with the balloon hysteroscope. A curved, blunt cannula was developed; it is 15 cm in length, 2 mm in diameter, and has a 4 mm rounded tip. A broad hub at the opposite end facilitates easy manipulation of the instrument. An 18-gauge needle was introduced through the lumen of the cannula, and a sliding lock was incorporated at the distal end; when the needle was withdrawn to the upper notch, it was entirely within the cannula. When it was forced forward to the distal notch, the tip of the needle protruded 2 mm beyond the end of the cannula. This instrument is shown in Figure 30-1. An attempt was made to locate the area of the cornu with this method. The needle then was advanced, and a staining solution was injected into the tissue. Twenty-nine uteri removed at surgery were explored through the cervical canal with this instrument; dye was placed in the region thought to be the tubal

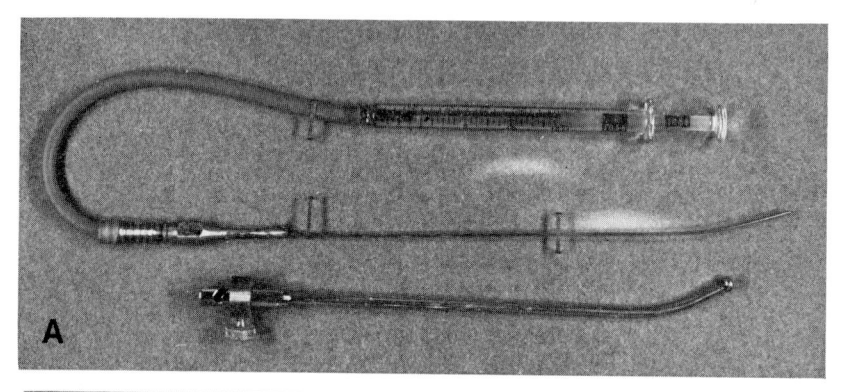

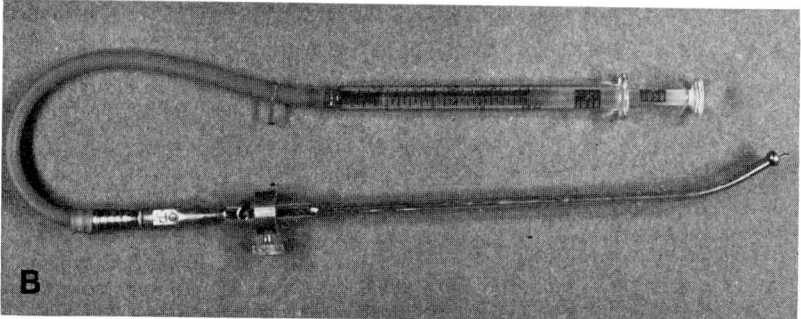

Figure 30-1. Intra-uterine cannula and syringe: a) cannula with needle withdrawn; b) cannula with needle in place.

orifice. Twenty-one of the uteri were injected with methylene blue and five with india ink. Both cornua were injected in each uterus. After the chemical was introduced into the cornua, a small polyethylene catheter was placed through the tubal lumen into the uterine cavity and the relationship of the dye to this catheter was observed. The following results were obtained:

1. *Methylene blue injection*
   a. Number of uteri injected 21
   b. Number of uteri where both cornua stained at ostia identified by catheter 18
   c. Failure of endometrium to take stain because of menses or concomitant D and C 3
2. *India ink injection*
   a. Number of uteri injected 5
   b. Number in which carbon particles were found within one high power field of ostia 4
   c. Number injected with no carbon particles found. ... 1

Figure 30–2 is a picture of a uterus opened after application of methylene blue into the cornual areas; a small polyethylene catheter was inserted through the tubal lumen on the left side. This demonstrates the close proximity of the point of dye application to the tubal orifice. The size of the methylene blue dot varied from 2 to 5 mm in diameter. In all of the 18 instances in which the dot was identified, the center of the dot was no more than 3 mm from the tubal orifice. This indicates that it is possible to identify the cornu of the uterus without difficulty and to inject a chemical solution into the area of tubal orifice in a high percentage of cases.

Since it was possible to identify the general area of the tubal orifice, an attempt was made to develop a means by which a sclerosing agent could be introduced into the tissue surrounding the tubal orifice in an area sufficiently wide and deep to cause occlusion of the tube as it courses through the uterine musculature. A jet injector* was modified by reducing the spring tension in the instrument. A known amount of india ink was injected

---

* This instrument is manufactured by the Scherer Corporation, Detroit, Michigan.

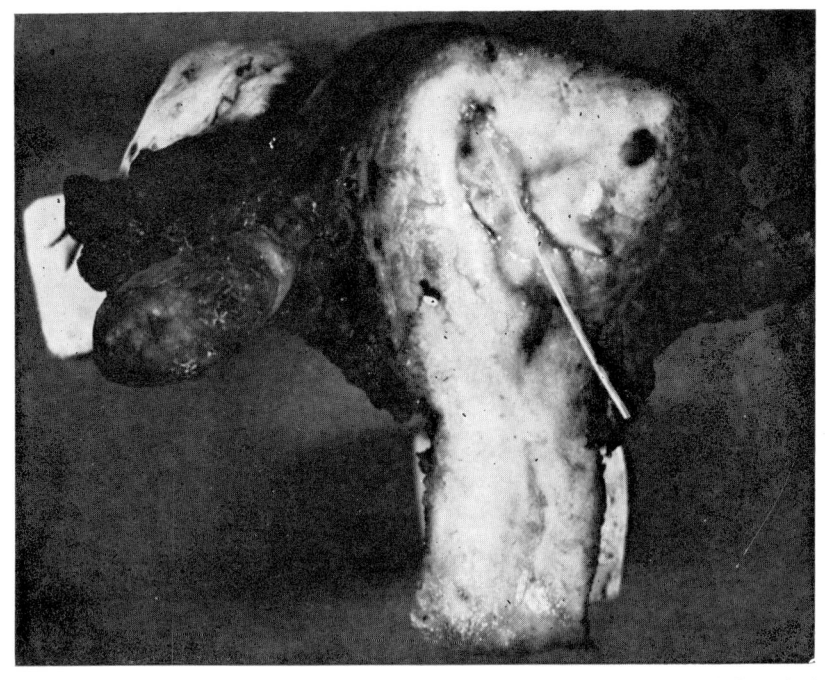

Figure 30-2. Open uterus with catheter protruding from the left tubal orifice, demonstrating the relationship of the methylene blue dot applied by the blind technique.

into the uterine wall in the area of the cornu in uteri removed at surgery. It was found that a small stream of carbon particles penetrated the full thickness of the uterine wall, although the bulk of the carbon particles did not penetrate more than 1 or 2 mm below the tissue surface. This phenomenon persisted even though the pressure in the instrument was reduced to a minimum. The depth of penetration in many instances was not consistent. Due to the inconsistency of the results and the fact that particles were found penetrating the full depth of the uterine wall, it was considered that it would be unsafe to use this instrument to deliver sclerosing agents which might penetrate the full thickness of the uterine wall and be deposited in the abdominal cavity, causing damage to other organs.

The balloon hysteroscope has been used in a limited number of cases in an attempt to identify the tubal orifices. In the small number of cases examined, the authors have been successful in most instances, but think further experimentation with this instrument is necessary. It is also considered that a new type of balloon will have to be developed if chemical agents are to be introduced into the cornual area by this technique. The elastic balloon currently in use obstructs the access to the tubal orifice. When the balloon is penetrated in order to apply the chemical agent, it can collapse before filling and cause distortion of the application. At the present time the authors are attempting to develop a plastic balloon-type bag without elastic recoil. When this membrane is perforated, the uterus will not collapse suddenly as the chemical is introduced into the cornu or tubal orifice.

Since it is possible to identify the cornu and the tubal orifice in most cases, either blindly or by direct vision, attempts to determine what sclerosing agent is best for tubal occlusion are being made. The rhesus monkey has been chosen as the experimental animal, since its uterus and fallopian tubes are very similar to those of a human. Cautery, sclerosing agents, and tissue adhesives have been applied to the cornua of six animals by hysterotomy, with no attempt to invade the canal of the fallopian tube. The following results were observed:

Monkey Number	Agent Used and Location	Results
1	Two second electrocautery right cornu; isopropyl-2-cyanoacrylate monomer left cornu.	no reaction
2	Sotradechol 1% right cornu; methyl-2-cyanoacrylate monomer left cornu.	no reaction
3	Methyl-2-cyanoacrylate monomer both cornua.	no reaction
4	Electrocautery 10 sec. both cornua.	no reaction
5	Cross-linked gelatin adhesives (14% of 37% formalin) both cornua.	superficial necrosis
6	Cross-linked gelatin adhesives (50% of 37% formalin) both cornua.	superficial necrossi

Obviously, this work is in its embryonic stage and no firm conclusions can be drawn at this time. However, the authors believe that since it is possible to identify the tubal orifice in most instances, the application of an effective sclerosing agent or adhesive compound can be accomplished if and when the ideal agent is identified. Future research will attempt to find an agent that will, when applied to the cornual area, occlude the tubal orifice. If this is unsuccessful, an attempt will be made to introduce sclerosing and adhesive agents into the tubal lumen, thereby producing a more selectively located lesion.

REFERENCES

1. Corfman, P.A., and Taylor, H.C., Jr.: An instrument for transcervical treatment of the oviducts and uterine cornua. *Obstet Gynec*, 27: 800, 1966.
2. Dickinson, R.L.: Simple sterilization of women by cautery stricture at the intra-uterine tubal openings. *Surg, Gynec Obstet*, 23:203, 1916.
3. Froriep, R.: Zur vorbeugung der notwendigkeit des kaiserschnitts und der perforation. *Not Gabiente Nature and Heilkunde*, 221:10, 1849.
4. Hefnawi, F., Fuchs, A.R., and Laurence, K.A.: Control of fertility by temporary occlusion of the oviduct. *Amer J Obstet Gynec*, 99:421, 1967.
5. Hyams, M.N.: Sterilization of the female by coagulation of the uterine cornu. *Amer J Obstet Gynec*, 28:96, 1934.
6. Kocks, J.: Eine neue methode der sterilisation der frauen. *Centralblatt Gynak*, 2:617, 1878.
7. Nishizaki, S.: Tubal sterilization through uterine cavity. Report II. *Jap J Obstet Gynec*, 12:285, 1929.
8. Porter, J.O.: Sutherland, C.G., and Brown, W.E.: Transuterine tubal cautery for sterilization. *Amer J Obstet Gynec*, 74:341, 1957.
9. Rakshit, B.: Experiments on tubal blocking for sterilization without laparotomy. *J Obstet Gynaec. India*, 18:1, 1968.
10. Sheares, B.H.: Sterilization of women by intra-uterine electro-cautery of the uterine cornu. *J Obstet Gynaec Brit Emp*, 65:419, 1958.

Chapter 31

EXPERIMENTAL STUDIES OF FALLOPIAN TUBE OCCLUSION*

RALPH M. RICHART, ROBERT S. NEUWIRTH AND HOWARD C. TAYLOR, JR.

Most population control programs offer a variety of techniques for the prevention of conception. Contraception using oral hormonal medications and intra-uterine devices is effective, the agents can be administered to large segments of the population with relative ease and apparent safety, and the programs can be carried out with relatively unskilled personnel. Vasectomy also can be accomplished on a large scale; it does not require expensive or sophisticated facilities and, because of its simplicity and relatively low risk, it can be introduced effectvely to the population by specially trained paramedical personnel. The termination of pregnancy by abortion has proved to be an effective population control technique in a number of countries; but it remains essentially unavailable to the developing nations for a number of reasons, including the requirement for expensive and sophisticated hospital facilities and the need for a large number of physicians to carry out the procedures in order to care properly for unforeseen complications. The last major technique of population control is that of fallopian tube occlusion, usually accomplished by operative interruption and ligation. The customary methods of tubal ligation require a hospital and operating suite, general or spinal anesthesia, and a trained gynecological surgeon. More simplified techniques recently have been used; these include laparoscopy, culdoscopy, and ligation under local anesthesia. Each of these, however, requires the services of a skilled physician and none of the techniques are suitable for application on a mass basis.

* From the International Institute for the Study of Human Reproduction and the Departments of Pathology and Obstetrics and Gynecology, College of Physicians and Surgeons of Columbia University; and the Obstetrical and Gynecological Service (The Sloane Hospital for Women) of the Presbyterian Hospital, New York City.

Because motivation is a major factor in the control of reproduction, and women are generally more easily motivated to accept sterilization procedures than are men, female sterilization should be an important part of population control programs. There is a need for an acceptable technique of tubal occlusion which can be administered on a mass basis. The ideal technique should be the following: applied to the fallopian tube through the cervix; inexpensive; simple; safe; relatively painless; foolproof enough to permit its application by trained paramedical personnel; and have an effectiveness approaching a hundred percent after a single application. Several attempts to fulfill these criteria have been made utilizing cornual cauterization, cornual cryotherapy, and the application of various physical and caustic chemical agents to the uterine cavity, cornu, and fallopian tube. Although the techniques have met with varying rates of success, skilled physicians were required for their application and two or more applications were required in order to obtain satisfactory results.

The authors thought that if an appropriate chemical agent could be found that would produce permanent obliteration of the tubal lumen, such an agent might be introduced readily through the cervix and provide an acceptable method for a rapid and inexpensive sterilization procedure which could be used in large populations.

For this reason, research has been done with a variety of agents that are known to produce severe tissue damage and fibrosis; and an attempt has been made to compare systematically various classes of agents and individual agents with regard to their effectiveness in producing tubal obliteration. This paper is a report of work in progress utilizing rabbits, and rhesus and pigtail monkeys as experimental animals.

MATERIALS AND METHODS

In all experiments utilizing rabbits, a ventral incision was made in the lower abdomen; the uterus, fallopian tubes, and ovaries were mobilized and delivered into the wound; and a small scissor incision was made in the antimesometrial wall of the uterus approximately 5 mm proximal to the uterotubal junction. A Teflon or polyethylene catheter was introduced into the fallopian tube through the uterine incision. The agent under study was injected into the tubal lumen until, by direct vision, it approached the fimbriated end. In other experiments in the rabbit, an attempt was made to infiltrate the uterine and tubal musculature as well as the peritubal fat and connective tissue. This was accomplished utilizing a specially designed tip attached to a commercially available cocked-spring injector used for intracutaneous or subcutaneous injections. Several different tips were used, but all produced a needlelike stream of chemical from one or more orifices which effectively permeated the tissues. In addition, gelfoam sponges and gauze strips were soaked in solutions of zinc chloride, silver nitrate, and salicylic acid and were placed in the uterine lumen at the uterotubal junction.

In the monkeys, the chemicals were introduced after the abdomen was opened with a ventral-midline lower abdominal incision; the uterus, fallopian tubes, and ovaries were delivered into the wound, and a catheter was passed a short distance into the fallopian tube through the fimbria. Infiltration of various agents into the myometrium, particularly the cornual region, also was done with the injector gun and by needle infiltration.

After the agents were applied, the animals were sacrificed at intervals. The reproductive tracts were removed, fixed in Bouin's solution, sectioned, stained, and examined histologically.

RESULTS

The agents utilized in these experiments, the concentrations used, the number of applications, and the results obtained are summarized in Tables 31-I to 31-VII. Zinc chloride, silver nitrate, phenol, and a variety of strong acids and bases all produced consistent and severe necrosis of the tubal epithelium and the muscular wall. Salicylic acid also was effective in higher concentrations. Atabrine®, sodium morrhuate, and Sotradecol® were ineffective and produced no discernible tubular damage. The sponges and gauze strips produced massive necrosis with all of the agents used, but permanent damage was not observed in any

Fallopian Tube Occlusion

TABLE 31-I
CHEMICAL APPLICATIONS TO RABBIT FALLOPIAN TUBES

Compound	Fallopian Tube Applications	Died	3–6 wk Damage	3–6 wk Occlusion	8–10 wk Damage	8–10 wk Occlusion
Ag NO$_3$ 5%	2	0	1	1	0	0
Ag NO$_3$ 10%	2	0	0	2	0	0
Ag NO$_3$ 20%	3	1	1	1	0	0
Salicylic Acid 5%	3	1	2	0	0	0
Salicylic Acid 10%	3	1	1	1	0	0
Phenol	8	4	2	0	2	0
H$_2$SO$_4$ Concentrated	6	4	1	0	0	1
NAOH 5N	6	0	2	0	4	0
Sodium Morrhuate	4	0	0	0	0	0
Sotradecol	4	0	0	0	0	0
Methyl Cyanoacrylate	12	4	4	4	0	0
Ethyl Cyanoacrylate	14	4	6	0	4	0
Isobutyl Cyanoacrylate	18	6	6	2	4	0

TABLE 31-II
CAUSTICS IN GAUZE AND GELFOAM APPLIED TO RABBIT FALLOPIAN TUBES

Compound	Fallopian Tube Applications	Died	No. Sacrificed at weeks 3	6	Damage	Occlusion
ZnCl$_2$ 100% in Gelfoam	6	6	0	0	0	0
ZnCl$_2$ 100% in Gauze	6	2	2	2	4	0
ZnCl$_2$ 10% in Gelfoam	8	0	4	4	0	0
Salicylic Acid 10% in Gelfoam	6	2	2	2	Minimal	0
ZnCl$_2$ 100% in Gelfoam	6	6	0	0	0	0
ZnCl$_2$ 40% in Gelfoam	4	0	2	2	4	0
ZnCl$_2$ 20% in Gelfoam	4	0	2	2	4	0
ZnCl$_2$ 10% in Gelfoam	8	0	4	4	0	0
AgNO$_3$ 20% in Gelfoam	4	0	2	2	4	0
AgNO$_3$ 10% in Gelfoam	4	0	2	2	4	0

TABLE 31-III
ZINC CHLORIDE AND ATABRINE APPLIED TO RABBIT FALLOPIAN TUBES

Compound	Fallopian Tube Applications	Died	No. Sacrificed at Weeks 3	6	3 Week Damage	3 Week Occlusion	6 Week Damage	6 Week Occlusion
Zn Cl$_2$ 200%	3	3	0	0	0	0	0	0
Zn Cl$_2$ 100%	3	2	1	0	1	0	0	0
Zn Cl$_2$ 50%	4	0	2	2	2	0	2	0
Zn Cl$_2$ 25%	2	0	1	1	1	0	1	0
Zn Cl$_2$ 10%	2	0	1	1	1	0	1	0
Zn Cl$_2$ 5%	2	0	1	1	1	0	1	0
Atabrine 2%	4	2	1	1	0	0	0	0
Atabrine 4%	4	1	2	1	0	0	0	0
Atabrine 1%	3	0	2	1	0	0	0	0

TABLE 31-IV
GRANULOMA PRODUCING AGENTS APPLIED TO RABBIT UTERINE MUSCLE

Compound	Rabbit Muscle Infiltrations	Died	No. Sacrificed at Months 1.5	4	5	6	Damage	Occlusion
Talc	4	1	1	1	1	0	3	0
Asbestos	4	1	1	1	1	0	3	0
Cellobiose	6	3	1	1	0	1	3	0
Be NO$_3$ 40%	2	1	0	1	0	0	1	0
Be NO$_3$ 10%	2	2	0	0	0	0	0	0
Be SO$_4$ 11%	4	4	0	0	0	0	0	0
Silica	5	2	1	0	0	2	3	0
Diatoms	5	0	2	0	0	3	5	0

TABLE 31-V
CAUSTICS AND ADJUVANT APPLIED TO RABBIT FALLOPIAN TUBES

Compound	Fallopian Tube Applications	Died	No. Sacrificed at Weeks 3	6	Damage	Occlusion
Freund's adjuvant	4	0	2	2	Slight—3 wks.	0
Freund's adjuvant with 10% AgNO$_3$	3	0	2	1		0
Freund's adjuvant with 5% ZnCl$_2$	3	0	2	1	Extensive at 6 wks.	0

TABLE 31-VI
CYANOACRYLATE APPLIED TO MONKEY FALLOPIAN TUBES

Compound	Applications	No. Sacrificed at Months 1.5	3	4	6	Damage	Occlusion
Methyl Cyanoacrylate	13	1	1	5	6	0	0
Ethyl Cyanoacrylate	11	1	1	5	4	Slight	0

TABLE 31-VII
INFILTRATION OF MONKEY MYOMETRIUM

Compound	Myometrium Applications	No. Sacrificed at Months 1.5	3	4	6	Granuloma
Silica	4	0	0	1	3	0
Cellobiose	2	0	0	0	2	0
Diatoms	5	0	0	1	4	2
Atabrine 2%	1	0	0	1	0	0
Raw Cellulose	1	0	0	1	0	0
Dissociated Plant Cells	1	0	0	1	0	1
Fine Talc	2	0	0	1	1	0
Quartz	1	0	0	0	1	0
Methyl Cyanoacrylate	2	1	0	0	1	0
Ethyl Cyanoacrylate	1	0	0	0	1	1

of the gelfoam applications after 6 weeks. Zinc chloride in gauze produced some fibrosis at 3 and 6 weeks, but not enough to occlude the lumen of the uterus or fallopian tube. The tissue adhesives, methyl, ethyl, and isobutyl cyanoacrylate produced tubal necrosis, fibrosis, and tubal occlusion in the rabbit, although at varying rates. All were ineffective, even after prolonged contact with the tubal epithelium, in producing total anatomical tubal closure in the monkey. The granuloma-producing agents elicited a granulomatous response with fibrosis, but, in all instances, the granulomata were of only microscopic size and failed to affect the size of the tubal lumen. Deaths consistently were produced by phenol, the higher concentrations of zinc chloride, and the beryllium compounds.

The most striking conclusion to be derived from this series of experiments is the singular capacity of the fallopian tube to repair itself after what can only be described as acute massive injury. With virtually all of the effective compounds (including zinc chloride, silver nitrate, salicylic acid, and other necrosis-producing agents), large sections of fallopian tube appeared to be completely necrotic in animals sacrificed during the early stages of the reaction. Despite this massive necrosis, islands of tubal epithelium and submucosa and fields of smooth muscle apparently survived the acute insult and, as the necrotic tissues were cleared away, epithelial repair began. In many instances, an obviously damaged, but intact, fallopian tube with a patent lumen was found 6 to 8 weeks following the original injury. Both the monkey and the rabbit appeared to be capable of reconstituting the tubal lumen following severe injury. In the monkey, because of the more complex structure of the primate fallopian tube, residual damage was more obvious than it was in the rabbit.

It should be emphasized that the end point in these studies has been total anatomical occlusion of the tubal lumen. A functional end point was thought to be too difficult to define.

The fertility of these animals has not been studied and it may be that, despite the patency of the tubal lumen, the tubal damage could be so severe as to prevent conception. The desired goal, however, is total occlusion, both to be certain of sterility and to preclude a high incidence of complications (e.g. ectopic pregnancy), which might occur in a damaged but patent fallopian tube.

In order to block the reestablishment of tubal patency following extensive damage, it may be necessary to devise a means of chronically applying an epitheliotoxic substance to the lumen so that fibrosis can occur without accompanying epithelial repair. Some of the cytotoxic agents might be appropriate for this type of application, but, because of their toxicity and possible carcinogenicity, they may not be applicable clinically. The cyanoacrylates consistently are effective in producing tubal occlusion in the rabbit and appear both to damage tubal epithelium and to promote fibroblast formation. The methylcyanoacrylate compound is the most effective and produces total occlusion of the fallopian tube in virtually all successful applications, as we have reported previously.[1] The ethyl and isobutyl derivatives also are effective in producing occlusion, but do so at a slower rate and with less reliability. Unfortunately these agents, which appeared to be so promising in the rabbit, do not elicit a similar response in the rhesus or pigtail monkey. The mechanism of action of the cyanoacrylates in producing epithelial necrosis and stimulating fibrosis is not known, but there appears to be considerable interspecific variation. The cyanoacrylates should be tested in human fallopian tubes in order to determine whether they should be studied further or abandoned. It seems futile, because of the species-specificity of response, to continue to use these agents in laboratory animals until their effect on human fallopian tubes has been ascertained. Because of the problems relating to the rapid polymerization of the cyanoacrylates, an effective delivery system would probably be difficult and expensive to design. This should probably not be undertaken until human trials have been completed. The design of such trials necessarily will be complex.

It is interesting to note that, although Zipper has reported that atabrine produces blockade upon lavage in the human uterus,[2] this substance produced no effect in rabbits or monkeys. These differences also may be attributable to species variation in tubal response. The lack of response to sodium morrhuate and Sotradecol, despite their sclerosing properties when applied to the vascular system, indicates the differences in the response of different epithelia to the same agents.

The granuloma-producing agents failed to produce the massive granulomatous response in the smooth muscle that they produce in fat and fibrous tissues. This may be ascribed to the relatively low fibroblast content of the tissues in the female reproductive tract. It probably is not possible to enhance the granuloma-producing properties of these agents in smooth muscle. Attempts were made to do so by injecting a mixture of granuloma-producing agents and caustic chemicals, but the mixture failed to elicit any greater response than did the granuloma-producing agents alone.

REFERENCES

1. Corfman, P.A., Richart, R.M., and Taylor, H.C.: The response of the rabbit tubo-uterine junction to a tissue adhesive. *Science*, 1348–1349, 1965.
2. Zipper, J., Medel, M., Stachetti, E., Pastene, L., Rivera, M., and Prager, R.: Chemical Agents for Transvaginal Sterilization. Presented at the Conference on Human Sterilization, Cherry Hill, New Jersey, October, 1969.

DISCUSSION: NONSURGICAL STERILIZATION

Sheldon Segal, *Moderator*

Dr. Segal opened discussion on Dr. Martens' paper on cryosurgery for tubal sterilization.

Dr. Southam asked if any of the tubes which were demonstrated to be closed by hysterogram reopened and whether any pregnancies resulted.

Dr. Martens said he did not know of any such cases.

Dr. Thompson wanted to know the depth of the lesion and if it went through the uterine wall.

Dr. Martens stated that they really did not know the extent of the lesion produced in each patient. It became a matter of judgment in determining the temperature to be used. An attempt was being made to produce as great a lesion as possible; by the time cryosurgery was done on the later patients, it was known that the initial attempts had not been successful. Some risks may have been taken, for there was some adherance to the frozen surface. Observation showed that no damage had been done, so there was no real concern about causing damage by freezing.

Mr. Pontarelli asked if the procedure were done under general or local anesthesia.

Dr. Martens explained that it had been done both ways. It can be accomplished when the patient is awake; the only painful part is the dilation of the cervix to 8 mm.

Dr. Garcia wanted to know if there was an increase in discharge.

Dr. Martens said that, with the amount of freeze employed, a tremendous outpouring of a watery discharge ensued, but there were no problems with either long-term or short-term bleeding. Cooper used freezing to operate in a bloodless field, for apparently the vessels do freeze. Most of the patients who were awake complained of nothing but an annoying discharge; there was no pain following the procedure.

Discussion: Nonsurgical Sterilization

Mr. Pontarelli wanted an explanation of the histological picture after eight or twelve weeks.

Dr. Martens stated that they had very few specimens; there was some missing tissue in the cornual regions but there was very little change. He did not think there had been any problem in misplacing the probe; he really believed that they were close enough to get the tubal ostia frozen for a satisfactory period of time.

Dr. Rakshit explained that there was someone in India working with the heat coil; the ostia could not be located in the research. He wanted to know if Dr. Martens had any such problems.

Dr. Martens said there were no problems with their procedures and Dr. Lyons had tried the heat coil technique in the United States a number of years ago.

Dr. Segal explained that the tissue was both frozen and thawed. It is possible, if not likely, that more tissue damage occurs during thawing than during freezing. He wanted to know if studies had been done with hysterectomy samples or with more than two thawings.

Dr. Martens stated that they had not done such work. He stated that there had been much discussion that the path of the tube through the intramural portion is not straight; many times it turns at almost a complete right angle, and it would be impossible to thread anything through the oviduct at that site.

Dr. Richart stated that there was a great deal of experience with the use of the cold technique on a surface. For example, even a single freezing and thawing can prove successful in the treatment of neoplastic cervical lesions. It was his opinion that repeated freezing and thawing in the lower part of the uterus produced tissue necrosis; he thought it obviously resulted in tissue death.

Dr. Martens explained that, in the hysterograms of the closed tubes, a defect was seen which suggested that a great deal of the tissue had been destroyed. But in spite of the destruction and the subsequent scar formation, some tubes were still patent.

Dr. Richart thought that one of the problems was that when there was benign tissue destruction, there was little scar formation and little tissue reaction.

Dr. Segal then opened Dr. Hulka's paper on cauterization for tubal sterilization for discussion.

Dr. Clyman wanted to know in what form the silver nitrate was delivered.

Dr. Hulka explained that it was delivered in a sheath through a small plastic cannula; as it is brought to the uterotubal area, nothing along the way is burned. When the site is reached, the tip is pushed out of the plastic, and the burn is accomplished. Some of the cauterization extends to about half way up the tube and about 1 or 2 cm into the uterus; essentially, the reaction is localized.

Dr. Tietze asked how the silver nitrate was put back into the sheath.

Dr. Hulka said he just pulled it back through the tube.

Dr. A.S. Lee commented that one of the problems involved was locating the correct position for cauterization, but that this could be done with some effort. He thought that the second problem involved the nature of the burn; the present efforts had been directed towards burning the tissues in order to produce damage that would create necrosis. When, for example, a finger is burned, scar tissue is formed when it is dirty or inflamed; however, there is no scar formation when the finger has been prepared. If simple burning is done and thin scar tissue is formed, no complications arise; the body absorbs some of the destroyed tissue, and the thin scar does not give the necessary blockage. He thought the object was not only to destroy the tissue, but to introduce another agent, e.g. a form of plastic, that would form a protective tissue. After this site is burned, connective tissue could grow in and form a block.

Dr. Hulka explained that the problem should be visualized schematically; one section being the tube and the other the opening into the uterus. If a lesion is induced, there is an initial disruption of epithelium and the production of an exudate. When this stream comes through, it will create a fistula; eventually epithelial healing will be produced. He thought Dr. A.S. Lee was suggesting some sort of plastic block to direct the site of the healing in order to produce an obstruction; he did not know if it were possible to insert such a material or if it would remain long enough to have any obstructive effect.

Dr. A.S. Lee thought that the first requirement was the destruction of some surface tissues; then the adhesive material or the plastic could be inserted. If a small cavity formed on the right side, a forming plastic would adhere to that corner and connective tissue would possibly start to grow in one or two days. This would remain in place.

Dr. Neuwirth said that he followed up on Hyams' experience within the last two years by contacting Dr. Hyams' wife and his office nurse. Dr. Neuwirth said that Hyams attempted to solve the localization problem with an attached cannula through which dye was injected under fluoroscopic control. After localization electrocoagulation was carried out. He continued to use the procedure until his death, but the results were not published. His wife said that the method apparently was successful.

Dr. Hulka commented that if fluid were injected into the uterus without obstructing the cervix, the tendency would be for the fluid to flow out; you could see it leaking out. There may be an advantage in injecting fluid and making sure it leaks out; it can do so if there is no perforation.

Dr. Neuwirth said that Hyams was interested in that, not so much from the point of view of risk of perforation, but because he wanted to deliver the electrocautery to the angle at which the tube joins the uterine cavity.

Dr. Corfman noted that Hyams' technique was different because the instrument he used had a tip that would permit the advancement to an additional centimeter into the cornu; the intent was to penetrate into the cornua as far as possible.

Dr. Segal opened Dr. Hayashi's paper on tubal sterilization under hysteroscopy for discussion.

Dr. Richart wanted to know if the hysteroscope employed was the plastic type or the balloon type. He also asked for comments on the ease of use and wanted to know if visualization of the ostium was a problem because of the redundancy of the endometrium, which might tend to obscure the view.

Dr. Hayashi said that it is possible to visualize the ostium such as quinacrine is introduced into the human a low injection pressure is sufficient to force it into the tube. A chemical is being introduced into a tube where high pressure is produced. Quinacrine penetrates the cells in the form of microcrystals. They have not been observed in humans, but have been seen two or three months after instillation in rats; they appear to produce something like a booster effect. In the portion of the tube that is wide-angled, the low pressure is maintained. The very thick endometrium is not affected.

Dr. Segal said that this meant that there were no differences in the effect quinacrine produced on whatever cells it reached, but that it did reach all the functional layers of the epithelium of the intramural portion of the tube. However, it does not reach deeply enough into the endometrium.

Dr. Zipper thought that research in the baboon, the monkey, and the rabbit had been successful; he considered this to be a very specific type of binding.

Dr. Segal mentioned that he had not shown the difference in binding to tubal versus endometrial epithelium.

Dr. Zipper explained that they were just starting work on the biochemical reaction of the rat.

Dr. Martens asked if it were possible to speak in terms of pregnancy risk and risk factors. He wanted to know how the variables were handled; for example, the exposure of the patient to the potential for conception and the frequency of intercourse. Other factors were the fertility of her sexual partner and the patient's own ovulation rate.

Dr. Zipper said that if Dr. Martens wanted to know if they were dealing with a group of infertile individuals the answer was no. The patients were a group of highly fertile women; they knew them to have a pregnancy rate of eighty to a hundred per ovulation year. At least half a dozen poor contraceptives had been used with these cases and the women became pregnant. In other words, they are highly fertile.

Dr. Martens inquired if Dr. Zipper knew the women were specifically mating at the time.

Dr. Zipper said they were mating.

Dr. Segal thought that the fact that the normal population

was unprotected was taken for granted in studying the clinic population.

Dr. Tietze stated that it was important to know when these women had had their last child. The possibility of postpartum infertility has to be considered in studies of this type. He thought that some of these women would be in the postpartum stage, for otherwise they would be pregnant.

Dr. Zipper explained that the sample was almost a hundred percent postpartum. In Chile, authorization is needed for sterilization; generally, women can be sterilized after their second child.

Dr. Segal wanted to know the effects of that condition.

Dr. Tietze thought that maximum fecundability would be higher somewhere just before the first postpartum menstrual cycle. If allowances were made for 2 ovulatory cycles, he thought that a pregnancy rate of between 80 and 90 percent could be expected within one year. He said that there was another problem that Dr. Zipper had not considered, one which no one has been able to consider. If there is a sample of women who are not using contraceptives and a time interval elapses between the return of menstruation (and presumably ovulation) and the beginning of the use of contraception, the more highly fecund couples will be selected out of the population. No one has paid attention to this, although it is known.

Dr. Segal asked if Dr. Tietze was speaking about reducing a theoretical pregnancy rate of 120 to 80; here the discussion was of a pregnancy rate reduction down to 12.

Dr. Tietze agreed and said he was very much impressed by portions of Dr. Zipper's paper and considered the results comparable to those obtained with the less successful intra-uterine contraceptive devices.

Dr. Clyman pointed out that in many instances hysterosalpingography reveals nonpatency but the tubes are open.

Dr. Zipper said that this was well-known, but there was no other method with which to determine tubal patency. When insufflation is used, the diagnosis can be incorrect. He was not previously aware of the fact that repeated hysterosalpingography could cause tubal obstruction. They had attempted to develop simpler techiques with which to demonstrate tubal patency. They were not aware of all the possible factors involved when the research was started; the next project was going to be of better design.

Dr. Rakshit asked why the dosages were 2 or 4 ml and he also wanted to know up to which point the liquid was instilled.

Dr. Zipper explained that they had done previous studies before attempting this series. In a study which involved the instillation of pure ethanol in a sample of 20 women, almost a hundred percent of them were pregnant after three or four months. He thinks that there is a difference between a dosage of 2 ml and a dosage of 4 ml for the use of any caustic under conditions that cannot be controlled can be dangerous. When 4 ml are introduced, pressure must be utilized; it is better to be on the safe side and use 2 ml, which is a very small volume.

Dr. Hulka noted that the mechanical means of tubal occlusion that had been discussed were mainly single application procedures. He suspected that the program was devised to include subsequent treatments; in that case, mechanical and chemical occlusion efforts might not differ so much.

Dr. Southam asked how long the procedure took and what discomfort was associated with it.

Dr. Zipper said that it took as long as it did to insert an intrauterine device. The only complication that resulted was excitation. Rochlin suggested the use of quinacrine because it is potent against some tumors and is almost nontoxic in humans. Dosages as high as 1 gm have been introduced into the peritoneal cavity for cancer therapy. Transvaginal chemical sterilization is a recommended procedure because it does not need anesthesia or any special skill in performance; the procedure is inexpensive and safe. Even if perforation ensues or the drug is introduced into the peritoneal cavity, no side-effects result.

Dr. Segal wanted to know the toxicity level for quinacrine.

Dr. Zipper said they had introduced as much as 250 milligrams without any problems.

Dr. Segal asked if their dosages were far below the toxicity level or at the margin of toxicity production.

Dr. Zipper explained that they considered their dosages to be far below the toxicity level. Increasing dosages had not produced any animal deaths. Quinacrine has been used for the treatment of human malaria in dosages as high as 80 mg per day for long periods of time.

Dr. Neuwirth noted that he had had experience with the use of quinacrine in the peritoneal cavity for cancer therapy, but he did not know of any experience with quinacrine in the normal peritoneal cavity. He wanted to know if Dr. Zipper had any information on this subject.

Dr. Zipper said they did not have any information on the subject, but they thought that quinacrine could enter the patient's peritoneal cavity without producing either secondary effects or subjective complaints.

Dr. Clyman asked if there was any evidence of carcinogenicity or any long-term effects.

Dr. Zipper stated that he did not have data relating to that.

Dr. Zipper questioned Dr. Richart on the concentrations of quinacrine that he had employed.

Dr. Richart said that he had used both 150 and 250 mg per animal.

Dr. Hulka wanted to know if the gauze that was soaked in the chemical agents was left in long enough to form a matrix.

Dr. Richart said that one of the problems in introducing a foreign body into the uterus was the production of infection and death. The battle was drawn between fibrosis and death.

Dr. Rakshit asked if the $Ag\ NO_3$ employed had produced any renal effects.

Dr. Richart explained that they had not studied the effects on the kidneys. In clinical use, the agent was applied to the cervix.

Dr. Hulka stated that silver nitrate was used frequently in cervical cauterization; it is left and absorbed and no renal effects are produced. He did not think that the relatively small amount used would be toxic.

Dr. Clyman returned to Dr. Thompson's problem with visualization of the tubal ostium. He said that he was never able to see it with the balloon technique. However, with lavage and the Normal hysteroscope, visualization of the ostium is possible.

Dr. Thompson wanted to know the extent of the problem with bleeding and the obstruction of the view.

Dr. Clyman explained that if the procedure was performed close to the menstrual period, there was not too much bleeding. After that, visualization was difficult.

Dr. Thompson said that they had had very little experience with the procedure.

Chapter 32

SUMMARY AND DIRECTIONS FOR THE FUTURE

Anna L. Southam

This meeting provided the opportunity for gynecologists, urologists, program directors, and biomedical engineers from all over the world to meet in both formal and informal sessions. The current status of vasectomy and tubal ligation was defined, and exciting new possibilities for simplifying these methods were discussed.

From the material presented in this conference, it is apparent that surgical occlusion of the vasa deferentia or the fallopian tubes is a widely used method of birth control throughout the world. When evaluated against the standard criteria for contraception, (acceptability, effectiveness, reversibility, safety, and cost) surgical sterilization, even as it is performed today, appears to be one of the best methods now available.

ACCEPTABILITY

Vasectomy and tubal occlusion are used widely in most countries and are the methods chosen by more physicians and accepted by more couples in India and in East Pakistan than any other type of birth control. In India alone, 6 million couples have chosen sterilization. In South Korea, 3 percent of eligible males have had vasectomies, and in Bombay, 20 percent. In the United States, 12 percent of women have been surgically sterilized by the end of their reproductive life, and an unknown but large number of men have had vasectomies.

Most candidates learn of the method from protected couples or from family planning workers. In East Pakistan, for example, a *grass roots* demand for vasectomy developed at a time when intra-uterine contraception was officially advocated and encouraged. Although centers to reverse vasectomies and tubal ligations have been established in India and South Korea and the availability of the reanastomosing surgery publicized, few individuals request repair.

A number of papers presented during this meeting reported progress in developing occlusive methods that could be reversed easily and thus increase their acceptability among couples with small families. The perfection of technical innovations, some on the horizon and others already in limited use, would make sterilization the ideal method of birth control. Sterilization merely inserts a barrier between the eggs and the sperm and provides the most acceptable of all mechanisms for the prevention of pregnancy.

EFFECTIVENESS

The reported failure rates are variable and difficult to determine. Less than one percent of the males with standard vasectomies become fertile again. The standard Pomeroy technique for tubal ligation is associated with a similarly low failure rate. If these percentages could be translated into pregnancies per hundred years of use, the failure rate would be insignificant, since the continuation rate extends to the end of reproductive life. The effectiveness of sterilization procedures could be evaluated more accurately if the age and parity of the women protected by either vasectomy or tubal ligation were known.

Attempts to occlude the tubal ostia by the trans-uterine approach using heat or cold are associated with high failure rates. Other physical agents such as ultrasound and laser beams have not been evaluated as yet. A number of chemical agents show promise, and while research is still in its early stages, pregnancy rates no greater than those associated with intra-uterine contraception have been reported.

REVERSIBILITY

The statistics presented at this meeting indicate that the standard surgical interruption of either the vas deferens or the fallopian tube can be reversed by experienced surgeons in perhaps seventy-five percent of the cases. The experience is sparse, since few individuals seek restoration of fertility. Research in progress on animals suggests that tubal occlusion produced by quinacrine may be reversed simply by the administration of large doses of estrogen. Development of removable plugs for obstruction of the vas deferens has just reached the stage of clinical trial, and the promising results obtained so far in animals have not yet been confirmed in man.

SAFETY

Since vasectomy is always done under local anesthesia, anesthetic complications are rare. Vasa deferentia are easily accessible to the surgeon, and there are no vital structures in the operative area. Complications are limited to those of infection and hematoma formation. No exact figures are available on rates, but they appear to be low. The reversible methods of vasectomy now being investigated do not promise to decrease complications. Tubal ligation is done under general or spinal anesthesia in most parts of the world, often through a laparotomy incision. The frequency of serious complications or anesthetic deaths is not known, but in India, where the experience is very great, not a single death has come to the attention of the Ministry of Health. Two deaths, both avoidable, occurred in a series of ten thousand operations in Japan. Morbidity associated with postpartum tubal ligation is more frequent following difficult labors and in the presence of severe anemia. Tubal ligation even during the antepartum period is well tolerated by pregnant women. The use of a laparoscope for interval ligations avoids a laparotomy incision, but not the anesthetic hazards. The culdoscopic method as taught in Mexico City and Miami requires only local anesthesia and should reduce complications further. The use of transuterine cornual cautery has been associated with severe complications, including uterine perforation and bowel injury. The use of chemical and physical agents for occlusion of either the vas or the tube would avoid surgical trauma, but would introduce possible other risks which remain to be evaluated.

COST

Vasectomy is the cheapest method of birth control available today. Only a few minutes of the scarcest commodity, surgical time, is required, since such requirements as information, dispensing and postoperative care can be carried out by trained nonmedical personnel. Physical or chemical methods might even bypass the medical establishment.

Tubal ligation as done in most of the world today is more expensive than vasectomy, but undoubtedly is less costly than providing for the constant and continued supervision that intrauterine and oral contraception require. The simpler techniques now available eliminate the need for hospitalization and general anesthesia, but considerable skill is required to use the culdoscope. Postpartum tubal ligation adds little to the hospitalization time, but it does put a strain on operating room facilities.

The development of safe chemical occlusive agents requiring no more time and no more skill than the insertion of an IUD and eliminating the need for continued medical surveillance, would revolutionize national family planning programs. Birth control would become one of the cheapest and simplest of all health services.

There seems to be a consensus among members of this group that a low motivation method such as sterilization is necessary. There is also optimism, shared by clinical investigators, program administrators, and biomedical engineers, concerning the feasibility of the proposed technical developments.

NAME INDEX

Aguero, O., v, 12–22
Alexander, A.M., 100
Ambrose, J., 153
Anderson, E.T., 115
Angello, S.J., 292
Arronet, G., 128
Averkin, E.C., 293

Banner, E.A., 128
Barker, D.W., v, 166–174
Barnard, J.W., 165
Barnes, H.C., 115
Baum, G., 153
Bergan, A., 36
Berhman, S.F., 127
Bernhard, W.F., 253
Berry, E., 262
Bierman, H., 282
Bliss, R.W., 153
Botella-Lluisia, J., 127
Bowers, C.J., 332
Bowers, M.K., 332
Boysen, H., 100
Brackett, B.G., 127
Bredemeir, H., 262
Brennan, J.F., 165
Brindley, G.S., 293
Brown, W.E., 333, 369
Bunge, R.G., v, 204–211
Burkhart, J., 262

Caballero-Gardo, J.A., 127
Cacares, C.A., 293
Cameron, J.L., 275
Campbell, C., 262
Cardenas-Conde, L., 18–22
Carpuk, O., 228
Castallo, M.A., 127
Chan, G., 262
Chez, R.A., v, 48
Chiara, A., 128
Clark, E.W., 36
Clarke, A., 263
Clavero-Nunez, S.A., 127

Clyman, M.J., v, 93–99, 100
Cooper, J.K., 293
Coover, H.W., Jr., 275
Corfman, P.A., iii, v, xi, 100, 274, 351, 359, 367
Crane, M., 127
Croley, H.T., 23–36, 37
Curtice, V., 262
Czernobilsky, B., 127

Dafoe, C., 353–359
Darbari, B.S., vi, 12–22
Dasmahapatra, T., 213
David, A., 127
Delgado, J.M.R., 293
De Vilbiss, L.A., 332
Dickinson, R.L., 332, 333, 359

Eduljee, S.Y., 128
Eggleton, R.C., 165
Eisenberg, L., 293

Fine, S., 262
Fort, A.T., 100
Frick, H.C., 203
Froriep, R., 351, 359
Fry, F.J., vi, 160–164, 165
Fry, R.B., 165
Fry, W.J., 164, 165
Fryer, T.B., 293
Fuchs, A.R., 228, 359
Gallegos, D.A., 127
Gamble, C.J., 333
Gamble, W.J., 253
Garb, A.E., 100
Garcia, C.-R., vi, 116–127
Garg, B., 293
Garrett, J.J., 153
Gellhorn, A., 352
George, A., 36
Gerraets, W., 262
Gioia, J.D., 333
Green-Armytage, V.B., 128
Greenwood, I., 153

Griffiths, W., 36
Gross, R.E., 253
Guerrero, C.D., 128
Guerry, D., 262, 263

Haggerty, P.E., 293
Haider, S.J., 36
Ham, W., 263
Hanton, E.M., 128
Harnstein, A., 128
Harrison, J.H., 159
Hasel, K., 211, 228
Hayashi, M., vi., 128, 201–203, 334–338
Haynes, M.A., 36
Hefnawi, F., 228, 359
Herrmann, J.B., 274, 275
Herwald, S.W., 292
Hittinger, W.C., 293
Howry, D.H., 153
Hrdlicka, J.G., 211, 228
Hulka, J.F., vi, 99, 312–332
Huq, R., 36
Hyams, M.N., 259, 333, 338

Immerwahr, G.E., 36
Innis, R.E., vi, 245–253, 262, 263
Ishikawa, H., 338
Islam, A.I.M.M., 37

Jabocs, J.E., 154
Jaffee, S.R., 253
Joyner, C.R., 153
Joyner, F.P., 275

Kamboj, V.P., 211
Kar, A.B., 211
Katz, A.R., 275
Kister, R.W., 127
Klein, E., 262
Ko, W.H., vi, 276–292, 293
Kocks, J., 359
Koenjian, E., 292
Koester, C.J., 253, 262
Kossoff, G., 153
Kothari, M.L., 212
Koya, T., 333
Kroener, W.F., Jr., 100, 128
Krumins, R.F., 165
Kusumoto, M., 333

Lah, S.C., 213
Lahiri, R.K., 213
Laurence, K.A., vii, 222–228, 359
Lee, H.Y., vii, 38–47, 71–75, 193–200
Leichner, G.H., 165
Leininger, R.I., 159
Leonard, F., vii, 155–159, 159, 275
Lettvin, J.Y., 164
Lewin, W.S., 293
Lin, W.C., 293
Lindgren, N., 292
Lisa, J.R., 333
Lobdell, D.D., 154

McLeod, F.C., vii, 143
McRae, L.A., 100
Mansukhani, G., 213
Marcus, S.M., 292
Martens, F.W., Jr., vii, 30–312
Massey, G.A., 154
Mason, W.P., 153
Mastroianni, L., 127
Mastroianni, L.M., 128
Mazziotta-Mirbal, R.L., 128
Mcdel, M., 339–351, 367
Melton, C., 164
Meyers, R., 165
Miller, R.A., 36
Mirkovitch, V., 159
Moon, K.H., vii, 204–211
Moore-White, M., 128
Moitra, A., 213
Mortimer, J.T., 293
Mosberg, W.H., Jr., 165
Moulding, T., 353–359
Mueller, H., 263
Mukherjee, S.R., 213
Mullison, E., 213
Mutch, M.G.J., 128

Nayar, P.S.J., 36
Neumann, H.H., 203
Neuman, M.R., 293
Neustadt, B., 128
Neuwirth, R.S., viii, 101–114
Nishizaki, S., 338, 359
Noyori, K., 262

O'Brien, J.R., 128
Okuyama, D., 165

Name Index

Omran, K.F., 313-332
Osterhaut, D., 275
Osterling, D.L., 353-359

Pai, D.N., viii, 5-11
Pal, R.K., 213
Palmer, R., 115, 128
Pardenani, D.S., 212
Pasricha, K., 333
Pastene, L., 339-351, 367
Peel, J., 128
Perugini, M.M., 292
Phatak, L.V., viii, 86-92
Pitkin, R.M., 221
Platt, M., 128
Porter, J.O., 333, 359
Potter, R.J., 253
Pous-Puigmacia, L., 128
Power, F.H., 115
Prager, D.J., iii, viii, xv-xvi, 141, 175-189, 243, 294-302
Prager, R., 339-351, 367
Pratt, J.H., 128

Quddus, A.H.G., 23-36, 37

Rakshit, B., viii, 221, 359
Ramseth, D., 293
Ranganathan, K.V., 99
Ratcliffe, J.W., viii, 23-36, 37
Reid, J.M., 153
Reiner, L., 352
Repetto, O., 36
Reswick, J.B., 293
Richart, R.M., iii, viii, xv-xvi, 69, 120-140, 191, 229-241, 274, 367
Ritala, A.M., 128
Rittler, C., 262
Rivera, M., 339-351, 367
Roberts, B.J., 36
Robinson, D.E., 153
Rabrock, R.B., 293
Rochlin, D.B., 352
Roy, D.K., 213
Rubin, I.C., 333

Sadik, N., 36
Saha, H.L., 213
Saiker, S., 213

Salzado, C., 351
Sataloff, J., 263
Schmidt, S.S., ix, 76-85
Schultz, D.F., 165
Schwartzman, W.A., 211, 228
Scott, D.A., 153
Segal, S., ix, 303, 368-378
Segal, S.J., 212
Shafiullas, A.B.M., 36
Shearly, C.N., 293
Shearer, N.H., Jr., 275
Sheares, B.H., 333, 359
Shimodaira, K., 333
Shiner, W., 262, 263
Shirodkar, V.N., 128
Shubeck, F., 221
Siddiqui, K.A., 36
Siegel, S., 275
Siegler, A.M., 128
Siegmund, W.P., 253
Slater, L., 293
Smith, J.W., 128
Snaith, L.M., 128
Southam, A.L., ix, 379-382
Sparks, N., 293
Stachetti, E., 339-351, 367
Stack, J.M., 127
Starbuck, D.L., 293
Stephens, R., 164
Steptoe, P.C., 115
Sutherland, C.G., 333, 359
Swope, C.H., ix, 254-262

Taylor, H.C., 3, 367
Taylor, H.C., Jr., 53-67, 274, 359
Thompson, H.E., ix, 153, 353-359
Tietze, C., 333
Tucker, D., 164

Vande Wiele, R.L., iii, xiii
Vara, P., 128
Vilar-Dominguez, E., 127
Vodovnik, L., 293

Wainer, A., 127
Wall, P.D., 164
Wallace, R., 262
Wallmark, J.T., 292

Wicker, T.H., Jr., 275
Williams, R., 263
Wilpizeski, C., 263
Winget, C.M., 293
Woodruff, J.D., 127
Woodward, S.C., ix, 264, 274, 275
Wulff, V.J., 164

Yasui, S., 333, 338
Yaukey, D., 36
Yin, E., 293

Zaidi, W.H., 36
Zinsser, H.O., 211, 228
Zipper, J., ix, 339–351, 367

SUBJECT INDEX

A

A scan system, 144
  ultrasonic echoes, 168
Abdominal
  hernia and sterilization by laparoscopy, 102
  instillation of liquid plastics, 218, 221
  wall
    distention of, 103
    punctures and laparoscopy, 102
Abortions
  acceptability of, 238, 239
  and reanastomosis, 137
  therapeutic and cornual cauterization, 317
  and tubal ligation, 239–240
Acceptance see Sterilization, acceptance of
Acetic acid, 185
Acoustic holograms, 178
Adhesions
  liquid plastics, effects, 218
  and polymerization, 184
  and vaginal procedures, 134
Adhesives
  cyanoacrylates, 181, 264–274
  use in fallopian tube occlusion, 354, 358, 365
  tissue reaction to, 98–99
Age
  impotence and, 41
  and sexual potency, 40–47, 62
  of tubectomy patients in India, 13, 237
  and tubal sterilization with clips, 201–203
  of vasectomy patients in East Pakistan, 27
Agglutinin, sperm, 233
Aldrige method of temporary surgical sterilization, 15
Alkyl cyanoacrylates, 181
Alpha cyanoacrylates, 264–265
Amenorrhea, 90, 343
Amplification process of laser radiation, 254
Amplifier, microelectronics, 283
Ampulla, 40
Anastomosis procedures
  end-to-end, 118-122
  hydrotubation, 118
  oviduct, 116–127
  snorkel procedure, 124
  uterotubal implantation, 122–124
Anemia, and sterilization surgery, 89
Anesthesia, 54–55, 103, 114, 132
Animal experiments
  with intravasal thread, 193–199
  with liquid plastics, 217–218
Anovulatory drugs, 137
Antepartum tubal ligation, 239–240
Anterior approach in tubal sterilization, 235
Antibiotics, preoperative, 89
Antibodies, sperm, 232–233
Antimetabolites use in nonsurgical sterilization method, 339
Antioxidants, 159
Antispermatic antibodies, 233
Argon ion laser, 255, 259(T)
Atabrine, 366
Audio-visual equipment, learning aid in sterilization programs, 50
Auto-immunity to sperm, 78, 232
Auxiliary fibers, 260

B

B Coulter Counter, 223
B scan, 145–147, 169
Bacterial cells, mutations of during quinacrine treatment, 373–374
Balloon hysteroscope, 355, 357–358
Bank, sperm, 234
Belgium, tubal ligation data, 21(T)
Beta polymers, 272
Bilateral
  distension, 321
  occlusion, 316

reanastomosis, 21
vasectomy, 204
Bioengineering technology, 175–189
Bioinstrumentation, 281–284
Biostable polymers, 156
Biotelemetry, 281
  implant, 284–285
Biowax, 193
Birth control
  methods, legal aspects, 56
  pills, amenorrheal incidence in cornual implantation, 137
Bladder injuries during surgery, 235
Blocking
  material, adherence of, 228–230
  tubal, with heat, 240–241
Bonding, cyanoacrylates, 265
Bowel damage, 317
Brain
  lesions, ultrasound technique, 178
  ultrasonic scanning, 175, 176
Burn, tissue
  cauterization, 370
  electric current, 186–187
  laser energy, 299

C

Cancer destruction with laser energy, 298
Cannula, internal, permanent, 80
Carbon dioxide laser, 255, 259(T)
  use in fallopian tube occlusion, 298
  lesion size, 300
Carcinogenicity of quinacrine, 376–377
Cardiac endoscopy, fiber optic, 251–253
Cardioscope, experimental, 251, 252 (Figs.)
Castration, 40
Catheter
  fiber optics, 296
  ureteral transilluminating, 251
Caustics
  applied to fallopian tubes (rabbit), 363(T), 364(T)
  in uterine cavity, 339
Cauterization
  coagulating current, 104
  and pregnancy rate, 316, 372
  and tissue damage, 318
  tubal, 15, 313–332, 370
  uterine hemorrhage and, 317
Cautery, 313–332
  coagulation, 101
  culdoscopic tubal sterilization, 97–98
  probe for tubal occlusion, 314(Fig.)
Cavitation lesion, 178
Cells, quinacrine effect on, 374
Center for Population Research, xi
Cervical cauterization with silver nitrate, 377
Cervical instillations of liquid plastics, 219
Cesarean section
  and Irving procedure, 14
  and tubal ligation, 93
  and tubectomy, 18, 20
Chain scission, 158
Chemical
  blockage of fallopian tubes, 213–221
  for burning lumen, 189
  contraceptives, 166
  curettage, 343
  transvaginal sterilization, 339–351, 353–359
  tubular damage, 362–363
Chip, silicon, 279
Christians, sterilization acceptance, 9, 13
Cicatricial lesions and sterilization reversibility, 339
  see also Scar tissue formation
Clips
  silver, 234
  for tubal sterilization, 201–203
Coagulating current, 104
Coagulation
  cautery, 101
  cornual, 334–338
  fallopian tubes, 97
  lesion, controlled, 318–319
Coitus, frequency and sterilization, 44–45
Cold light, fiber optic illuminator, 250–251
Cold technique, 366

Subject Index

Collagen
  content, 270
  substrate, fragmentation of, 265
Colpotomy approach, 93
  in vaginal tubal ligation, 132
Complications
  tubal sterilizations with clips, 201–203
  uterotubal cautery, 317–318
  vasectomy, 11, 33, 36
Compound scans, 170, 171, 172
Compounding ingredients, 158–159
Computer, implant, 301
Conception
  and uterotubal implantation, 122
  after vasectomy, 40
  see also Pregnancy
Consent form for vasectomy, 71
Contraceptives
  chemical, 166
  oral, 17, 20
Core-coating interface, 245, 246
Corkborer resection technique, 124 (Fig.)
Cornual
  agglutination by cryosurgery, 305
  cauterization, 317, 361
  coagulation under hysteroscopy, 334–338
  cryotherapy, 361
  resection, 15, 122
Cryoprobe freezing, 320, 322
Cryosurgery, 97–98, 305–312
  and fertility, 330
  healing, 329
  and laparoscopy, 111
  and Parkinsonism, 305
  probe temperature, 321–322
  tubal ligation, 308, 368–369
Cryosurgical closure of fallopian tubes, 305–312
Cul-de-sac approach, 235
Culdoscope, 93
Culdoscopic
  tubal sterilization with tissue adhesives, 98–99
  vaginal technique, 134

Culdoscopy
  methods, 93–97, 203
  and tubal sterilization, 93–99
Culdotomy and clip method, 203
Curettage
  chemical, 343
  dilatation, 308
cw lasers, 260
Cyanoacrylates, 158
  effect on fibroplasia, 267–274
  as hemostatic agents, 266–267
  applied to fallopian tube (monkey), 364 (T)
  resorption of, 182
  skin graft fixation, 265
  tissue response to, 181, 264–274
  toxicity study, 269–274
  in tubal occlusion, 366
Cytotoxics, 329
  carcinogenicity of, 366

D

Dacron, adherence, 230
De-esterification, hydrolytic, 158
Dickinson technique for uterotubal cautery, 313, 315, 316
Dilatation and curettage, 308
Dilation of lumen of vas, 76–78, 229
Diode lasers, 225, 259 (T)
Doppler effect, 147
Double freezing, 332
Ductus deferens
  congenital absence of, 234
  occlusion of, temporary, 204–211

E

East Pakistan
  IUCD, 23
  male sterilization, 23–36
East Pakistan Research and Evaluation Centre (EPREC), 25, 32, 34
Echoes, ultrasonic pulse, principle, 147–148
  intensity, 168
  time separation, 148
Effectiveness of sterilization procedures, 380

Ejaculations
    after insertion of intravasal thread (IVT), 199
    after sterilization surgery, 40, 45, 74, 130
Elastomers, vas occlusion with, 222–228
    See also Plastic, Silastic, Silicon
Electrical impulse stimulation, 282
Electrocautery, 371
Electrocoagulation, 104, 106, 111, 371
    high-frequency, 315
    Hyams technique, 316
    tubal, 15
Electrode
    occlusion of the vas, 186
    placements, 288
Electromagnetic radiation, 180
Electromyographic signals, 288
Electronic circuits
    implant transmitter, 285, 288
    lifetime, 288
    M-series telemetry units, 288–289
    multiplex systems, 290
    packaging density, 276
    single-channel telemetry systems, 285–288
    transistorized, 277, 278 (Fig.)
    vacuum tubes, 277
Electronic devices, solid state, 285
Electronic implant, 281–284
Electronic stimulation level, 282
Electronic transmitters, 285–288
End-to-end anastomosis, 118–122, 125
Endometrial biopsy, 90
Endometritis, chronic, 90
Endosalpingeal destruction, 98
Endoscope, fiber optic, 251
Endosplint, 80, 82
    migration, 131
    and sexual intercourse, 84
    silastic, 81 (Fig.)
Epididymal obstruction, 79
Epididymis
    dilation of, 78
    and reanastomosis, 120
    silastic plug, effect on, 228
    spermatic granuloma, 85
Epididymitis, bacterial, 74
Epididymovasostomy, 78

Epithelial repair, 365
Epithelium regeneration, 182, 183
Estrogen, quinacrine injected in, 373
Ethanol formalin, 339, 340–344
    instillation technique, 240

F

Fabric grafts, 156-157
Fallopian tubes
    blocking with plastics, 213–221
    caustics application, 363 (T)
    chemical applications, 363 (T)
    coagulation of, 97
    cryosurgical closure of, 305–312
    histopathological examination, 90–91
    occlusion
        and carbon dioxide laser, 289
        experimental studies of, 360–367
        with sclerosing agents, 344
        with tissue adhesives, 354, 358, 365
    after quinacrine instillation, 346 (Fig.)
    self-repair, 365
Family planning
    programs
        in East Pakistan, 23–36
        in India, 5–11, 12–17
        in Venezuela, 18–22
    and religion, 9
    see also Religion
    sterilization camps, 8
Federal Communication Commission, and electronic implants, 285
Fees paid to vasectomy patients, 23–26, 31
    see also Incentive fee
Fertility
    cryosurgery and, 328–332
    rate in India, 16
    regulating techniques, xi
    restoration, 63, 116, 139, 241, 243
        hydrotubation, 118
        end-to-end anastomosis, 118–121
            technique, 119
        and use of liquid plastics, 220
        mechanical obstruction, 204–211
        snorkel procedure, 124
        uterotubal implantation, 122–124

Name Index

see also Recanalization, Reversibility
Fiber
  auxiliary, 260
  bundle
    flexible, 248–249
    transmittance of, 247, 248
  laser, 260
  probe, 261
  materials
    flint glass, 27
    transmission loss, 247
    refractive indices of, 246
  optics, 245–253
    endoscope, 251
    hysteroscope, 372
    illuminators, 220–251
    laser energy, 260, 261
    laser probe, 297
    multifiber construction technique, 249
  plastic, 294–292
  quartz, 295
  rod, 249
  size, 248
  ultraviolet-transmitting, 295
Fibroplasia, cyanoacrylates effect, 267–274
Fibrous tissue, and electric current, 186
Filiform threads, 193, 194, 196
Fimbrial reaction, 116
Fimbriectomy
  Kroener, 97
  surgical sterilization by, 93
Financial gain by vasectomy, 23–26, 31, 3
  see also Incentive fee
Fistula formation, 327
  permanent and filiform threads, 196
Flint glass fibers, 247, 295
Fluoroscopy, 318
  coagulation, 335
Foreign sterilization programs, 53–67
Free vasectomies, 39
Freezing
  damage by, 368
  lesion with nitrous oxide, 332
  repeated, and tissue necrosis, 369
  unit, 305, 306 (Fig.), 307 (Fig.)

uterine wall, 308
Freon, 328
  cryoprobe, 331
Fulguration of vs, 131–132

G

Gas lasers, 255
Gastroscope, 297
  -bronchoscope, 372
Gelatin block, 186
Gelfoam applications to fallopian tubes, 362, 365
Germany, tubal ligations in, 21 (T)
Glass multifibers, 295
Government free vasectomy service, 39
Grafts, plastic, 156, 157
Granulation
  external, 189
  tissue, resection, 268 (Fig.)
Granuloma
  formation, 182
  producing agents, 364

H

Heat coil technique, 369
Helium-neon laser, 255, 259 (T), 300
Hematoma, vasectomy and, 11
Hemoglobin levels, 89
Hemorrhage, uterine, 317
Hemostasis, cyanoacrylate use, 266–267
High density packaging, 277, 278 (Fig.), 285
Hindus
  sterilization acceptance, 9
  tubal ligation, 13
  vasectomy patients, 26
Holografs, acoustic, 178
Holographic techniques, 143, 178
Holography, 153
  optical, 179
Hormone
  male, vasectomy effect, 40
  ovarian and sterilization reversal, 340
Hyams technique of electrocoagulation, 316
Hybrid integrated electronic circuit, 279, 285

Hydrosalpinx, 91, 202
Hydrotubation for occlusion reversal, 118
Hydroxyproline, 181
　content, 270
Hypomenorrhea, 343
Hysterectomy, libido effect, 64
Hysterograms
　cryosurgical sterilization, 309
　postoperative, 110
Hysterosalpingograms
　and cornual cautery, 372
　after cornual coagulation, 336
　after cryosurgery, 308–310
Hysteroscope, 354
　balloon, 355
　glass, 372
Hysteroscopy
　cornual coagulation, 334–338
　and menstrual cycle, 372
　before ovulation, 373
　during secretory stage, 373–373
　tubal sterilization, 371–372

I

Illumination, fiber optics for, 245–253
Illuminators, fiber optics, 250–251
Image conduit, 249
Imaging technique, 144–147
Implant
　biotelemetry, 284–285
　computer, 301
　electronics, 281–284
　instruments and microelectronics, 276–292
　polymer, 155–159
　　cyanoacrylates, tissue responses to, 264–274
　　experimental results, 272(T)
　stimulation, 290–292
　telemetry, 281–282
　transmitters, 285
　　power, 286
Implantation
　electronic transmitter, 288
　gelatin block, 186
　plastics, 157 (T)
　radioactive polymer, 158
　uterotubal, 122–124

Impotency, 41
Incentive fee for sterilization in East Pakistan, 23–26, 35, 58–59, 60
Incident light, 247, 248
Incision, vasectomy, 72
　length, 40
India
　birth rate, 16
　fertility rate, 16
　occupational distribution of vasectomy patients, 10
　oral contraceptives, 17
　sterilization
　　facilities, 15
　　number of, 5 (T), 9
　tubal ligation program, 12–17
　vasectomy camps, 5–11
Indian vasectomy camps, 5–11
　temporary, 9
Infections
　post-tubectomy, 135
　vasectomy, 11
Infertility, postpartum, 375
Inflammation
　and cyanoacrylates, 182, 266, 272, 273
　spermicidal solution, 120–121
Insufflation
　after instillation of ethanol formalin, 341
　and plastic injection, 216
　and quinacrine treatment, 349
　Rubin's 320–321
　tubal patency evaluation, 341
Integrated circuits, 278, 279
　cost, 281
　performance, 281
　reliability, 278–281
Intercourse see Sexual intercourse
Interfaces
　optical fibers, 245–246
　specular reflection properties of, 169
Internal reflection, 245–246
International Institute for the Study of Human Reproduction, xi, xiii
Interval tubal ligations, 133
Intra-abdominal hematomas, 202
Intracardiac illumination, 250–251

Subject Index

Intraligamentous hematomas, 202
Intraperitoneal air, expressed, 97
Intravasal thread (IVT)
  dimension of, 194
  insertion site, 198
  removal, 196, 197 (Fig.)
  reversibility, 196
    vas occlusion, 193–200
      semen analysis, 196
    vasal dilatation, 199
Intra-uterine contraceptive devices (IUCD), 6–7
  see also IUCD
Intra-uterine tubal cauterization, 15
Involuntary vasectomies, 233
Irradiation
  laser, 256
  ultrasound, 180
Irving procedure, 14–15
Isobutyl-2-cyanoacrylate and tubal occlusion, 98
Isotherms, 328
IUCD
  use in East Pakistan, 23, 24 (Fig.)
  use in Venezuela, 20
  insertion rates in India, 7, 16
  materials, 159

J

Jet injector, 356–357

K

Korean vasectomy program, 38–47
Kroener fimbriectomy sterilization, 97, 99
Krypton laser, 225, 259 (T)
K-series transmitters, 285–286
Kymograph, 305

L

Labor, type of, and sterilization results, 88
Lactic acid, 158
Laparoscope, 102
Laparoscopy
  instruments, 103 (Fig.)
  local anesthetics, 132
  nonpuerperal sterilization, 101–114
  contraindications for, 102
  technique, 102–109
Laser
  energy
    cancer destruction, 298
    and fiber optic delivery system, 262
  fibers, 260
  flexible, 260
  gas, 254
  lesions, 256, 257, 258, 260, 261
  size, 300
  operation, methods, 255
    long-pulsed laser, 255
  photocoagulator, 255
  probe, fiber optics, 297
  radiation, 254–262
  tissue damage, 256, 299
Lasers, commercial, 254–255, 259 (T)
Lavage, vas, 45
Learning aids in sterilization programs, 48–52
Lee's vasetomy hook, 72, 73
Legal aspects of sterilization in Venezuela, 56
Lesion
  laser, 256, 257, 258, 260, 261, 299, 300
  and quinacrine, 351
  ultrasound, 161, 162, 164, 173–174
  of the vas, 176, 179
Lesioning transducer, 174
Libido
  and hysterectomy patients, 64
  in tubal sterilization with clips, 202
  and vasectomy, effect on, 33
Life Table Method, 241
Ligation see Tubal ligation
Light conduction by optical fibers, principle, 245–248
Light guides, 248
Liquid plastics see Plastics
Loop see IUCD
  chemicals for burning, 189
  size and reanastomosis, 138
  tubal, in anastomosis procedures, 120–121
  vas, dilatation of, 76–78, 69, 80, 229

M

Madlener, technique, 15, 17
  and tubal sterilization with clips, 201–203
Male hormone production, 62–63
  see also Hormone, male
Male sterilization
  in East Pakistan, 23–36
  principles of, 39–40
  reversal, 53–54
    see also Recanalization, Sterilization reversal with ultrasound, 177
Mapping, ultrasonic, 167–173
Marital counseling, 65
Marital relations, postoperative side effects, 36
Marriage, length of and vasectomy surgery, 42
Mating, fertility, and silastic occlusion of vas deferens, 224
Mechanical sterilization
  obstructions and temporary sterilization, 204
  techniques, 166–167
Medroxy progesterone, 329
Membrane transmission, 178
Menopause, tubectomy reconstruction, 14
Menorrhagia, 90, 91
Menstrual cycle
  endometrial biopsy, 90
  flow, 137
  and hysteroscopy, 372
  and instillation of ethanol formalin, 340
  tubal ligation, irregularities, 91
Menstruation
  postcoagulation, disturbances, 335
  reflux type, 137
Mercury cells, 288
Meridional ray, 246, 247 (Fig.)
Mesosalpinx
  clamps, 95
  ligament, 95
Methyl compounds, epithelial tissue and, 182, 183

Methyl cyanoacrylates, 181
  and fallopian tube occlusion, 366
  multiple applications, 183
  polymerization rate, 184–185
  toxicity and resorption, 270 (T)
Microelectronics
  circuits, 282
    example, 278 (Fig.)
  implant instruments, 276–279
Micrometer screw-thread advancement device, 98
Microsurgical approach to oviduct anastomosis, 121
Microvolts, 285
Microwatts, 285
Midline technique, 130–131
Monochromatic light, 255
Monolithic semiconductor, integrated circuits, 279
Monomer
  cyanoacrylates, 158
  tissue adhesives, 98
Mucosal destruction, 118
Multifiber, 249
  bundles, 249
  construction, techniques, 249
  glass, 295
Multiparity
  tubal sterilization with clips, 201–203
  tubectomies performed, 20–21
Multiple-chip silicon, integrated circuit, 285
Multiplex systems, 290
Muslims
  sterilization acceptance, 9
  tubal ligation, 13
  vasectomy patients, 26
Mutations in bacterial cells with use of quinacrine, 373
Myometrium, infiltration of, 364 (T)

N

National Institute of Child Health and Human Development, xi
National population control, xv
Necrosis, 183
Neodymium lasers, 225, 256, 259 (T)
  lesions, 257
Neurosis, and sterilization, 46–47

Subject Index

Neurotic tendencies in vasectomy patients, 71
Nitrogen, liquid, 305
Nitrous oxide method of freezing lesions, 332
Nonpatency, tubal, 342
Nonpuerperal sterilization by laparoscopy, 101–114
Nonreactive polymers, 264
Nonreactive suture methods for reversible vas occlusion, 193
Nonsurgical sterilization method, 339, 368–378
Numerical aperture (N.A.), 246, 250, 251
nominal, 247
Nylon
splints, 80, 81 (Fig.)
sutures, use in vasal blockage, 198
threads, filiform, 193–194
tissue reaction from, 196

O

Obstetrical hospitals and tubal ligation data, 18–22
Occlusion
devices for, 230
ductus deferens, temporary, 204–211
reversal and intravasal thread insertion, 193–200
with silastic, 222–228
tubal
with adhesives, 98–99
reversal, 118
vas, with electrode, 186
Oligomenorrhea, 343
Optic endoscope, 251
Optical
energy interaction with tissue, 225–256
fibers, 245–253
composition, 294
flexibility and size, 294
light conduction by, principles, 245–248
holography, 179
insulation, 246
Oral contraceptives, 17, 20
Oral horomonal medication, 360

Organometallic compounds, 159
Oscilloscope, 144
Ostium, visualization of, 371
Ovarian hormone, and sterilization reversal, 340
Ovary, intra-uterine relocation, 126 (Fig.)
Oviduct
anastomosis procedures, 116–127
laser lesions, 261
lumen blockage with liquid plastics, 220
occlusion with plastics, 235
Ovulation and hysteroscopy, 373
Oxygen saturation of blood, 296

P

Pacemaker, new, 283
Parectasis of the vas, 232
Patency
and silicone plugs, 231
tubal
clips, use of, 202
and insufflation, 341
vasal, 79–80, 193, 198
Penetration depth of ultrasonic image, 149, 150
Perforation, accidental, 329–330
Periadnexal adhesions, 116
Peritoneoscope, Ruddock, 101
Peritonitis, 137, 317
Peritonization, 121
Personality disorganization after sterilization, 46
Photochemical interaction of optical energy and tissue, 255–256
Photocoagulator, laser, 255
Photons in laser radiation, 254
Planned Parenthood Federation of Korea, 38
Plastic
clips, 203
device
removal, 207–208
temporary occlusion of the ductus deferens, 204–211
fibers, 294–295
injection method, 213–216

instillation in blocking fallopian tubes, 213–221
Plasticizers, 159
Plastics
 for blocking fallopian tubes, 213–221
 compounding ingredients, 158–159
 implantation and tensile strength, 156–157
 occlusion of vas deferens, 222–228, 230
 oviduct occlusion, 235
  temporary, 354
 temporary occlusion of ductus deferens, 203–211
 see also Silastic, Silicone
Plugging material
 dislodgement of, 224–225
 shrinkage, 231
 silastic, 213–221, 222–228
 temporary sterilization, 204–211
Pneumoperitoneum, 103
Poly-cyanoacrylates, degradation of, 158
Polyethylene splints, 80, 118–119
Polymer
 biodegradable, 158
 biostable, 158
 chemical reactions, 158
 degradation, 157
 stability, 156–158
 sutures, 185
 tubal reconstruction, 185
Polymer implants, 155–159
 cyanoacrylates, tissue response, 264–274
Polymerization
 and adhesions, 184
 partial, 185
 rate, methyl cyanoacrylates, 184–185, 265
Polyurethane implant, 157 (T)
Pomeroy technique, 14, 117 (Fig.)
 culdoscopic approach and tubal ligation, 99
 and puerperal state, 138
 transvaginal tubal ligation, 93
 tubal sterilization with clips, 201–203
Population control
 abortions, 238, 239
 fallopian tube occlusion, 360

female sterilization, 361
 national, xv
 sterilizations performed, 237, 238
 ultrasonics, application, 116–174
Postcoagulation, 335
Posterior fornix, 97
Postpartum cryosurgery, 312
Postpartum infertility, 375
Postoperative care, vasectomy, 74
Postoperative complications
 tubal sterilization with clips, 203
 vasectomy, 11, 33, 36
Postoperative pregnancies, 202
Postoperative side effects of vasectomy, 33, 36
Postpartum surgery, 14
Potassium permanganate
 tissue damage, 129, 130
 vas lavage with, 45, 73
Pregnancy
 abnormal, 137
 ectopic, 137
 after male sterilization reversal, 53
 rate
  and cauterization, 316
  and quinacrine treatment, 344
 reanastomosis, 125
 after restoration of tubal function, 137
 after tubal ligation, 234, 235
 tubal occlusion, 343
 and tubal sterilization with clips, 202
 uterotubal implantation, 122
Probe
 fiber laser, 261
 tip, temperature, 305, 311
Proctoscope, fiber optics, 296
Progestational agents, 328
Prostatic fluid, antigens in, 233
Protein denaturation, 178
Pseudopregnancy, 224
Psychiatric examination, postvasectomy, 46
Psychiatric screening, 39, 57
Psychosomatic disturbances following tubectomy, 14
Psychological screening, 57–58
Psychological side effects from vasectomy, 33, 36

Subject Index

Puerperal sterilization, 87, 88
  late effects of, 89-91
Pulmonary disease and sterilization by laparoscopy, 102
Pulmonary tuberculosis and tubal ligation, 19 (T)
Pulse doppler, arterial determination with, 188
Pulse echo principle, 147-148, 153
Pulse laser, 300
Pulse, sonic, 144
  width, 148
Pulse laser energy, 256
Pyogenic membrane, 271

Q

Quartz fibers, 295
Quinacrine chlorhydrate, 340, 349
  effect on cells, 373-374
  cumulative effect, 350-351
  injected in estrogen, 373
  instillations, number of and effects, 345 (T)
  toxicity level, 376-377
  treatment patterns, 344, 345 (T)
  and insufflation, 344
Quinine, fallopian tube blockage with, 213

R

Radial velocity, 148
Radiation
  electromagnetic, 180
  laser, 254-262
Radioactive polymer, implantation of, 158
Reanastomosis
  bilateral, 121
  oviduct, 116-122
  and pregnancy, 125
  reoperation, 120
  of the vas, 45, 54, 63, 75
Recanalization, 53-54, 63, 111
  intravasal thread, 198
  spontaneous, 45-46, 73, 75
  after ultrasonic therapy, 180
Reconstruction after tubectomy, 14
Recruiting agents, vasectomy, 31-32, 35, 59

Reflection, ultrasonic, 144-145
  and pulse echo principle, 147-148
Rejection, plastics, 218
Religion
  sterilization acceptance, 9
  tubal ligation, 13
  and vasectomy patients, 26
Reproductive processes, contraception of, 166
Resection
  granulation tissue, 268 (Fig.)
  tubal and polyethylene splinting, 118-119
Resolution scanning, 172
Reversibility, 236, 380-381
  intravasal thread, use of, 193-200
  mechanical obstructions, 204-211
  reoperation, 120
  tissue adhesives, 99
  tubal ligation, 139
  vasal occlusion, 193-200, 204, 211, 380
  vasectomy, 45, 54, 63, 75, 187
Reversible sterilization, 229-241
  see also Reversibility, Recanalization, Fertility restoration
Reversible vasal occlusion
  intravasal thread use, 193-200
  use of plastic device, 204-211
Rivanol, vas lavage with, 45
Rubin's insufflation, 320-321
Rubin's test, 316
Ruby laser, 255, 259 (T)
  lesion, 256-257
Ruddock peritoneoscope, 101

S

Saddle block, 136
Salicylic acid, tubal sterilization with, 362
Salpingectomy, total, 15
Salpingitis, 91
Scan transducer, rotating, 171
Scanning techniques, 147
  A scan system, 144, 168
  B scan system, 145-147, 169
  compound, 170
  high-speed, 171
Scar tissue formation, 370

Sclerosing agents
  and fallopian tube occlusion, 354, 358
  nonspecific, 339
Screening, preoperative for vasectomy patients, 71
Scrotal wound, suture, 74
Secretory phase, 90
Self-castration, 47
Semen
  analysis after insertion of intravasal thread, 196, 199
  plastic device, removal of, 208–209
  positive for sperm, 75
  and sperm agglutinin studies, 233
  see also Seminal fluid
Seminal fluid
  sperm count, 130
  and vasectomy effect, 40
Seminal plasma, 63
Sexual desire
  and hysterectomy patients, 64
  vasectomy, postoperative effects, 33, 36, 44
Sexual intercourse, after vasectomy, 40, 44–45, 74
Sexual potency, and aging, 40–47, 62
Sexual response and tubectomy, 14
Sexual weakness, 65
Shirodkar method, 15
Side effects, vasectomy, postoperative, 33, 36
Silastic
  blockage of fallopian tubes, 218–219
  occlusion of vas deferens, 222–228
  plug, 223
    dislodgement of, 224–225
  splints, 80, 81 (Fig.), 131
  see also Plastics
Silicon
  chips, 279
  photocell, 286
Silicone
  degeneration, 230
  fallopian tube blockage, 213–221
  occlusion of vas, temporary, 210
  plugs and patency, 231
  thread, 230
  see also Plastics

Silk suture technique, occlusion of vas with, 210
Silver clip, 234
Silver nitrite
  cervical sterilization, 377
  destruction, 321, 324, 325, 362
  transvaginal sterilization, 353
  tubal sterilization, 370
Sims perineal retractor, 97
Spin graft fixation and cyanoacrylates, 265
Snorkel procedure for oviduct anastomosis, 124
Sodium morrhuate, 217–218
Solid-state circuits, 276
Sonar techniques, 144
Sonic energy
  rate of attenuation, 151
  reflection, 147
Sonic imaging systems, 143
Sonic pulse, 144
Sonification, 180
Sound waves, 169
Specular reflection properties of interfaces, 169
Sperm
  agglutinin, 233
  antibodies, 232–233
  autoimmunity, 78, 232
  bank, 234
  clearance technique, 75, 78, 232
  storage, 234
Sperm count
  electronic method, 223
  in intravasal thread studies, 199
  after recanalization, 53
  reduction of, 130
Sperm-free ejaculate, 45, 130
  after use of intravasal thread, 199
  and silastic occlusion of vas deferens, 224
Sperm granuloma, 74
Sperm lavage, 45, 73
Sperm leakage, 84
Sperm passage, blocked and use of intravasal thread, 199, 200
Sperm production after recanalization, 54

Subject Index

Spermatic artery
  damage to, 189
  differentiation, 188
Spermatic fluid, 78
  spillage, 82
Spermatic granuloma
  and anastomosis failure, 82
  of the epididymis, 78, 85
  formation, 46, 54
  sperm leakage, 84
  and vasal occlusion reversibility, 232
Spermatozoa, vasectomy effect on, 40
Spermicidal solution
  inflammation, 129
  vas lavage with, 45
Spinal anesthesia and tubectomy, 54–55
Splints, 80–82
  migration of, 131
  nylon thread, 197
  polyethylene, 118–119, 120
Stabilizers, 159
Staining, tubal orifice, 356
Sterility duration, culdoscopy patients, 203
Sterilization
  acceptance, 9, 12, 17, 379
  cautery, 97–98, 313–323
  cryosurgery, 97–98, 305–312
  culdoscopic, with tissue adhesives, 98–99
  laparoscopy, 101–114
    contraindications, 102
  laser, 256
  mechanical technique, 166–167, 204–211
  neurosis, 46–47, 71
  nonpuerperal by laparoscopy, 101–114
  permanent, 120–140
  puerperal, 87, 88
  reversal procedures, 116–127
  temporary, 204–211
  time and morbidity, 88
  transvaginal, 339–351
  tubal, 14–15
    with clips, 201–203
  ultrasonic, 176–177
Sterilization programs
  in East Pakistan, 23–36
  in India, 5–11, 12–17
  in Korea, 38–47
  learning aids, 48–52
  in Venezuela, 18–22
Sterilization reversal, 53–54
  and use of ovarian hormone, 340
Sterilization chemical, transvaginal delivery, 353–359
Storage, sperm, 234
Sulfur dioxide, polymers, 185
Surgical procedure
  ultrasonic, 160–164
  vasectomy, 72–74
Sutures
  and cyanoacrylates, 264–266
  intravasal thread, 193–200
  microsurgical approach, 121
  nylon, 193–194, 196, 198
  oviduct anastomosis, 119–121
  silk and vas occlusion, 210
  vasectomy, 73, 74, 82, 83

T

Tattoo removal, 298
Teflon
  adherance, 230
  tubing, 98
Telemetry systems, 281
  application, 292
  implant, 284-285
  M-series, 288–290
  single-channel, 285–288
Temporary occlusion
  of ductus deferens, 204–211
  of fallopian tubes, 213–221
Testicular
  changes in vasal blockage, 234
  hormone production, 63
  spermatogenesis, 193
  tenderness and vasetomy, 11
Testosterone, 63
Thawing, tissue damage during, 369
Thermal
  conduction, 258, 260, 299
  energy, 256
  interaction of optical energy and tissue, 256
  method, ultrasound, 178

Thermocouple, 305
  multiple, 306
Thermopile, 287
Thermoreaction, 298
Thin-film integrated circuits, 278, 285
Tissue adhesives, 98–99
  cyanoacrylates, 99
  and occlusion of fallopian tubes, 354, 358, 365
  and sterilization reversibility, 99
Tissue coagulation and electrocautery, 318–319
Tissue compatibility with surgical implant, 155
Tissue damage
  by cautery, 318
  intravasal thread, 198
  by thawing, 369
Tissue glue, 185
  see also Adhesives
Tissue interface, depth of, 144
Tissue laser effect, 299
Tissue responses to polymeric implants, 264–274
Tissue structure, visualization of, 143–153
Transcervical approach to sterilization, 353
Transection, tubal, at laparoscopy, 104–107, 111
Transillumination, 104, 251
  with ureteral catheter, 297
Transistor, electronic circuit, 277, 278 (Fig.)
Transmitters
  implant, 285, 288
  performance specification, 286 (T)
  power supply, 286, 288
Transplantation of human oviduct, 125
Transuterine cornual sterilization, 98
Transvaginal
  sterilization with chemical agents, 339–351, 353–359, 376
  tubal ligation, 93, 135, 136
Trifluoroisopropyl cyanoacrylates, toxicity and resorption, 270
Tubal
  blockage, by heat, 240–241
  cauterization, 15, 313, 332

electrocoagulation, 15
epithelium, chemical use and necrosis, 362
function restoration and pregnancy, 137
insufflations, 341
  after quinacrine treatment, 344
ligation
  antepartum, 239–240
  interval, 133
  oviduct anastomosis, 116–127
  plastics, 216
  pregnancy after, 234, 235
  reversal, 139
  vaginal, 132
obstruction, accidental pregnancies, 343
occlusion
  reversal, 118
  safety, 381
  with tissue adhesives, 98–99
  transvaginal, 353
orifice
  identification of, 358
  staining, 356
patency
  cytotoxic agents, 366
  ethanol formalin treatment, 342
  insufflation, 341, 375
  and use of liquid plastics, 220
  restoration, 202
pregnancies and uterotubal implantations, 122
reconstruction and periadnexal adhesions, 116
sterilization
  cauterization, 313–332
  with clips, 201–203
  by cornual coagulation, 334–338
  by laparoscopy, 101–114
  methods, 14–15
  operative culdoscopy, 93–99
  reversal, 139
  with ultrasound, 177
  transection, 104–107
Tube, necrosis, 113
Tubectomy camps, 67
Tubectomy
  anesthesia, 54–55

Subject Index

and cesarean section, 18
legal aspects in Venezuela, 18
reversal, 116–127
surgery, 14–15
Tuboperitoneal fistula, 110 (Fig.)
Tubular damage with chemical agents, 362–363

U

Ultrasonic
  echoes, 168
  energy
    range, 146–153
    reflection of, 144–145
  frequencies and increased absorption, 172
  image technique, 143, 145–147
    interpretation of, 175
    penetration depth, 149, 151
    pulse width, 148
  lesions, 161, 162, 164, 173–174, 176, 180
  mapping, 167–173
  pulse width, 148
  sterilization, 176–177
  surgical techniques, 160–164
  tissue visualization, 168–169
  transducer, beam, 169
  visualization, 167–173, 177
Ultrasonics application in population control, 166–174
Ultrasound 143
  destruction mechanism, 178
  irradiation, 180
  surgical techniques, 160–164
  toxicity, 18–181
Ultraviolet transmission of, 295
Ultraviolet-transmitting fibers, 295
Ureteral transilluminating catheter, 251
Uterotubal cautery, 317–318
Uterotubal junction, occlusion by cautery, 318–328
Urethane solutions and fallopian tube blockage, 211–213
Uterine casts, 354
Uterine cavity, caustic agents, injections of, 339
Uterine perforation, 218
Uterine probe, 308

Uterine sound, 340
Uterine wall
  carbon particles in, 357
  freezing, 308
Uterotubal
  implantation, 122, 123 (T), (Fig.), 124 (Fig.)
  occlusion by cautery, 315 (Fig.), 316
  pregnancy results, 122
Uterus, secretory stage and hysteroscopy, 372–373
USA, tubal ligation in, 21 (T)

V

Vaginal
  culdoscopic technique, 134
  tubal ligation, 132
  instillation of liquid plastic, 218
  Pomeroy sterilization, 93, 95
  preparation for culdoscopy, 94
  route of sterilization, 14
Vas
  acoustic lesion of, permanent, 176
  anastomosis, 78
  fulguration of, 131–132
  lavage, 45
  occlusion
    with electrode, 186
    with plastic device, 204
  patency of, 79–80
  reanastomosis, technique, 78–84, 131–132
  resection of, 76
  splinting, 80
  sutures, 84
Vas deferens
  laser lesions, 261
  lavage, 45
  occlusion with silastic, 222–228
Vasa, closing of, 40
Vasal
  dilatation, and intravasal thread use, 199
  occlusion reversibility
    intravasal thread insertion, 193–200
    and use of plastic device, 204–211
  patency restoration, 193, 198
  repair with cyanoacrylates, 185

Vascular granulation tissue, 271
Vasectomy
  conception after, 40
  contraindications, 71
  financial gain by, 23–36, 31
  free government service, 39
  indications for, 71
  intercourse after, 40
  involuntary, 233
  marriage, length of, 42
  operative technique, modified, 71–75
  postoperative care, 74
  principles, 39–40
  procedure, 40
  reversibility, 187
  sexual changes, 33
  side effects, 33
  surgical procedure, 72–74
  ultrasonic lesions, 179–180
Vasectomy camps, 5–11
Vasectomy hook, 73
Vasectomy programs
  in East Pakistain, 23–36
  in India, 5–11
  in Korea, 38–47

Vasovasotomy, 63
  and nonmotile sperm, 78
Venezuela, tubal ligations, 18–22
Venous obstruction, 236
Visualization
  fiber optics for, 245–253
  ultrasonic, 167–173

W

Walthard modification, 15
Wash out technique, 75
Wavelength
  fiber, 296
  laser, 255–258
West Pakistan, population control, 57
Wire splint, 80
Work, return to after vasectomy, 74
Wound
  -closure agents *see* Adhesives, Cyanoacrylates
  nonsuture closure, 158

Z

Zinc chloride, use in fallopian tubes, 362, 363 (T), 365

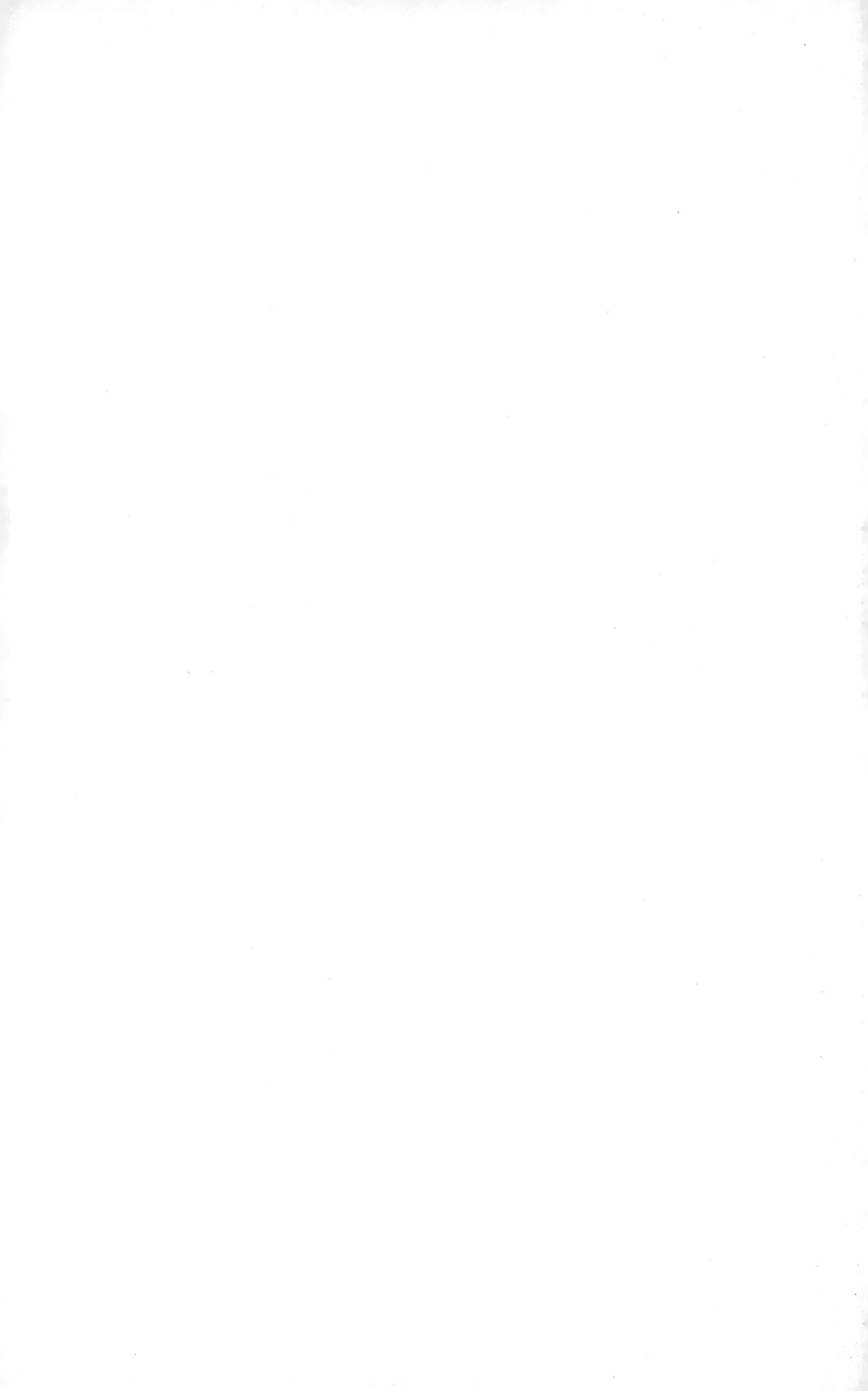

RD 571
C66
1969